Melanoma

CRITICAL DEBATES

Melanoma

CRITICAL DEBATES

EDITED BY

Julia A. Newton Bishop

MB ChB MD FRCP
Consultant Dermatologist
Honorary Reader in Dermatological Oncology
ICRF Senior Clinical Scientist
St James's University Hospital
Leeds
UK

Martin Gore

MB BS PhD FRCP
Consultant Cancer Physician
Royal Marsden Hospital
London
UK

Blackwell
Science

Editorial Offices:
Osney Mead, Oxford OX2 0EL, UK
Tel: +44 (0)1865 206206
Blackwell Science Inc., 350 Main Street, Malden, MA 02148-5018, USA
Tel: +1 781 388 8250
Blackwell Science Asia Pty, 54 University Street, Carlton, Victoria 3053, Australia
Tel: +61 (0)3 9347 0300
Blackwell Wissenschafts Verlag, Kurfürstendamm 57, 10707 Berlin, Germany
Tel: +49 (0)30 32 79 060

First published 2002

Library of Congress Cataloging-in-Publication Data

Melanoma: Critical Debates /edited by J. A. Newton Bishop, M. Gore.
p. cm.
ISBN 0-632-05772-6
1. Melanoma. I. Bishop, J. A. Newton (Julia A. Newton) II. Gore, Martin
[DNLM: 1. Melanoma.
QZ 200 C437 2001]
RC280.M37 C48 2001
616.99′477—dc21

2001035202

ISBN 0-632-05772-6

A catalogue record for this title is available from the British Library

Set in 10/13½ Sabon by SNP Best-set Typesetter Ltd, Hong Kong
Printed and bound in Great Britain by MPG Books Ltd, Bodmin, Cornwall

For further information on Blackwell Publishing, visit our website:
www.blackwell-science.com

Contents

List of contributors

EDITORS

Julia Newton Bishop MB ChB MD FRCP, *Consultant Dermatologist, Honorary Reader in Dermatological Oncology, ICRF Senior Clinical Scientist, ICRF Cancer Medicine Research Unit, St James's University Hospital, Beckett Street, Leeds LS9 7TF, UK*

Martin Gore MB BS PhD FRCP, *Consultant Cancer Physician, Royal Marsden Hospital, Fulham Road, London SW3 6JJ, UK*

CONTRIBUTORS

Phillipe Autier MD MPH, *Deputy Director, Division of Epidemiology and Biostatitics, European Institute of Oncology, 1135 Ripamonti, Milan, Italy*

Wilma Bergman MD PhD, *Department of Dermatology, Leiden University Medical Center, PO Box 9600, 2300 RC Leiden, The Netherlands*

Marianne Berwick PhD, *Division of Epidemiology and Biostatistics, Box 44, Memorial Sloan Kettering Hospital, 1275 York Ave, New York, NY10021, USA*

Alexander Eggermont MD PhD, *Surgical Oncologist, Department of Surgical Oncology, Daniel Den Hoed Cancer Centre, 301 Groene Hilledijk, 3075 EA, Rotterdam, The Netherlands*

Tim Eisen PhD MRCP, *Senior Lecturer and Consultant Medical Oncologist, Department of Medicine, Institute of Cancer Research, The Royal Marsden Hospital, Downs Road, Sutton, Surrey SM2 5PT, UK*

Mark Elwood MD DSc FFPHM, *Director, National Cancer Control Initiative, 1 Rathdowne Street, Carlton (Melbourne), Victoria, 3053, Australia*

Judy Evans MA FRCSEd (PLAST) FRCS, *Nuffield Hospital, Derriford Road, Plymouth, Devon PL6 8BG, UK*

Andrew Goodman MRCP FRCR, *Lead Clinician, Department of Oncology, Devon and Exeter Hospital, Barrack Road, Exeter, EX2 5DW, UK*

Rudolf Happle MD, *Professor of Dermatology, Department of Dermatology and Allergology, Phillipp University of Marburg, Deutschhausstraße 9, 35033 Marburg, Germany*

Peter Hersey FRACP D.Phil, *Room 443, David Maddison Building, Cnr King & Watt Street, Newcastle NSW 2300, Australia*

Stephen Johnston MA MRCP PhD, *Consultant Medical Oncologist, Department of Medicine, Royal Marsden Hospital, Fulham Road, London SW3 6JJ, UK*

Richard Kefford MB BS (Syd) PhD FRACP, *Professor of Medicine and Director, Westmead Institute for Cancer Research, University of Sydney at Westmead Millenium Institute, Westmead, NSW 2145, Australia*

Ulrich Keilholz MD PhD, *University Hospital Benjamin Franklin, Free University Berlin, Hindenburhdamm 30, D-12200 Berlin, Germany*

Nigel Kirkham MD FRCPath, *Consultant Pathologist, Department of Histopathology, Royal Sussex County Hospital, Brighton BN2 5BE, UK*

Sewa Legha MD FACP, *8501 Hawaii Lane, Houston, Texas, 77040, USA*

Ferdy Lejeune MD PhD, *Professor of Oncology and Director of Centre Pluridisciplinaire d'Oncologie, Centre Hospitalier Universitaire Vaudois, Rue du Bugnon 46, CH-1011 Lausanne, Switzerland*

Danielle Liénard MD, *Medecin Associe and Consultant, Centre Pluridisciplinaire d'Oncologie and Principal Clinical Investigator, Ludwig Institute for Cancer Research, Centre Hospitalier Universitaire Vaudois, Rue du Bugnon 46, CH-1011 Lausanne, Switzerland*

Jacqueline Newby MA MRCP MD, *Senior Registrar in Medical Oncology, 18 Barncroft Way, St Albans, Hertfordshire AL1 5QZ, UK*

Poulam Patel MD MRCP, *Consultant Medical Oncologist and ICRF Clinical Scientist,* ICRF *Cancer Medicine Research Unit, St. James's University Hospital, Beckett Street, Leeds LS9 7TF*

Razvan Popescu MD MRCP, *Department of Oncology, Centre Hospitalier Universitaire Vaudois, Rue du Bugnon 46, BH06, CH-1011 Lausanne, Switzerland*

Jonathan Rees FRCP FMedSci, *Department of Dermatology, University of Edinburgh, Royal Infirmary Lauriston Building, Lauriston Place, Edinburgh EH3 9YW, UK*

David Ross MD FRCS (PLAST), *Department of Plastic Surgery, 3rd Floor, Lambeth Wing, Lambeth Palace Road, London, SE1 7EH, UK*

Merrick Ross MD FACS, *Professor of Surgery, Chief of Melanoma and Sarcoma Division, Department of Surgical Oncology, The MD Anderson Cancer Center, 1515 Holcombe Boulevard, Houston, Texas, USA*

John Spencer MD FRCR, *Consultant Radiologist, Department of Radiology, St James's University Hospital, Beckett Street, Leeds LS9 7TF, UK*

Michael Timmons MA MChir FRCS, *Consultant Plastic Surgeon, Department of Plastic Surgery, Bradford Royal Infirmary, Duckworth Lane, Bradford BD9 6RJ, UK*

Antony Young PhD, *Department of Environmental Dermatology, St John's Institute of Dermatology, Guy's, King's and St Thomas' School of Medicine, King's College London, University of London, St Thomas' Hospital, London SE1 7EH, UK*

Introduction

The treatment of melanoma is indeed a debate and this book is intended to address the major areas of controversy in a practical way. It is written with the health care professional in mind who is part of the multidisciplinary team which manages the disease from screening to palliative care.

The incidence of melanoma has increased dramatically in North America, Europe and Australasia this century [1] which is attributed to changed patterns of behaviour of white-skinned peoples in the sun [2–4]. The first chapter by Marianne Berwick addresses the issues which remain to be resolved, concerning the critical patterns of sun exposure and the age at which it occurs. Artificial ultraviolet light (UV) exposure allows individuals in colder climates to expose their skin to UV doses hitherto unprecedented, which has potentially grave effects on the incidence of melanoma in these populations. The issue of sunbeds is addressed by Philippe Autier in Chapter 2. Protection from the carcinogenic effects of UV is clearly important. There has been concern however, that although sunscreens demonstrably reduce the ill-effects of UV light [5,6], that the general public has become too reliant on sunscreens. There has even been the suggestion that over-reliance on sunscreens may encourage children to stay out in the sun for longer which might even increase their susceptibility to melanoma [7–9]. Antony Young discusses these issues in Chapter 3.

The white population is the primary group at risk of developing melanoma and there is clear variation in susceptibility to skin cancer within this population. Epidemiological studies established the increased susceptibility of sun susceptible phenotypes such as red hair to skin cancer [10] and understanding of the molecular basis of this has been developed by Jonathan Rees who describes this progress in Chapter 4. The presence of multiple melanocytic naevi, or moles, is however, a more potent risk factor for melanoma [11,12]. Those who manifest this so-called atypical naevus phenotype (or dysplastic naevus phenotype) are a challenge, particularly to dermatologists and primary health care physicians, not least because the phenotype is common, occurring in at least 2% of the population [13] (chapter 5).

It is postulated that the sun susceptible phenotype and the atypical mole syndrome are due to low penetrance melanoma susceptibility genes. Much more rarely, families can carry germ-line high-penetrance susceptibility genes and have a strong family history of melanoma. These families were initially described in the 19th century by Norris [14] but first explored in the 1980s [15,16]. A significant proportion of the largest of these families, are now shown to be caused by germline mutations in the CDKN2A gene which codes for the protein p16. In Chapter 6, Richard Kefford discusses familial predisposition to melanoma in general terms and the specifics of genetic testing.

One of the great challenges is the early detection of melanoma, particularly perhaps in areas of relatively low incidence, such as Europe and some parts of the USA. In the UK primary health care teams see very few early tumours in their working lifetime and the population perceives the risk of melanoma to be low. In the skin cancer screening clinic, often named the pigmented lesion clinic, the challenge is to diagnose melanomas at the *in situ* stage when cure is the result of excision, in a cost-effective way. This challenge is considerable, as the appearances are subtle and difficult to distinguish from the common atypical naevus. Wilma Bergman discusses approaches to this problem in Chapter 8. Management problems do not end at excision, there are difficulties in the histopathological diagnosis of early melanocytic lesions which are discussed by Nigel Kirkham in Chapter 7. The pigmented lesion clinics represent opportunist screening and allow expertise to be concentrated in one place. In areas of high incidence of melanoma, it is possible that active screening might be a cost-effective exercise. In Chapter 9, Mark Elwood discusses different approaches to screening at different latitudes and therefore within different backgrounds of melanoma incidence.

Patients with congenital naevi, particularly the giant pigmented type, are at increased risk of melanoma [17,18] but there is uncertainty about the magnitude of that risk. In clinical practice a balance is needed between the potential value of surgery for these naevi and any potential cosmetic deficit. This issue is discussed by Julia Newton Bishop and Rudolf Happle in Chapter 13.

The treatment of melanoma is still essentially surgical but there remains considerable controversy about the optimal margins of excision of the primary tumour. There are randomized clinical trial data to support a 1 cm margin for tumours less than 2 mm in Breslow thickness [19] and some data concerning the safety of margins for thicker tumours [20]. There are also different approaches to excision margins for tumours thinner than 1 mm with some clinicians choosing to remove these with a 0.5 cm margin and others considering that this is only appropriate when the lesion is in radial growth phase [21], as the likelihood of recurrence is thought to be low in such circumstances [22,23]. There is a particular lack of trial data on what constitutes safe margins of excision for lentigo maligna and nail bed/subungual melanomas. These issues are discussed by Michael Timmons in Chapter 10.

In patients at risk of relapse there is no evidence that intensive staging procedures, or follow up involving regular imaging in order to diagnose early relapse, alters survival. In Chapter 11, John Spencer, Razvan Popescu and Poulam Patel discuss the need to balance the radiation dosage of computerized tomography, the relatively high false positivity of scans and the resulting anxiety that can be caused. They also discuss the value of different staging strategies. The absence of effective systemic therapy for melanoma means that most guidelines recommend follow up should be predominantly clinical [24]. However, there is some controversy as to whether fit patients who might contemplate aggressive therapy with IL-2 based treatments benefit from early intervention and thus a more aggressive follow-up policy. The organization of clinical follow up is discussed by Judy Evans in Chapter 19.

The surgical treatment of lymph node relapse remains controversial. Several trials have failed to show any survival benefit of elective lymph node excision [25,26]. Sentinel node biopsy is a modification of the approach which uses lymphoscintigraphy and dye to localize the principal draining lymph nodes [27]. The technique is undoubtedly of value as a staging procedure but it remains to be seen whether it impacts on survival. David Ross and Merrick Ross discuss the issues that are evolving around this technology in Chapter 12.

The treatment of patients with advanced melanoma is as yet ineffective in terms of impacting survival, although chemotherapy has a valuable palliative role and this is discussed by Tim Eisen and Jaqueline Newby in Chapter 14. There is hope that the biological response modifiers, immunotherapy and some of the newer agents with novel mechanisms of action may offer more hope in both the adjuvant setting and for the treatment of metastatic disease. Alexander Eggermont, Ulrich Keilholz and Sewa Legha discuss these topics in Chapters 15 and 18. It is recognised that patients and the health care team are somewhat emotionally invested in vaccines for cancer therapy and this important area of research is reviewed by Peter Hersey in Chapter 16.

Sometimes disease recurs in a limb and in this situation surgery or CO_2 laser therapy is the treatment of choice. However, isolated limb perfusion is of great value when control is being lost and its role is outlined by Ferdy Lejeune and Danielle Liénard in Chapter 17. The use of radiotherapy in palliation and its limitations are described by Andrew Goodman in Chapter 20 and finally Stephen Johnston discusses the possible role of female hormones and pregnancy in melanoma in the last chapter of the book.

Melanoma is a disease that engenders much negativity in many therapeutic circles. However, it is a cancer which requires great care and attention if patients are to be managed optimally. Expertise is required at every stage of the patient's journey from early diagnosis to the palliation metastatic disease. It is a tumour that is increasing in frequency, but so is our knowledge of its biology and it is only a matter of time before we will make a significant impact on the survival of patients.

References

1 Parkin D, Muir C, Whelan SEA. Cancer incidence in five continents. *IARC. Sci Publ* 1992; (120): 45–173.
2 Armstrong B. Epidemiology of malignant melanoma: intermittent or total accumulated exposure to the sun? *J Dermatol Surg Oncol* 1988; **14**: 835–49.
3 Armstrong B, Kricker A. *Sun exposure causes both nonmelanocytic skin cancer and malignant melanoma*. Proceedings on Environmental UV Radiation and Health Effects 1993: 106–13.
4 Armstrong BK, Kricker A. How much melanoma is caused by sun exposure? *Melanoma Res* 1993; **3** (6): 395–401.
5 van Praag MCG. *et al*. Determination of the photoprotective efficacy of a topical sunscreen against UVB-induced DNA damage in human epidermis. *J Photochem Photobiol B* 1993; **19**: 129–34.
6 Roberts L, Beasley D. Commercial sunscreen lotions prevent ultraviolet radiation induced immune suppression of contact hypersensitivity. *J Invest Dermatol* 1995; **105**: 339–44.
7 Autier P. *et al*. Melanoma and use of sunscreens: an EORTC case-control study in Germany, Belgium and France. *Int J Cancer* 1995; **61**: 749–55.
8 Autier P. *et al*. Sunscreen use, wearing clothes, and number of nevi in 6- to 7-year-old European children. European Organization for Research and Treatment of Cancer Melanoma Cooperative Group. *J Natl Cancer Inst* 1998; **90** (24): 1873–80.
9 Autier P. *et al*. Sunscreen use and duration of sun exposure: a double-blind, randomized trial. *J Natl Cancer Inst* 1999; **91** (15): 1304–9.
10 Gallagher R. *et al*. Sunlight exposure, pigmentation factors, and risk of non melanocytic skin cancer. *Arch Dermatol* 1995; **131**: 164–9.
11 Bataille V. *et al*. Risk of cutaneous melanoma in relation to the numbers, types and sites of naevi: a case-control study. *Br J Cancer* 1996; **73**: 1605–11.
12 Swerdlow AJ. *et al*. Benign melanocytic naevi as a risk factor for malignant melanoma. *Br Med J* 1986; **292**: 1555–60.
13 Newton JA. *et al*. How common is the atypical mole syndrome phenotype in apparently sporadic melanoma? *J Am Acad Dermatol* 1993; **29**: 989–96.
14 Norris W. A case of fungoid disease. *Edinb Med Surg J* 1820; **16**: 562–5.
15 Lynch HT. *et al*. Family studies of malignant melanoma and associated cancer. *Surg Gynaecol Obstet* 1975; **141**: 517–22.
16 Clark W. *et al*. Origin of familial malignant melanoma from hereditable melanocytic lesions: the BK mole syndrome. *Arch Dermatol* 1978; **114**: 732.
17 Illig L. *et al*. Congenital nevi ≤10 cm as precursors to melanoma. 52 cases, a review, and a new conception. *Arch Dermatol* 1985; **1** (121): 1274–81.
18 Swerdlow AJ, English JSC, Qiao Z. The risk of melanoma in patients with congenital nevi: a cohort study. *J Am Acad Dermatol* 1995; **32**: 595–9.
19 Veronesi U. *et al*. Thin stage I, primary cutaneous malignant melanoma. Comparison of excision with margins of 1 versus 3 cm. *N Engl J Med* 1988; **318** (18): 1159–62.
20 Balch C. *et al*. Efficacy of 2 cm surgical margins for intermediate thickness melanomas (1–4 mm): results of a multi-institutional randomized surgical trial. *Ann Surg* 1995; **218**: 262–7.
21 Roberts D. *et al*. The UK guidelines for the management of malignant melanoma. *Br J Derm* (in press).
22 Elder DE. Prognostic Guides to Melanoma. In: Mackie R, ed. *Clinics in Oncology*. London: WB Saunders, 1984: 457–76.
23 Elder DE, Murphy G. Malignant tumors (melanomas and related lesions). *Atlas of Tumor Pathology: Melanocytic Tumors of the Skin*, 2 (3rd series). Washington DC:

Armed Forces Institute of Pathology, 1991: 103–205.

24 Newton Bishop J. *et al.* UK guidelines for the management of cutaneous melanoma. *Brit J Plast Surg* 2001.

25 Cascinelli N. *et al.* Immediate or delayed dissection of regional nodes in patients with melanoma of the trunk: a randomized trial: WHO melanoma programme. *Lancet* 1998; **351**: 793–6.

26 Sim F. *et al.* Lymphadenectomy in the management of stage I malignant melanoma: a prospective randomized study. *Mayo Clin Proc* 1986; **61**: 697–705.

27 Morton D. *et al.* Technical details of intraoperative lymphatic mapping for early stage melanoma. *Arch Surg* 1992; **127**: 392–9.

Julia Newton Bishop
Martin Gore

Part 1: Aetiology

1: Patterns of sun exposure which are causal for melanoma

Marianne Berwick

Role of sun exposure

Sun exposure is generally equated with ultraviolet (UV) radiation exposure, although the evidence does not rule out other unmeasured exposures associated with the sun. The alarming rise in skin cancer incidence has led to numerous attempts to explain why there has been such an increase. In the public mind, a major correlation exists between increased outdoor activity and increased skin cancer rates. In fact, there are no data available to substantiate such a relationship; although there has been a dramatic increase in melanoma incidence over the last 50 years, no data show that has been an increase in outdoor activity during the past 50 or so years although the trend toward wearing less clothing is self-evident.

The data to support an association between sun exposure and the development of melanoma are indirect. There has been a latitude gradient for the incidence of melanoma among white people, such that the highest rates are nearest the equator. In Europe this gradient has been confounded by the fact that those with darker pigmentary phenotype live in the southern areas of Europe and those with lighter phenotype in the northern, so that the gradient in Italy, for example, was actually reversed. However, cutaneous phenotype does not explain the higher melanoma rates in Norway than in Sweden. Furthermore, new data suggest that trends for mortality are levelling off in terms of latitude [1]. Armstrong & Kricker [2] estimate that between 68 and 90% of all melanomas are caused by sun exposure. Most would not dispute this estimate; however, it is likely that *intermittent lifelong* sun exposure among *susceptible* individuals leads to melanoma. The rest of this chapter will examine the data supporting this statement.

Patterns of sun exposure

Intermittent, chronic and cumulative sun exposure

While there is no standard measure of sun exposure in research, it can be generally classified as intermittent or chronic, and the effects may be considered as acute or cumulative. *Intermittent sun exposure* is that obtained sporadically, usually during recreational activities, and particularly by indoor workers who have only weekends or vacations to be outdoors and have not adapted to the sun. *Chronic sun exposure* is incurred by consistent sun exposure, usually by outdoor work, but also among those people who are outdoors a great deal for other reasons. *Cumulative sun exposure* is the additive amount of sun exposure that one receives over a lifetime. Cumulative sun exposure may reflect the additive effects of intermittent or chronic sun exposure, or both.

Indeed, different patterns of sun exposure appear to lead to different types of skin cancer among susceptible individuals. In Europe, Rosso *et al.* [3] quantified suggestions by Kricker *et al.* [4] that basal cell carcinoma and squamous cell carcinoma have *different* patterns, such that squamous cell carcinoma appears to have a threshold at approximately 70 000 h of exposure to the sun after which incidence increases sharply, regardless of whether it is chronic or intermittent sun exposure. This is highly consistent with the molecular genetic evidence [5] where combined analysis of skin cancer mutations from several laboratories found the p53 tumour suppressor gene mutated in 90% of human squamous cell carcinomas and approximately 50% of basal cell carcinomas. Approximately 70% of tumours exhibited the characteristic UVB footprint; a C to T or a CC to TT mutation at specific codons.

Basal cell carcinoma appears to share some risk factors with melanoma, as pointed out by Urbach many years ago [6]. Some basal cell carcinomas may be caused by chronic sun exposure, but a large portion (one-third or more) is apparently caused by intermittent sun exposure, similar to that implicated in melanoma. In the study by Rosso *et al.* [3], basal cell carcinoma incidence was increased twofold at a lower cumulative exposure than squamous cell carcinoma (8000–10 000 cumulative hours) with a subsequent plateau in risk followed by a decrease in risk for higher exposures. Occupational exposures are thus associated with squamous cell carcinoma risk and recreational exposures with basal cell carcinoma risk. This exposure–response pattern is consistent with the results from a recent randomized trial of sunscreen efficacy that found statistically significant protection from the development of squamous cell carcinoma, but no evidence at all for protection from the development of basal cell carcinoma [7]. It is unlikely that such a trial could be carried out for melanoma, because of a lack of statistical power. Therefore, the similarities between basal cell carcinoma and melanoma are all the more critical to under-

Table 1.1 Comparison of holiday beach sun exposure for melanoma and basal cell carcinoma in the same European population in childhood and adulthood. After [8]

Lifetime sun exposure	CMM OR (95% CI)	BCC OR (95% CI)
Holidays at beach during childhood		
Never	1.00	1.00
1–1600 h	2.4 (1.1–1.4)	1.2 (0.8–1.8)
>1600 h	1.8 (1.2–2.6)	1.8 (1.0–3.1)
P-value for linear trend	0.03	0.04
Holidays at beach during adulthood		
Never	1.00	1.00
1–1600 h	1.1 (0.7–1.7)	1.9 (1.3–2.8)
>1600 h	2.1 (1.4–3.1)	1.7 (1.2–2.4)
P-value for linear trend	0.04	0.05

Abbreviations: BCC, basal cell carcinoma; CI, confidence interval; CMM, cutaneous malignant melanoma; h, hours; OR, odds ratio.

stand. Data from Europe support the suggestion that intermittent sun exposure has similar effects on melanoma and basal cell carcinoma (Table 1.1).

Perhaps surprisingly, analytic epidemiologic studies have shown only modest risks at best for the role of sun exposure in the development of melanoma incidence, and two recent systematic reviews have demonstrated extremely similar estimates of effect for the role of intermittent sun exposure; an odds ratio of 1.57 [9,10]. It is important to note that chronic sun exposure, as in those occupationally exposed to sunlight, is protective for the development of melanoma, with an odds ratio of 0.70, equivocal for the development of basal cell carcinoma, and a risk factor for squamous cell carcinoma (Table 1.2).

Intermittent sun exposure

The studies in Table 1.2 show odds ratios ranging from 0.6 to 8.4 for intermittent sun exposure, with a summary odds ratio calculated by Elwood & Jopson [10] for the first 23 studies of 1.71 (95% CI = 1.54–1.90). As Elwood & Jopson point out, the measurement of sun exposure is complex and the discrepancies in Table 1.2 could be sorted out by conducting new studies using compatible protocols in different populations with different levels of sun exposure.

Chronic sun exposure

A clearer explanation for the rise in melanoma incidence that takes into account the different effects of chronic and intermittent sun exposure, proposed

Table 1.2 Studies of intermittent sun exposure and melanoma. After [10]

Reference	Place	Number of cases	Odds ratio (95% CI)
Klepp & Magnus [11]	Norway	78	2.4 (1.0–5.8)
Mackie & Aitchison [12]	Scotland	113	0.6 (0.2–1.2)
Lew *et al.* [13]	USA	111	2.5 (1.1–5.8)
Rigel *et al.* [14]	USA	114	2.4 (1.2–5.0)
Elwood *et al.* [15]	Canada	595	1.7 (1.1–2.7)
Sorahan & Grimley [16]	UK	58	6.5 (1.0–42.0)
Dubin *et al.* [17]	USA	1091	1.7 (1.2–2.3)
Green *et al.* [18]	Australia	183	1.9 (0.5–7.4)
Holman *et al.* [19]	Australia	267	1.1 (0.7–1.8)
Osterlind *et al.* [20]	Denmark	474	1.8 (1.2–2.5)
Beitner *et al.* [21]	Sweden	523	1.8 (1.2–2.6)
Dubin *et al.* [22]	USA	290	1.5 (1.0–2.4)
Grob *et al.* [23]	France	207	8.4 (3.6–19.7)
Zanetti *et al.* [24]	Italy	256	2.3 (1.3–3.8)
Zaridze *et al.* [25]	USSR	96	3.4 (0.6–17.4)
Herzfeld *et al.* [26]	USA	324	2.0 (1.3–3.3)
Autier *et al.* [27]	Belgium, France, Germany	420	6.1 (1.8–20.3)
Nelemans *et al.* [28]	Netherlands	128	2.4 (1.3–4.2)
Westerdahl *et al.* [29]	Sweden	400	1.2 (0.8–1.8)
Holly *et al.* [30]	USA	452 females	0.8 (0.6–1.1)
Rodenas *et al.* [31]	Spain	105	4.9 (2.2–10.9)
Berwick *et al.* [32]	USA	650	2.7 (1.3–5.5)
Walter *et al.* [33]	Canada	583	
Arranz *et al.* [34]	Spain	113	1.5 (1.0–2.4)

Abbreviation: CI, confidence interval.

by Gallagher *et al.* [35], is that as people have replaced outdoor occupations with indoor, they have engaged in more intermittent sun exposure. Gallagher *et al.* showed that the decrease in outdoor occupations, or chronic exposure which is inversely associated with melanoma, could explain the increase in melanoma incidence in Canada (Table 1.3).

Elwood & Jopson [10] calculated an overall odds ratio for chronic sun exposure, after excluding studies with heterogeneous results, of 0.76 (95% CI = 0.68–0.86). This estimate is similar to that reported by Nelemans *et al.* [9] and Walter *et al.* [33].

The major hypotheses for the role of chronic and intermittent sun exposure as causal in the development of melanoma are the following.

1 Intermittent sun exposure leads to the development of melanoma because the skin (melanin, thickness) never has the opportunity to adapt. It is the burst of UV on unadapted skin that leads to the development of tumours.

2 Chronic sun exposure leads to the development of melanoma because the DNA damage sustained to the melanocyte is not repaired and increases the mutation rate.

Table 1.3 Results of case control studies on occupational sun exposure and melanoma. After [10]

Reference	Country	Cases	Odds ratio (95% CI)
Klepp & Magnus [11]	Norway	78	1.4 (0.6–3.5)
Mackie & Aitchison [12]	Scotland	113	0.4 (0.1–0.7)
Elwood *et al.* [15]	Canada	595	0.9 (0.6–1.5)
Graham *et al.* [36]	USA	218 males	0.7 (0.3–1.3)
Dubin *et al.* [17]	USA	1096	2.5 (1.4–4.4)
Elwood *et al.* [37]	UK	83	1.7 (0.3–8.6)
Cristofolini *et al.* [38]	Italy	103	0.9 (0.5–1.7)
Osterlind *et al.* [20]	Denmark	474	0.7 (0.5–0.9)
Zanetti et al. [24]	Italy	73	2.1 (0.6–6.8)
Garbe *et al.* [39]	Germany	200	5.5 (1.2–2.8)
Beitner *et al.* [21]	Sweden	523	0.6 (0.4–1.0)
Dubin *et al.* [22]	USA	283	1.8 (0.9–4.0)
Grob *et al.* [23]	France	207	2.5 (1.2–5.1)
Herzfeld *et al.* [26]	USA	321	0.7 (0.5–1.0)
Autier *et al.* [27]	Belgium, France, Germany	420	0.3 (0.1–0.9)
Westerdahl *et al.* [29]	Sweden	400	0.8 (0.6–1.0)
White *et al.* [40]	USA	256	0.6 (0.3–1.2)
Holly *et al.* [30]	USA	452 females	0.8 (0.5–1.5)
Rodenas *et al.* [31]	Spain	100	3.7 (1.7–7.5)
Chen *et al.* [41]	USA	650	0.5 (0.2–1.1)
Wolf *et al.* [42]	Austria	193	1.1 (0.7–1.6)
Arranz *et al.* [34]	Spain	116	0.5 (0.3–0.7)

3 An alternative hypothesis is that chronic sun exposure leads to adaptation by increasing the thickness of the skin and inducing melanin in the keratinocytes that then protects the melanocytes.

At this time there is no animal model, or suitable biological alternative, that can be used to understand better the mechanism of melanoma. Therefore we need to rely on observational epidemiological studies to gain insights as to the way in which solar exposure interacts with genetic susceptibility to lead to cutaneous melanoma.

Cumulative sun exposure

The evidence for cumulative exposure comes from two sources to date: migrant studies and studies of lifetime exposure, controlling for intermittent and occupational exposure.

Data from Australia [43] and Israel [44] show that individuals who migrate at a young age from areas of low exposure, such as the UK, to areas of high exposure, such as Australia or Israel, have a lifetime risk of developing melanoma that is similar to that of the new country. On the other hand, individuals who migrate later in life—adolescence or older—from areas of low solar exposure to areas of high solar exposure, have a risk that is quite reduced. These data have often been cited to indicate that childhood sun exposure is more important than adult sun exposure in the development of melanoma. However, they can also be interpreted to indicate that the length of exposure is critical rather than the time of exposure: those who migrate early in life have a longer period for intense exposure compared to those who migrate later in life.

Individual susceptibility

Effect varies by skin type

The pattern of sun exposure that appears to induce melanoma development is complex and clearly differs according to skin type (propensity to burn, ability to tan). Armstrong [45] proposed a model consistent with data from other epidemiological studies [30,40,46,47] where risk for melanoma increases with increasing sun exposure among those who tan easily but only by a small amount, after which risk decreases with increasing exposure. Among subjects who are intermediate in their ability to tan, risk continues to increase slowly and then at some point declines with increasing exposure. On the other hand, those subjects who have great difficulty tanning have an almost linear increase in risk with increasing sun exposure. This model recognizes that individuals are differentially susceptible to sun exposure and have different levels of risk based on skin type. Moreover, it supports the idea that different *types* or *patterns* of sun exposure are associated with different levels of risk for melanoma.

All studies of melanoma do not support the idea that the patterns differs among individuals, because most studies of sun exposure and the development of melanoma have collected data using different questions and analysed them differently, so it is difficult to obtain consistency of effects. One study that illustrates this distinction quite clearly was a cohort study assessing swimsuit use outdoors during adolescence (ages 15–20) in relation to the risk of melanoma [47]. In this study Weinstock *et al.* found that swimsuit wearing among sun-resistant phenotypes was statistically significantly protective for the risk of developing melanoma (RR = 0.3, 95% CI = 0.1–0.8) whereas among sun-sensitive phenotypes risk was statistically significantly elevated (RR = 3.5, 95% CI = 1.3–9.3). These data in women are consistent with data reported by Holly *et al.* [30] showing that women who maintain a tan year-round are at reduced risk for developing melanoma (OR = 0.5, 95% CI = 0.3–0.9). It is likely that sun-sensitive women are not in this category, as they are unlikely to be able to maintain a year-round tan. A striking example of the critical importance of skin type in relationship to sun exposure as a risk factor for melanoma is seen in the recent study from Spain [34] where, *without adjusting for skin type*, farmers were at a significantly increased risk for developing melanoma (OR = 3.3, 95% CI = 1.4–7.8). *When adjusted for skin type and age*, farmers were at a significantly reduced risk for developing melanoma (OR = 0.5, 95% CI = 0.3–0.8).

Importance of sunburn in development of melanoma

While sunburn is the most visible and immediate effect of overexposure to UV, it is also the one that the public is most likely to associate with the development of melanoma. However, the emerging consensus is that it is unlikely that sunburn is *causally* associated with melanoma; it is more likely that sunburn is a clear indicator of the interaction between too much sun exposure and a susceptible phenotype, *or* severe solar exposure to skin unaccustomed to it.

The role of sunburn in the development of melanoma is a critical consideration. This aspect of sun exposure is the one most often cited as key to determining melanoma risk. Numerous articles in the lay media as well as dermatology journals stress the importance of a specific number of sunburns in increasing risk for melanoma. However, a critical look at these studies will show that the relative risk for developing melanoma, when adjusted for host characteristics, is often not statistically significant and is not always impressive.

Sunburn creates 'sunburn cells' which are damaged keratinocytes, are apoptotic and do not replicate [48]. Therefore, sunburn is not likely a surrogate for skin cancer, but rather sunburn is a 'marker' of the combination of intense intermittent sun exposure and sun sensitivity. The studies of sunburn and melanoma in Table 1.4 support this idea. The univariate estimates for the association of sunburn with melanoma are all positive. However, when the estimates are adjusted for potential confounders, such as skin type, age and sex, they almost uniformly become smaller and lose statistical significance. If sunburn were on the causal pathway for the development of melanoma, then this adjustment would actually strengthen the estimates.

Measurement error

Measurement error is a more serious problem in evaluating sunburn history than other sun-associated variables [54–56]. At least three studies have conducted test–retest reliability studies and concluded that sunburn history is poorly recalled with only a little over half the subjects giving the same answer at two points in time to the question: 'Have you ever been sunburned severely

Table 1.4 Studies of sunburn and melanoma, showing change from unadjusted to adjusted rates

Reference	Number of subjects	Unadjusted OR (95% CI)	Adjusted OR (95% CI)
MacKie & Aitchison [12]	113 adults	4.7 (2.5–8.8)	2.8 (1.1–7.4)
Lew *et al.* [13]	111 teens	2.1 (1.1–7.4)	Not given
Elwood *et al.* [49]	595 children	1.9 (not given)	1.3 (0.9–1.8)
Sorahan & Grimley [16]		7.0 (not given)	2.0 (not given)
Green *et al.* [50]	183 adults	3.4 (1.7–6.1)	2.4 (not given)
Holman *et al.* [19]	507 adults	Not given	1.6 (0.8–3.0)
Elwood *et al.* [37]	83 adults	3.2 (1.6–6.3)	1.5 (0.7–3.5)
Cristofolini *et al.* [38]	103 teens	1.2 (0.7–3.2)	0.7 (0.4–1.2)
Holly *et al.* [51]	121 adults	4.4 (1.8–10.9)	3.8 (1.4–10.4)
Osterlind *et al.* [20]	474 all	3.7 (2.3–6.1)	2.7 (1.6–4.8)
Weinstock *et al.* [52]	123 women	2.4 (1.3–4.4)	2.2 (1.2–3.8)
Dubin *et al.* [22]	132 adults	1.8 (1.2–3.8)	0.9 (not given)
Elwood *et al.* [53]	195 children	3.6 (1.3–11.2)	2.4 (0.8–7.3)
Zanetti *et al.* [24]	254 children	8.9 (3.5–26.8)	3.8 (2.3–6.4)

Abbreviations: CI, confidence interval; OR, odds ratio.

enough to cause pain or blisters for two days or more?' Other sun-associated variables, such as time spent outdoors during recreation, appear to be more reliably remembered [54].

Furthermore, the relationship between sun exposure, sunscreen use and the development of skin cancer is confounded ('negative confounding'), by the fact that subjects who are extremely sun-sensitive often engage in fewer activities in the bright sun and wear sunscreen when they do. These subjects are genetically susceptible to the development of skin cancer, and they may develop skin cancer regardless of the amount of sunlight exposure or the sun protection factor of the sunscreen.

Indeed, a great deal of research is currently being focused on suberythemic exposures (doses of UV radiation that do not cause an actual burn), but that may have biological significance. Certainly, exposures to the UVA portion of the UV spectrum may lead to the development of melanoma [57].

Relevance of age in development of melanoma

Much has been made of the critical time of sun exposure in the development of melanoma. This concept has not yet been proven and it is highly likely that all stages of development are important.

Not only is intermittent sun exposure the critical factor in epidemiological analyses, but lifetime intermittent sun exposure is also critical—both in early and later life. One can also interpret these data to suggest that sun exposure patterns are consistent throughout life. Individuals who receive a great deal of intermittent sun exposure during early life are also likely to receive a great deal of intermittent sun exposure during later life. The implication remains; long exposure to an intermittent pattern of sun exposure increases risk for the development of melanoma.

It is worthwhile looking at the estimates of effect of sun exposure on the development of melanoma in tandem with the other major risk factors for the development of melanoma: naevi number and pigmentary phenotype. Work is ongoing to determine the interrelationship of genetic susceptibility and these phenotypical characteristics [58]. In data from our large population-based study in Connecticut [37], we estimated the risk for developing melanoma for naevus number, pigmentary phenotype and sun exposure in early life as well as sun exposure 10 years prior to the diagnosis of melanoma, adjusting for age and sex. The risk for melanoma with numerous naevi in this study is six times that of someone with few naevi. The risk for melanoma with the most sensitive pigmentary phenotype is almost six times that of someone with the least sensitive phenotype. However, the risk for melanoma with increasing early life sun exposure or increasing later life sun exposure is only twice that of someone with the least sun exposure. Clearly, genetically determined characteristics, such as naevi and pigmentary phenotype, are more powerful determinants of melanoma risk than sun exposure.

The argument that 70% of an individual's sun exposure is likely to be obtained before the age of 20 may be true; however, this often-quoted statistic is merely an estimate [59]. With the changes in lifestyle of the 1990s and the early 21st century, it is quite possible that individuals in the latter half of life receive a very substantial amount of sun exposure as a result of early retirement and flexible work schedules. At the same time, there are numerous forces at work to diminish the outdoor experiences of young people; the tremendous increase in video games and computers as well as the increasing atomization of neighbourhoods, so that 'pick up' ball games are no longer as easy to organize.

The preponderance of data show that excessive intermittent sun exposure at any age increases risk for melanoma. Although the public and many researchers feel that sun exposure during early childhood is the critical period for melanoma induction, there are no empirical data to support this view. It surely is an attractive view.

Autier & Dore [60] attempted to address the issue as to whether early life or later life sun exposure was the critical factor in determining melanoma risk. They found that both time periods were important. An interesting comparison shows the joint effect of sun exposure during childhood and adulthood (Table 1.5). They find, as one might expect, that the highest risk among adults is for those who had high intermittent sun exposure as children. Conversely, those who had low sun exposure during childhood and high sun exposure in adulthood had a similar risk to those who had high exposure during childhood and

Table 1.5 Joint effect on melanoma risk of sun exposure during childhood and during adulthood in Europe

Indice of sun exposure during adulthood	Indice of sun exposure during childhood		
	Low	Moderate	High
Low	16/37	92/180	11/11
	1.0	1.1	2.0
		0.6–2.0	0.7–5.6
Moderate	25/41	103/66	27/13
	1.4	3.4	4.2
	0.6–3.0	1.7–6.6	1.7–10.3
High	28/33	93/56	17/8
	2.0	3.6	4.5
	0.9–4.5	1.8–7.1	1.6–12.5

Table 1.6 Joint effect on melanoma risk of sun exposure during childhood and during adulthood in Connecticut

Indice of sun exposure during adulthood	Indice of sun exposure during childhood		
	Low	Moderate	High
Low	37/68	58/50	29/34
	1.0	2.1	1.6
		(1.2–3.7)	(0.8–2.9)
Moderate	14/32	104/103	80/67
	0.8	1.9	2.2
	(0.4–1.7)	(1.2–3.0)	(1.3–3.7)
High	15/21	139/73	174/101
	1.3	3.5	3.2
	(0.6–2.9)	(2.2–5.7)	(1.9–5.0)

low exposure during adulthood. These authors have suggested that their analysis may well underestimate childhood exposure as a result of the long period of recall required.

Our own data from Connecticut (Table 1.6) are similar to those shown by Autier & Dore [60], who point out the difficulties of comparing sun exposure among different countries such as Australia and Canada at varying latitudes. Other data support the idea that intermittent sun exposure leads to increased risk at any age. Holly *et al.* [30] showed that more than seven painful sunburns during elementary school increased risk twofold (OR = 2.0, 95% CI = 1.4–2.9) and that more than seven sunburns after the age of 30 (the age of women in this study ranged from 18 to 59) increased risk twofold (OR = 2.0, 95% CI = 1.1–3.8).

In conclusion, data from very different settings seem to suggest that intermittent sun exposure is critical to the risk for developing melanoma. In the published studies that looked at both early life and adult sun exposure, there is very little difference between the effect of sun exposure at either stage, but lifelong intermittent sun exposure is indeed cumulative.

The message for the public should thus be: 'Be cautious *all* your life. Enjoy the sun in moderation.'

References

1 Lee JA. Declining effect of latitude on melanoma mortality rates in the United States: a preliminary study. *Am J Epidemiol* 1997; **146**: 413–7.

2 Armstrong BK, Kricker A. How much melanoma is caused by sun exposure? *Melanoma Res* 1993; **3**: 395–401.

3 Rosso S, Zanetti R, Martinez C, *et al*. The multicentre south European study '*Helios*'. II. different sun exposure patterns in the aetiology of basal cell and squamous cell carcinomas of the skin. *Br J Cancer* 1996; **73**: 1447–54.

4 Kricker A, Armstrong BK, English DR, Heenan PJ. A dose–response curve for sun exposure and basal cell carcinoma. *Int J Cancer* 1995; **60**: 482–8.

5 Kraemer KH. Commentary. Sunlight and skin cancer: another link revealed. *Proc Natl Acad Sci USA* 1997; **94**: 11–4.

6 Urbach F, Rose DB, Bonnem M. Genetic and environmental interactions in skin carcinogenesis. In: *Environmental Cancer.* Baltimore, MD: Williams and Wilkins, 1972: 356–71.

7 Green A, Williams G, Neale R, *et al*. Daily sunscreen application and betacarotene supplementation in prevention of basal-cell and squamous-cell carcinomas of the skin: randomised controlled trial. *Lancet* 1999; **354**: 723–9.

8 Rosso S, Zanetti R, Pippione M, Sancho-Garnier H. Parallel risk assessment of melanoma and basal cell carcinoma: skin characteristics and sun exposure. *Melanoma Res* 1998; **8** (6): 573–83.

9 Nelemans PJ, Rampen FHJ, Ruiter DJ, Verbeek ALM. An addition to the controversy on sunlight exposure and melanoma risk: a meta-analytical approach. *J Clin Epidemiol* 1995; **58**: 1331–42.

10 Elwood JM, Jopson J. Melanoma and sun exposure: an overview of published studies. *Int J Cancer* 1997; **73**: 198–203.

11 Klepp O, Magnus K. Some environmental and bodily characteristics of melanoma patients: a case–control study. *Int J Cancer* 1979; **23**: 482–6.

12 MacKie RM, Aitchison T. Severe sunburn and subsequent risk of primary cutaneous malignant melanoma in Scotland. *Br J Cancer* 1982; **46**: 955–60.

13 Lew RA, Sober AJ, Cook N, Marvell R, Fitzpatrick TB. Sun exposure habits in patients with cutaneous melanoma: a case–control study. *J Dermatol Surg Oncol* 1983; **12**: 981–6.

14 Rigel DS, Friedman RJ, Levenstein MJ, Greenwald DI. Relationship of fluorescent lights to malignant melanoma: another view. *J Dermatol Surg Oncol* 1983; **9**: 836–8.

15 Elwood JM, Gallagher RP, Hill GB, Pearson JCG. Cutaneous melanoma in relation to intermittent and constant sun exposure: the Western Canada Melanoma Study. *Int J Cancer* 1985; **35**: 427–43.

16 Sorahan T, Grimley RP. The aetiological significance of sunlight and fluorescent lighting in malignant melanoma: a case– control study. *Br J Cancer* 1985; **52**: 765–9.

17 Dubin N, Moseson M, Pasternack BS. Epidemiology of malignant melanoma: pigmentary traits, ultraviolet radiation, and the identification of high risk populations. In: Gallagher RP, ed. *Epidemiology of Malignant Melanoma: Recent Results in Cancer Research*. Berlin: Springer-Verlag, 1986: 56–75.

18 Green A, Bain C, McLennan R, Siskind V. Risk factors of cutaneous melanoma in Queensland. In: Gallagher RP, ed. *Epidemiology of Malignant Melanoma: Recent Results in Cancer Research*. Berlin: Springer-Verlag, 1986: 76–97.

19 Holman CDJ, Armstrong BK, Heenan RJ. Relationship of cutaneous malignant

melanoma to individual sunlight-exposure habits. *J Natl Cancer Inst* 1986; **76**: 403–14.
20 Osterlind A, Tucker MA, Stone BJ, Jensen OM. The Danish case–control study of cutaneous malignant melanoma. II. Importance of UV-light exposure. *Int J Cancer* 1988; **42**: 319–24.
21 Beitner H, Norell SE, Ringborg U, Wennersten G, Mattson B. Malignant melanoma: aetiological importance of individual pigmentation and sun exposure. *Br J Dermatol* 1990; **122**: 43–51.
22 Dubin N, Pasternack BS, Moseson M. Simultaneous assessment of risk factors for malignant melanoma and non-malignant melanoma skin lesions, with emphasis on sun exposure and related variables. *Int J Epidemiol* 1990; **19**: 811–9.
23 Grob JJ, Gouvernet J, Aymar D, *et al.* Count of benign melanocytic nevi as a major indicator of risk for nonfamilial nodular and superficial spreading melanoma. *Cancer* 1990; **66**: 387–95.
24 Zanetti R, Franceschi S, Rosso S, Colonna S, Bidoli E. Cutaneous melanoma and sunburns in childhood in a southern European population. *Eur J Cancer* 1992; **28A**: 1172–6.
25 Zaridze D, Mukeria A, Duffy SW. Risk factors for skin melanoma in Moscow. *Int J Cancer* 1992; **52**: 159–61.
26 Herzfeld PM, Fitzgerald EF, Hwang S, Stark A. A case–control study of malignant melanoma of the trunk among white males in upstate New York. *Cancer Detect Prev* 1993; **17**: 601–8.
27 Autier P, Doré JF, Le Jeune F, *et al.* and EORTC Malignant Melanoma Cooperative Group. Recreational exposure to sunlight and lack of information as risk factors for cutaneous malignant melanoma. Results of a European Organization for Research and Treatment of Cancer (EORTC) case–control study in Belgium, France and Germany. *Melanoma Res* 1994; **4**: 79–85.
28 Nelemans PJ, Rampen FHJ, Groenendal H, Kiemeney LALM, Ruiter DJ, Verbeek ALM. Swimming and the risk of cutaneous melanoma. *Melanoma Res* 1994; **4**: 281–6.
29 Westerdahl J, Olsson H, Ingvar C. At what age do sunburn episodes play a crucial role for the development of malignant melanoma? *Eur J Cancer* 1994; **30A**: 1647–54.
30 Holly EA, Aston DA, Cress RD, Ahn DK, Kristiansen JJ. Cutaneous melanoma in women. I. Exposure to sunlight, ability to tan, and other risk factors related to ultraviolet light. *Am J Epidemiol* 1995; **141**: 923–33.
31 Rodenas JM, Delgado-Rodriguez M, Herranz MT, Tercedor J, Serrano S. Sun exposure, pigmentary traits, and risk of cutaneous malignant melanoma: a case–control study in a Mediterranean population. *Cancer Causes Control* 1996; **7**: 275–83.
32 Berwick M, Begg CB, Fine JA, Roush GC, Barnhill RL. Screening for cutaneous melanoma by skin self-examination. *J Natl Cancer Inst* 1996; **88**: 17–23.
33 Walter SD, King WD, Marrett LD. Association of cutaneous malignant melanoma with intermittent exposure to ultraviolet radiation: results of a case–control study in Ontario. *Can Int J Epidemiol* 1999; **3**: 418–27.
34 Espinosa Arranz J, Sanchez Hernandez JJ, Bravo Fernandez P, *et al.* Cutaneous malignant melanoma and sun exposure in Spain. *Melanoma Res* 1999; **9**: 199–205.
35 Gallagher RP, Elwood JM, Yang CP. Is chronic sunlight exposure important in accounting for increases in melanoma incidence? *Int J Cancer* 1989; **44** (5): 813–5.
36 Graham S, Marshall J, Haughey B, *et al.* An inquiry into the epidemiology of melanoma. *Am J Epidemiol* 1985; **122**: 606–19.
37 Elwood JM, Williamson C, Stapleton PJ. Malignant melanoma in relation to moles, pigmentation, and exposure to fluorescent and other light sources. *Br J Cancer* 1986; **53**: 65–74.
38 Cristofolini M, Fraceschi S, Tasin L, *et al.* Risk factors for cutaneous malignant melanoma in a northern Italian population. *Int J Cancer* 1987; **39**: 150–4.
39 Garbe C, Kruger S, Stadler R, Guggenmoos-Holzmann I, Orfanos CE. Markers and relative risk in a German population for developing malignant melanoma. *Int J Dermatol* 1989; **28**: 517–23.
40 White E, Kirkpatrick CS, Lee JAH. Case–control study of malignant

melanoma in Washington state. I. Constitutional factors and sun exposure. *Am J Epidemiol* 1994; **139**: 857–68.

41 Chen Y, Dubrow R, Holfrod TR, *et al.* Malignant melanoma risk factors by anatomic site: a case–control study and polychotomous logistic regression analysis. *Int J Cancer* 1996; **67**: 636–43.

42 Wolf P, Quehenberger F, Mullegger R, Stranz B, Kerl H. Phenotypic markers, sunlight-related factors and sunscreen use in patients with cutaneous melanoma: an Austrian case–control study. *Melanoma Res* 1998; **8**: 370–8.

43 Khlat M, Vail A, Parkin M, Green A. Mortality from melanoma in migrants to Australia: variation by age at arrival and duration of stay. *Am J Epidemiol* 1992; **135** (10): 1103–13.

44 Iscovich J, Howe GR. Cancer incidence patterns (1972–91) among migrants from the Soviet Union to Israel. *Cancer Causes Control* 1998; January **9** (1): 29–36.

45 Armstrong BK. Epidemiology of malignant melanoma: intermittent or total accumulated exposure to the sun? *J Dermatol Surg Oncol* 1988; **14**: 835–49.

46 Dubin N, Moseson M, Pasternak BS. Sun exposure and malignant melanoma among susceptible individuals. *Environ Health Perspect* 1989; **81**: 139–51.

47 Weinstock MA, Colditz GA, Willett WC, *et al.* Melanoma and the sun: the effect of swimsuits and a 'healthy' tan on the risk of nonfamilial malignant melanoma in women. *Am J Epidemiol* 1991; **134**: 462–70.

48 Gilchrest BA, Eller MS, Geller AC, Yaar M. The pathogenesis of melanoma induced by ultraviolet radiation. *N Engl J Med* 1999; **340**: 1341–8.

49 Elwood JM, Gallagher RP, Hill GB, Spinelli JJ, Pearson JCG, Threlfall W. Pigmentation and skin reaction to sun as risk factors for cutaneous melanoma: the Western Canada Melanoma Study. *Br Med J* 1984; **288**: 99–102.

50 Green A, Siskind V, Bain C, Alexander J. Sunburn and malignant melanoma. *Br J Cancer* 1985; **51**: 393–7.

51 Holly EA, Kelly JW, Shpall SN, Chiu S. Number of melanocytic nevi as a major risk factor for malignant melanoma. *J Am Acad Dermatol* 1987; 17: 459–68.

52 Weinstock MA, Colditz GA, Willett WC, *et al.* Nonfamilial cutaneous melanoma incidence in women associated with sun exposure before 20 years of age. *Pediatrics* 1989; **84**: 199–204.

53 Elwood JM, Whitehead SM, Davison J, Stewart M, Galt M. Malignant melanoma in England: risks associated with naevi, freckles, social class, hair colour, and sunburn. *Int J Epidemiol* 1990; **19**: 801–10.

54 English DR, Armstrong BK, Kricker A. Reproducibility of reported measurements of sun exposure in a case–control study. *Cancer Epidemiol Biomarkers Prev* 1998; **7** (10): 857–63.

55 Westerdahl J, Anderson H, Olsson H, Ingvar C. Reproducibility of a self-administered questionnaire for assessment of melanoma risk. *Int J Epidemiol* 1996; **25** (2): 245–51.

56 Berwick M, Chen YT. Reliability of reported sunburn history in a case–control study of cutaneous malignant melanoma. *Am J Epidemiol* 1995; **141** (11): 1033–7.

57 Moan J, Dahlback A, Setlow RB. Epidemiological support for an hypothesis for melanoma induction indicating a role for UVA radiation. *Photochem Photobiol* 1999; **70** (2): 243–7.

58 Begg CB, Berwick M. A note on the estimation of relative risks of rare genetic susceptibility markers. *Cancer Epidemiol Biomarkers Prev* 1997; February **6** (2): 99–103.

59 Stern RS, Weinstein MC, Baker SG. Risk reduction for nonmelanoma skin cancer with childhood sunscreen use. *Arch Dermatol* 1986; May, **122** (5): 537–45.

60 Autier P, Doré JF. Influence of sun exposures during childhood and during adulthood on melanoma risk. EPIMEL and EORTC Melanoma Cooperative Group. European Organisation for Research and Treatment of Cancer. *Int J Cancer* 1998; **77**: 533–7.

2: Are sunbeds dangerous?

Philippe Autier

Introduction

Exposure to solar radiation has been recognized as a major environmental risk factor for cutaneous melanoma [1], and ultraviolet radiation (UV, 100–400 nm) is deemed to represent the part of the solar spectrum involved in melanomaogenesis. An epidemic of cutaneous melanoma has affected most fair-skinned populations in the last half century. This is increasingly considered to be a result of more exposure to sunlight for recreational or cosmetic purposes. Long-term exposure to ultraviolet radiation is also known to have a role in other health conditions such as cataracts, keratitis, skin photo-ageing and immunosuppression.

The fashion of using artificial sources of ultraviolet radiation (sunlamps, sunbeds, solaria) for cosmetic or recreational purposes is now widespread among fair-skinned communities, particularly in North European countries. The *precautionary principle* is frequently evoked in the shaping of European health policies, or when food or drug safety issues are debated. In brief, that principle consists of avoiding the general public use of, or exposure to, a substance whose safety remains open to question. However, even though the health hazards associated with sunbed use—potentially at least—are equivalent to those associated with intense recreational sun exposure, the commercialization and use of tanning devices remains poorly controlled.

From sunlamp to sunbed

Since the beginning of the last century, exposure to solar radiation has been regarded as beneficial for health, particularly because of its importance for vitamin D synthesis. Furthermore, sunlight or ultraviolet radiation is commonly used to treat various dermatological conditions such as psoriasis. In many areas populated by fair-skinned people, bright sunlight is available only during a few periods of the year. Therefore, alternative sources of ultraviolet radiation have been invented. In the 1950s and 1960s, mercury lamps emitting large proportions of ultraviolet C (UVC, 100–280 nm) and ultraviolet B radiation (UVB, 280–315 nm) were popular in Northern Europe and North America. Typically, they were portable devices equipped with a single UV lamp, sometimes accompanied by infrared lamps to heat the skin. Exposure to these lamps was of short duration but could lead to the development of erythema, burns and blistering. These UV lamps were primarily intended for domestic use and therefore many were still in use after most nations had put a ban on their commercialization.

In the 1970s, UVB was recognized as the most carcinogenic part of the solar spectrum, and a shift in usage occurred towards low-pressure fluorescent tubes emitting mainly in the ultraviolet A range (UVA, 315–400 nm). Body-sized tanning units, called sunbeds or solaria, became commercially available. UVB represents 0.5–4% of the spectrum of sunbeds equipped with fluorescent lamps [2–4]. UVB is far more efficient than UVA for inducing the synthesis of melanin and therefore the presence of UVB in sunbed output is critical for the induction of a deep persistent tan. In that respect the term 'UVA tanning', often used to designate the acquisition of a tan using artificial sources of ultraviolet radiation, is misleading.

As well as the traditional fluorescent tubes, high-pressure lamps producing large quantities of long wave UVA (>335–400 nm) per unit of time are sold, that can emit 10 times more UVA than is present in sunlight. Some sunbeds combine both high-pressure long-wave UVA lamps with classic low-pressure fluorescent lamps.

The UV output and spectral characteristics (amounts of UV in the UVB or UVA ranges) of sunbeds vary considerably. Surveys in the UK on sunbeds operated in public or commercial facilities revealed substantial differences in UV output, mainly for UVB, for which 60-fold differences in output were observed [3–4]. These differences occur because of sunbed design (e.g. the type of fluorescent tubes used as sources, the materials composing filters, the distance from canopy to the skin), sunbed power and tube ageing. Sunbeds in commercial facilities have a greater output in the UVB range [5], as consumers are more satisfied by the fast and deep tan they have paid for.

The indoor tanning fashion

Usage of sunbeds spread in the 1980s. Before then, less than 5% of the adult population in Belgium, France and Germany had ever used a sunlamp for tanning purpose [6]. Another 5% had been exposed to artificial UV sources for medical or occupational reasons. In 1995, about one-third of the adult population of these countries had ever used sunbeds. Numerous surveys in Europe and North America in recent years indicate that between 15 and 35% of women, and between 5 and 10% of men between 15 and 30 years have used sunbeds [6–10]. These figures may rise to 50% in countries such as Sweden [11,12]. A market survey carried out in Denmark in 1996 (AC Nielsen-AIM, Copenhagen, 1997) showed that 11% of subjects, aged 13 years or more, reported use of sunbeds less than once each month, 8% used sunbeds 1–3 times per month, and 5% used sunbeds at least once every week. The latter data indicate that a non-negligible proportion of the population may receive huge amounts of UV through sunbed use. A study has estimated that Swedish adolescents received annual total dosage of UV from sunbeds comparable to dosage received from the sun [13]. In the last few years, the indoor tanning fashion has rapidly extended in Mediterranean areas, such as the north of Italy, and in countries with an emerging economy, such as Argentina [14]. A substantial proportion of sunbeds are used in private facilities, and homemade solaria are not uncommon.

The popularity of indoor tanning is rooted in the perceived cosmetic and psychological benefits of acquisition or maintenance of a healthy, attractive look [15]. There is also a widespread belief that acquisition of a prevacation tan may protect against the harmful effects of the sun. There is a possibility that another strong motive for sunbed use would be the ability of UV exposure (especially high UVA doses) to induce a sensation of well-being, mediated by the synthesis of enkephalin in the skin, that enters the bloodstream and then influences the central nervous system [16].

Relationship between indoor tanning and skin lesions and melanoma

Clinical data

Numerous clinical reports have been published about the deleterious effects of exposure to sunlamps/sunbeds on the skin (for a review see Spencer & Amonette [17]) and on the eye [18]. Severe skin burns have be seen in subjects who used photosensitizing drugs or skin lotions to foster their tanning ability (e.g. the psoralens) [19].

In the absence of valid animal models for human melanoma, epidemiological studies are mandatory for producing the most convincing documentation of an association between sunbed use and melanoma.

Epidemiological data

Epidemiological investigation of the possible association between sunbed use and skin malignancy faces the challenging question of how to recognize *now* a current exposure that could become recognized as a major carcinogenic hazard in the future? Three aspects must be carefully born in mind when reading the epidemiological literature on this topic. First, the latency period between exposure to a potentially carcinogenic agent and melanoma occurrence may be 20 or 30 years. Sunbed use is an exposure that has become more frequent in the last 20 years, so the impact on melanoma incidence may not be detectable before the year 2000 or 2010.

Secondly, the existence of a latency period may lead to an underestimation of the actual association between indoor tanning and melanoma. Because the carcinogenic effect of more recent exposure is not yet detectable, a lack of distinction between ancient and recent exposures may mask the actual increase in risk. As shown in a theoretical example displayed in Table 2.1, the masking effect will be more pronounced if recent exposures are more frequent than ancient exposures. The disease–exposure association only appears when ancient and recent exposures are distinguished.

Thirdly, sunbed users have a greater propensity than average to enjoy recreational sun exposure [7]. Hence, statistical analysis of epidemiological data should always adjust risk estimates for recreational sun exposure.

Results from epidemiological studies

At least 19 epidemiological investigations have examined the association between cutaneous melanoma and exposure to sunlamps or sunbeds (reviewed by Swerdlow & Weinstock [20]). Most of these studies only examined whether at least one exposure to sunlamp/sunbed was associated with cutaneous melanoma, and produced negative answers. These results are not highly informative because of the masking effect of recent sunbed exposures (Table 2.1).

Since 1979, five epidemiological case–control studies have explored in more detail the relationship between exposure to sunlamps/sunbeds and cutaneous melanoma (Table 2.2) [6,11,21–23]. These studies mainly addressed the significance of the use of sunlamps or sunbeds during the 1980s, when the

Table 2.1 Theoretical example of masking effect of recent exposures that have no detectable impact on a disease

	Not exposed	Exposed	Ancient exposures	Recent exposures
Cases	300	90	30	60
Controls	300	90	15	75
Estimated risk*		1.00	2.00	0.80
95% Confidence interval		0.71–1.41	1.01–3.99	0.54–1.18

* Risk is calculated as an odds ratio, always using the 300 cases and 300 controls not exposed as the reference group.

Table 2.2 Sunlamp or sunbed use and risk of cutaneous melanoma

Study place, year of publication [ref] (number of cases–controls)	Study years	Estimated melanoma risk for ever vs. never exposed to sunlamp/ sunbed	95% Confidence interval
Scotland, 1988 [29] (180/120)	1979–84	2.9†	1.3–6.4*
Ontario, Canada, 1990 [30] (583/608)	1984–86	Males: 1.88† Females: 1.45†	1.20–2.98* 0.99–2.13
Sweden, 1994 [3] (400/640)	1988–90	1.3‡	0.9–1.8
Belgium, France, Germany, 1994 [2] (420/447)	1991–92	0.97†	0.71–1.32
Connecticut, 1998 [23] (624/512)	1987–89	1.13‡	0.82–1.54

* $P \leq 0.05$.
† Crude risk estimates.
‡ Adjusted for natural sun sensitivity, sunburn history and exposure to sunlight.

indoor tanning fashion was in its early phase. In the Scottish and Ontario studies, melanoma occurrence appeared more elevated among subjects who had ever exposed their skin to sunlamps/sunbeds. However, risk estimates were not adjusted for recreational sun exposure. The Swedish study [11] suggested a positive association between sunbed use and cutaneous melanoma among subjects less than 30 years old but, because of the small numbers of cases and controls in that age range, the association was not statistically significant.

An association between indoor tanning and cutaneous melanoma risk is suggested by the following data.

1 The five studies found some degree of increasing melanoma risk with increasing sunlamp/sunbed exposure (Table 2.3).

2 In four studies (Table 2.4), the melanoma risk associated with sunbed use was systematically higher in subjects who had their first exposure many years before the diagnosis of melanoma, than in subjects with more recent exposures (the Swedish study [11] did not explore that aspect).

3 In the EORTC study [6], subjects who reported skin erythemal reactions caused by tanning sessions and more than 10 h of accumulated exposure to sunlamp/sunbed displayed a sevenfold increase in melanoma, after adjustment for natural sun susceptibility and recreational sun exposure.

The possible role of sunbed use in the aetiology of ocular melanoma has been examined by three epidemiological studies [24–26]. These three studies produced results consistent with a two- to fourfold increased risk for uveal melanoma associated with sunlamp/sunbed use.

Table 2.3 Duration of exposure to sunlamp or sunbed and melanoma risk*

Study place, year of publication	Duration of exposure	Cases	Controls	Estimated melanoma risk	95% CI
Scotland, 1988	Never used	142	110	1.0§	–
	< 3 months	6	3	0.7	0.1–3.8
	3 months–1 year	24	5	3.1	1.0–9.9
	> 1 year	8	2	3.4	0.6–20.3
Test for linear trend: P = 0.0029					
Ontario, 1990					
Males	Never used	210	242	1.00‡	–
	< 180 min	25	20	1.44	0.75–2.82
	≥ 180 min	39	18	2.50	1.34–4.80
Test for linear trend in males: P = 0.0012					
Females	Never used	222	256	1.00‡	–
	< 180 min	39	39	1.17	0.70–1.95
	≥ 180 min	38	27	1.62	0.91–2.89
Test for linear trend in females: P = 0.070					
Sweden, 1994	Never used	282	479	1.0§	–
	1–3 sessions	44	67	1.1	0.7–1.9
	4–10 sessions	30	55	1.1	0.7–1.9
	> 10 sessions	41	33	1.8	1.0–3.2
Test for linear trend: P = 0.020					
Belgium, France, Germany, 1994†	Never used	310	327	1.00§	–
Exposure starts ≥ 1980	< 10 h	36	45	0.75	0.46–1.25
	≥ 10 h	19	18	0.99	0.49–2.00
Exposure starts < 1980	< 10 h	16	15	1.00	0.47–2.13
	≥ 10 h	18	7	2.12	0.84–2.12
Test for linear trend: P = 0.033 when start < 1980; P = 0.89 when start ≥ 1980					
Connecticut, USA, 1998	Never used	483	417	1.00§	–
	< 10 sunlamp uses	76	50	1.25	0.84–1.84
	≥ 10 sunlamp uses	63	40	1.15	0.60–2.20
Test for linear trend: P = 0.068					

* Duration of exposure, relative risk, and 95% confidences as in published reports. The Mantel χ^2 for trend was calculated by us.

† The 21 cases and 35 controls who were exposed to sunlamp or sunbed for non-tanning purpose are not reported in this table.

‡ Adjusted for age.

§ Adjusted for age, sex, natural sun-sensitivity and recreational sun exposure.

Discussion of epidemiological data

The studies we reviewed indicated the possibility of an association between sunlamp/sunbed use and melanoma.

The association could be the consequence of bias. For instance, melanoma patients might be more likely to remember past exposures to UV sources. The Ontario study performed a part of the interview before patients were told they

Table 2.4 Ancient and recent exposure to sunlamp or sunbed and risk of cutaneous melanoma. These results were not reported in the Swedish study [11]

Reference	Estimated melanoma risk (95% CI)	
	First exposure more ancient	First exposure more recent
Scotland, 1988 [29]†	9.1 (2.0–40.6)*	1.9 (0.6–5.6)
Ontario, Canada, 1990 [30]†		
Males	2.00 (1.21–3.34)*	1.52 (0.56–4.25)
Females	1.53 (0.96–2.46)	1.24 (0.67–2.31)
Belgium, France, Germany, 1994 [2]‡	2.12 (0.84–5.37)	0.99 (0.49–2.00)
Connecticut, USA, 1998 [23]§	1.33 (0.84–2.12)	1.15 (0.64–2.07)

* $P \leq 0.05$.
† Five years since last use, unadjusted odds ratio for ever exposed vs. never exposed.
‡ First exposure took place before 1980, odds ratio for 10 h of exposure or more vs. never exposed, adjusted for age, sex, natural sun-sensitivity and recreational sun-exposure.
§ Exposures ≤ 1970 are more ancient, and exposures after 1970 are more recent; adjusted for age, sex, natural sun-sensitivity, and recreational sun-exposure.

had a melanoma, and concluded that recall bias was not likely to explain their findings [22]. Unfortunately, the Ontario study did not adjust risk estimates for sun exposure. Similarly, the positive trends described in Table 2.3 would need adjustment for recreational sun exposure and natural sun sensitivity before making any firm conclusions. Also, timescales for expressing duration of sunlamp/sunbed exposure were variable between studies. Hence, methodological aspects may partly explain results from epidemiological studies on sunbed exposure and cutaneous melanoma.

Despite these limitations, the consistency in dose–response trends, the higher risk systematically found for most ancient exposures, as well as the melanoma risk associated with sunlamp/sunbed-induced skin erythema merit attention. These results are quite consistent with the hypothesis of a delayed impact of sunbed use on melanoma incidence because of the latency period of several decades between exposure to a carcinogenic agent and cancer occurrence.

Sunbed use is capable of causing skin erythema and blistering, and UV-induced skin erythemal reactions (sunburns) are known risk factors for cutaneous melanoma. Skin erythema or burns are reported by 18–44% of sunbed users, mainly by subjects with a poor ability to tan [6–8,11–12,17–27]. UVB is also known to be 1000 times more erythemogenic than UVA, and sunlamp/sunbed-induced erythemal reactions could be attributable to the UVB present in the tanning machine output [2]. In that respect, it could be argued that the higher melanoma risk observed with more ancient exposures (Table 2.3) could be attributable to the older type UV lamps that emitted significant amounts of UVB. However, in the EORTC and in other studies [6–8,10–12], skin erythema occurred after exposure to modern sunbeds. Also, high fluxes of UVA—commonly found in modern tanning machines—are capable of inducing skin erythemal reactions [28].

Because of the latency between exposure to carcinogenic agents and melanoma occurrence, epidemiological studies completed so far would have just been capable of examining the influence of exposures that took place when indoor tanning was less common. In that respect, only new studies will be able to reveal the eventual melanoma risk attributable to sunbed exposure that has became widespread after 1980.

Medical use of ultraviolet radiation

Ultraviolet radiation is used to treat a variety of skin diseases, such as psoriasis. UV-based therapies occur in controlled conditions within the frame of scheduled treatment protocols. The UV spectra emitted by tanning equipment are wider that those used for treating skin diseases and it is not known whether the cutaneous responses of the average sunbed user resemble those seen in the skin of patients suffering from severe psoriasis. Thus, experience derived from UV-treated patients can hardly be transposed to indoor tanning for cosmetic or leisure purposes.

One prospective study found an increased melanoma risk in patients suffering from severe psoriasis treated with a combination of UVA and psoralens (PUVA therapy) [29]. The increased risk was mainly apparent in psoriatic patients who had received 250 treatments or more. However, it was impossible to ascertain which treatment component was implicated in the higher melanoma risk, as psoralens are potent photocarcinogens, and a proportion of patients received various other potentially carcinogenic treatments (e.g. coal tar).

Is there a limit below which indoor tanning would be safe?

At present it is not possible to define the cumulative time of exposure that would lead to increased melanoma risk. If assessable, this limit would be highly variable according to the UV spectrum emitted by a tanning machine and the individual sensitivity to UV radiation. Although epidemiological studies provide clues to the amount of cumulative sunbed exposure possibly leading to significant melanoma risk (Table 2.3), results are quite heterogeneous. The breakdown of risk by skin phototype is not available, and the time period during which sessions took place was not always analysed. Several expert groups have suggested maximum numbers of tanning sessions, but these are ‘best guess’ not supported by human data. For instance, in 1990, the British

Photodermatology Group recommended not to exceed a cumulative amount of 10 h of indoor tanning per year [30]. A document entitled 'Outdoors and indoors: sun wisely', produced under the auspices of the Dutch Cancer Society [31], argues that sunbed exposure not exceeding 50 minimal erythemal doses (MED) per year is acceptable (1 MED corresponds to the UV dose triggering a minimal skin erythema in a moderately sun-sensitive subject). A 30-min sunbed session represents an exposure to 0.7–1 MED, and a 2-week summer holiday on the Mediterranean with regular sunbathing may represent a cumulative UV dose of 100 MED. Hence, limits suggested for duration of sunbed exposure are well above the levels of sunbed exposure found to be possibly associated with an increased melanoma risk (Table 2.3), and with sun exposure behaviours known to be associated with melanoma occurrence.

Arguments often evoked for the defence of indoor tanning

The sunbed industry, tanning enthusiasts and a fraction of the medical community exploit several lines of argument to defend the use of artificial tanning devices. A more subtle position is the recognition of the good and bad effects of indoor tanning but that, on balance, good effects outweigh bad effects. Arguments put forward by indoor tanning advocates are often speculative and of questionable scientific validity, but they represent the core of most documents backing the commercialization of sunbeds, and the justification that indoor tanning is not an unacceptable health threat. Daily experience shows that these arguments are often accepted as true science by many doctors, institutions active in cancer prevention and decision makers. We review and briefly discuss the most important of them.

The UV spectrum emitted by sunbeds is safer than the solar spectrum

This argument suggests that a tan acquired through sunbed use would be safer than a tan acquired through sunbathing on a beach. It is largely based on the fact that compared to the summer Mediterranean sun, the UV spectrum of a modern sunbed contains between one and two times more UVA, and about half the amount of UVB [4]. However, the concept of a 'safe tan' is ill-founded and tanning with either UVB or UVA conveys a carcinogenic risk of similar order of magnitude [28,32]. The UV wavelength(s) involved in melanoma occurrence remain(s) unknown. Nevertheless, UVA is no longer regarded as an innocent radiation. An increasing number of data indicate that UVA is able to induce skin erythema, genetic damage, local and systemic immunosuppression and skin malignancies in animals [1,28,33], and that it could be implicated in melanomaogenesis [34,35].

Recent studies suggest that tanning is a direct consequence of UV-induced DNA damage [36]. Substantial skin DNA damage is detectable after sunbed exposure, which is comparable to DNA damage induced by exposure to natural sunlight; this is chiefly caused by the UVB fraction present in the output of most sunbeds [37,38]. Thus, at present, the available scientific data hardly support the idea that an artificially acquired tan would be safer than a tan acquired through sun exposure.

Acquisition of a tan with sunbed use would achieve the maximum protective effect through a combination of pigmentation and skin thickening

Recent data show that acquisition of a prevacation tan offers only little protection against UV-induced DNA damage [39], and the moderate skin thickening induced by sunbed use would afford even less photoprotection than tanning [40]. Also, many uncertainties persist as to the role of melanin, and of the induction of melanin synthesis in skin carcinogenesis [41,42].

A prevacation tan confers protection against sunburn and other deleterious effects of the sun

This argument is a corollary of the former one. Surveys in various fair-skinned communities show that between 25 and 50% of sunbed users report that they want to 'prepare the skin for the holidays'. Because a prevacation tan offers some protection against sun-induced erythema, a prevacation tan may induce hazardous sun exposure behaviour, such as the promotion of prolonged sun exposure. Hence, the risk of melanoma eventually associated with indoor tanning would include not only the exposure to UV radiation emitted by tanning devices, but also the possibility of increased sun exposure at the start of the holiday [39].

Regulations

A number of reports from various scientific domains have triggered reactions intended to discourage use of sunbeds [43–46]. Norms for cosmetic use of UV-emitting devices have been published by official organizations [47–50]. Since 1990, several countries (e.g. Sweden, UK, France, Belgium, USA, Canada) have issued specific regulations for sunbed installation, with indications of which of the different types of tanning device can be made available to the general public, commercial facilities and health professionals. These regulations also include a series of recommendations covering a broad ranges of issues, such as how tanning units must be operated and the information operators must deliver to consumers. There is advice about what warning messages should be visible in the room where the sunbed is installed, the protection of eyes, the danger of taking photosensitizing medications or lotions, and many other aspects.

In some countries (e.g. UK and the Netherlands) lists of recommendations exist, formulated by, or in association with the sunbed industry. In the present state of controversy, only those regulations or recommendations originating from bodies working in total independence from commercial interests should be considered.

An important objective of these regulations is the requirement for better information for consumers. The impact of these regulations on potential health hazards associated with sunbed use is, however, difficult to estimate. On the positive side, these regulations are likely to protect consumers against the most dangerous UV devices. However, enforcement of regulations remains a challenge [8–17] and surveys repeatedly show the ignorance of both sunbed users and tanning facility operators of health hazards associated with indoor tanning.

Existing regulations do not apply to private use of sunbeds. Furthermore, they rarely reflect the body of knowledge available on the association between UV exposure and skin cancers or other UV-induced lesions, such as premature skin ageing. In that respect, most existing regulations could simply result in the provision of a false sense of security to both consumers and tanning parlour operators, and thus encourage indoor tanning.

Conclusions

Despite regulations and recommendations, the bottom line is that each time an individual desires to acquire a tan, or to feel a sensation of well-being, either through sunbathing or through sunbed use, there is exposure to biologically effective, potentially carcinogenic doses of UV. Hence, from a strict point of view—exposure to a hazardous health agent—the sunbed market remains largely unregulated.

If the latency period hypothesis is well grounded, the accumulating data from daily dermatological practice, and laboratory or epidemiological research provide good reasons to believe that the indoor tanning fashion may represent a time-bomb. Given the great number of subjects currently using sunbeds, even a moderate increase in risk may contribute to a significant extra number of melanoma patients in the next decades.

It is unlikely that public health control of indoor tanning will effectively take place in the absence of visible life-threatening conditions attributable to that fashion. With time, the melanoma risk eventually conveyed by indoor tanning will become more apparent, mainly in the northern areas of America and Europe. New epidemiological studies are needed to monitor the impact of sunbed use on the occurrence of skin and eye cancers, and to establish whether the latency period hypothesis is valid or not.

In the meantime, health prevention programmes should discourage sunbed use. Prevention messages should be targeted to adolescents and young adults, with the main objective of bringing correct information on health hazards possibly associated with indoor tanning, and to combat the numerous unverified beliefs accompanying the promotion of exposure to artificial sources of UV radiation.

References

1 International Agency for Research on Cancer (IARC). Solar and ultraviolet radiation. *IARC Monogr Eval Carcinog Risks Hum* 1992; **55**: 217–28.

2 Rivers JK, Norris PG, Murphy GM, *et al.* UVA sunbeds: tanning, photoprotection, acute adverse effects and immunological changes. *Br J Dermatol* 1989; **120**: 767–77.

3 Wright AL, Hart GC, Kernohan E, Twentyman G. Survey of the variation in ultraviolet outputs from ultraviolet A sunbeds in Bradford. *Photodermatol Photoimmunol Photomed* 1996; **12**: 12–16.

4 McGintley J, Martin CJ, MacKie RM. Sunbeds in current use in Scotland: a survey of their output and patterns of use. *Br J Dermatol* 1998; **139**: 428–38.

5 Wright AL, Hart GC, Kernohan EE. Dangers of sunbeds are greater in the commercial sector. *Br Med J* 1997; **314**: 1280–1.

6 Autier P, Doré JF, Lejeune F, *et al.* Cutaneous malignant melanoma and exposure to sunlamps or sunbeds: an EORTC multicenter case–control study in Belgium, France and Germany. *Int J Cancer* 1994; **58**: 809–13.

7 Autier P, Joarlette M, Lejeune F, Lienard D, Andre J, Achten G. Cutaneous malignant melanoma and exposure to sunlamps and sunbeds: a descriptive study in Belgium. *Melanoma Res* 1991; **1**: 69–74.

8 Oliphant JA, Forster JL, McBride CM. The use of commercial tanning facilities by suburban Minnesota adolescents. *Am J Public Health* 1994; **84**: 476–8.

9 Banks BA, Silverman RA, Schwartz RH, Tunnessen WW. Attitudes of teenagers toward sun exposure and sunscreen use. *Pediatrics* 1992; **89**: 40–2.

10 Rhainds M, De Guire L, Claveau J. A population-based survey on the use of artificial tanning devices in the province of Québec. *J Am Acad Dermatol* 1999; **40**: 572–6.

11 Westerdahl J, Olsson H, Masbäck A, *et al.* Use of sunbeds or sunlamps and malignant melanoma in Southern Sweden. *Am J Epidemiol* 1994; **140**: 691–9.

12 Boldeman C, Beitner H, Jansson B, Nilsson B, Ullen H. Sunbed use in relation to phenotype, erythema, sunscreen use and skin disease: a questionnaire survey among Swedish adolescents. *Br J Dermatol* 1996; **135**: 712–16.

13 Wester U, Boldemann C, Jansson B, Ullén H. Population UV-dose and skin area: do sunbeds rival the sun? *Health Phys* 1999; **77**: 436–40.

14 Chouela E, Pellerano G, Bessone A, Ducard M, Poggio N, Abeldano A. Sunbed use in Buenos Aires. *Photodermatol Photoimmunol Photomed* 1999; **15**: 100–3.

15 Arthey S, Clarke VA. Suntanning and sun protection: a review of the psychological literature. *Soc Sci Med* 1995; **40**: 265–74.

16 Nissen JB, Avrach WW, Hansen ES, Stengaard-Pedersen K, Kragballe K. Increased levels of enkephalin following natural sunlight (combined with salt water bathing at the Dead Sea) and ultraviolet A irradiation. *Br J Dermatol* 1998; **139**: 1012–19.

17 Spencer JM, Amonette RA. Indoor tanning: risks, benefits, and future trends. *J Am Acad Dermatol* 1995; **33**: 288–98.

18 Daxecker F, Blumthaler M, Ambach W. Keratitis solaris and sunbeds. *Ophthalmologica* 1995; **209**: 329–30.
19 Latarjet J, Tranchant P, Boucaud C, Robert A, Foyatier JL. Les brûlûres sévères dues aux psoralènes (severe skin burns due to psoralens). *La Lettre Du Brûlologue* 1993; **15**: 2–3 [in French].
20 Swerdlow AJ, Weinstock MA. Do tanning lamps cause melanoma? An epidemiologic assessment. *J Am Acad Dertamol* 1998; **38**: 89–98.
21 Swerdlow AJ, English JSC, MacKie RM *et al*. Fluorescent lights, ultraviolet lamps, and risk of cutaneous melanoma. *Br Med J* 1988; **297**: 647–50.
22 Walter SD, Marrett LD, From L, Hertzman C, Shannon HS, Roy P. The association of cutaneous malignant melanoma with the use of sunbeds and sunlamps. *Am J Epidemiol* 1990; **131**: 232–43.
23 Chen Y, Dubrow R, Zheng T, Barnhill RL, Fine J, Berwick M. Sunlamp use and the risk of cutaneous malignant melanoma: a population-based case–control study in Connecticut, USA. *Int J Epidemiol* 1998; **27**: 758–65.
24 Tucker MA, Shields JA, Hartge P, Augsburger J, Hoover RN, Fraumeni JF. Sunlight exposure as risk factor for intraocular melanoma. *N Engl J Med* 1985; **313**: 789–92.
25 Seddon JM, Gradoudas ES, Glynn RJ, Egan KM, Albert DM, Blitzer PH. Host factors, UV radiation, and risk of uveal melanoma: a case–control study. *Arch Ophthalmol* 1990; **108**: 1274–80.
26 Holly EA, Aston DA, Char DH, Kristiansen JJ, Ahn DK. Ocular melanoma in relation to ultraviolet light exposure and host factors. *Cancer Res* 1990; **50**: 5773–7.
27 Diffey BL. Use of UVA sunbeds for cosmetic tanning. *Br J Dermatol* 1986; **115**: 67–76.
28 Roza L, Baan RA, Van Der Leun JC, Kligman L. UVA hazards in skin associated with the use of tanning equipment. *J Photochem Photobiol B* 1989; **3**: 281–7.
29 Stern RS, Nichols KT, Vakeva LH. Malignant melanoma in patients treated for psoriasis with methoxsalen (psoralen) and ultraviolet A radiation (PUVA): the PUVA Follow-Up Study. *N Engl J Med* 1997; **336**: 1041–5.
30 Diffey BL, Farr PM, Ferguson J, *et al*. Tanning with ultraviolet A sunbeds. *Br Med J* 1990; **301**: 773–4.
31 Dutch Cancer Society. *Outdoors and Indoors: Sun Wisely*. Report on the 'Sensible Sunbathing' Consensus Meeting held under the auspices of the Dutch Cancer Society in Utrecht on October 6, 1995.
32 van Weelden H, de Gruijl FR, Van der Putte SCJ, Toonstra J, an der Leun JC. The carcinogenic risk of modern tanning equipment: is UVA safer than UVB? *Arch Dermatol Res* 1988; **280**: 300–7.
33 Lavker RM, Gerberick GF, Veres D, Irwin CJ, Kaidbey KH. Cumulative effects from repeated exposures to suberythemal doses of UVB and UVA in human skin. *J Am Acad Dermatol* 1995; **32**: 53–62.
34 Setlow RB, Woodhead AD. Temporal changes in the incidence of malignant melanoma: explanation from action spectra. *Mutat Res* 1994; **307**: 365–74.
35 Drobestsky EA, Turcotte J, Châteauneuf A. A role for ultraviolet A in solar mutagenesis. *Proc Natl Acad Sci USA* 1995; **92**: 2350–4.
36 Pedeux R, Al-Irani N, Marteau C, *et al.* Thymidine dinucleotide induce S phase cell cycle arrest in addition to increased melanogenesis in human melanocytes. *J Invest Dermatol* 1998; **111**: 472–7.
37 Woollons A, Clingen PH, Price ML, Arlett CF, Green MH. Induction of mutagenic damage in human fibroblasts after exposure to artificial tanning lamps. *Br J Dermatol* 1997; **137**: 687–92.
38 Woollons A, Kipp C, Young AR, *et al.* The 0.8% ultraviolet B content of an ultraviolet A sunlamp induces 75% of cyclobutane pyrimidine dimers in human keratinocytes *in vitro*. *Br J Dermatol* 1999; **140**: 1023–30.
39 Hemminki K, Bykov VJ, Marcuson JA. Re: sunscreen use and duration of sun exposure—a double-blind, randomized trial. *J Natl Cancer Inst* 1999; **91**: 2016–47.
40 Sheehan JM, Potten CS, Young AR. Tanning in human skin types II and III offers modest photoprotection against erythema. *Photochem Photobiol* 1998; **68**: 588–92.
41 Barker D, Dixon K, Medrano EE, *et al.* Comparison of the responses of human melanocytes with different melanin

contents to ultraviolet B irradiation. *Cancer Res* 1995; **55**: 4041–6.

42 Kvam E, Tyrell RM. The role of melanin in the induction of oxidative DNA base damage by ultraviolet A irradiation of DNA or melanoma cells. *J Invest Dermatol* 1999; **113**: 209–13.

43 Council on Scientific Affairs. Harmful effects of ultraviolet radiation. *J Am Med Assoc* 1989; **262**: 380–4.

44 European School of Oncology Advisory Board. Sun exposure, UVA lamps and risk of skin cancer. *Eur J Cancer* 1994; **30A**: 548–60.

45 World Health Organization. Environmental Health Criteria. *Ultraviolet Radiation: an authoritative scientific review of environmental and health effects of UV with reference to global ozone layer depletion*, Vol. 1, Geneva, 1994.

46 Boyle P, Veronesi U, Tubiana M, *et al.* European code against cancer. *Eur J Cancer* 1995; **31A**: 1395–405.

47 International Commission on Non-Ionizing Radiation Protection (ICNIRP). *Global Solar UV Index*. Publication ICNIRP–1/95, Germany: Oberschleibheim, 1995.

48 European Committee for Electrotechnical Standardization. *Safety of household and similar electrical appliances. Part 2: Particular requirements for ultraviolet and infrared skin treatment appliances for household and similar use*. International Electrotechnical Commission (IEC) 335-2-27: 1987 + amendement 1: 1989 modified, Brussels, 1992.

49 Food and Drug Administration. 1040, Sunlamps products: performance standards—final rule (21 CFR 1040). *Federal Register* 1985; **50**: 36548–52.

50 International Non-Ionizing Radiation Committee of the International Radiation Protection Association. Health issues of ultraviolet 'A' sunbeds used for cosmetic purpose. *Health Phys* 1991; **61**: 285–8.

3: Do sunscreens cause cancer or protect from a risk of melanoma?

Antony R. Young

Introduction

The use of topical sunscreens has increased during the latter part of the 20th century. This is a result of a combination of improved products, a greater public awareness of the health hazards of solar ultraviolet radiation (UVR), the possible effects of stratospheric ozone layer depletion and, almost certainly, better marketing by the sunscreen industry. Sunscreens are designed to prevent sunburn, but their use is widely advocated to reduce the risk of skin cancer [1] that is caused by exposure to solar UVR [2,3]. The claim to reduce skin cancer was critically evaluated by a working group of 23 international experts convened in Lyon, 11–18 April 2000, by the International Agency for Research on Cancer (IARC) [3]. The overall conclusion of this working group was:

> 'Topical use of sunscreens reduces the risk for sunburn in humans. Sunscreens probably prevent squamous cell carcinoma of the skin when used mainly during unintentional sun exposure. No conclusion can be drawn about the cancer-preventive activity of topical use of sunscreens against basal cell carcinoma and cutaneous melanoma. Use of sunscreens can extend the duration of intentional sun exposure, such as sunbathing. Such an extension may increase the risk for cutaneous melanoma.'

This chapter reviews some of the important issues about sunscreens and their role in the possible prevention of malignant melanoma and other types of skin cancer. This has become a controversial issue as some studies have reported a positive correlation between sunscreen use and malignant melanoma.

Terrestrial solar ultraviolet radiation

Ultraviolet radiation represents the part of the electromagnetic spectrum that spans wavelengths ranging from 200 to 400 nm. The UVR component is sub-characterized as UVC (200–280 nm), UVB (280–315 nm) and UVA (315–400 nm). UVA has also been divided into UVAI (340–400 nm) and UVAII (315–340 nm) because the shorter UVAII wavelengths interact with biomolecules by direct absorption mechanisms similar to that for UVB, whereas the longer UVAI wavelengths mediate damage via reactive oxygen species. There is no UVC in terrestrial sunlight as this is completely absorbed by stratospheric ozone (the ozone layer) and atmospheric oxygen. The ozone layer significantly attenuates UVB but has virtually no effect on UVA. Thus, the emission spectrum of terrestrial solar UVR contains UVB (~295–315 nm) and UVA as shown in Fig. 3.1(a). The ratio of UVB : UVA varies, depending on latitude, season, altitude and time of day. However, there is always very much more UVA than UVB, which never reaches more than 10% of total UVR content even under extreme conditions. Typically, in noon UK summer sun the UVB content is in the region of 5%.

Epidermal chromophores

The effects of UVR and visible radiation on living systems are caused by the absorption of energy by specific molecules, or parts of molecules, known as chromophores. Chromophores have very characteristic absorption spectra and the absorption of energy excites the chromophore and makes it prone to molecular reorganization or interaction with adjacent molecules. Important endogenous epidermal chromophores include DNA, aromatic amino acids (and therefore proteins), stratum corneum bound urocanic acid and melanin and its precursors and metabolites [4]. Urocanic acid normally exists in the *trans* form but, with UVR exposure, undergoes a photoisomerization to the *cis* form that initiates immunosuppressive effects. UVR exposure induces adjacent DNA pyrimidines to form chemical links (dimers) that cause mutations that lead to non-melanoma skin cancer. Thus, all photobiological effects including skin cancer are, by definition, initiated by the absorption of UVR or visible radiation energy by chromophores.

Action and hazard spectra

Intensity of UVR is expressed as irradiance using the unit W/m^2. Dose, expressed as J/m^2, is the product of irradiance and exposure time(s). Different wavelengths require different doses to induce the same photobiological effect. For example, the median minimal erythema dose (MED) of 300 nm radiation is 0.025 J/m^2 in fair-skinned people. However, the median MED at 360 nm is 32 J/m^2 [5]. This means that 300 nm is 1280 times more effective per unit physical dose at erythema induction compared with 360 nm. An action spectrum is a plot of biological efficacy vs. wavelength. Very few action spectra

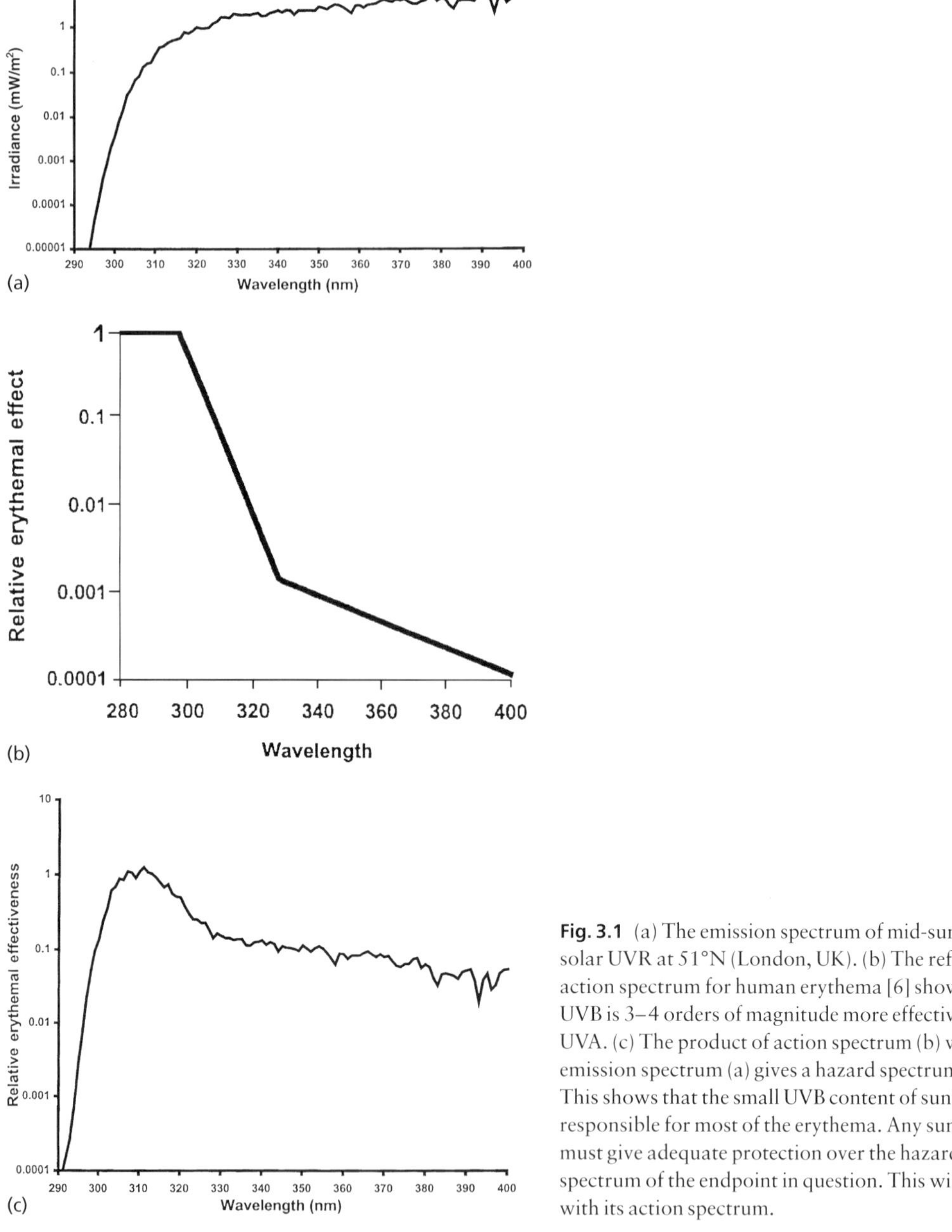

Fig. 3.1 (a) The emission spectrum of mid-summer solar UVR at 51°N (London, UK). (b) The reference action spectrum for human erythema [6] shows that UVB is 3–4 orders of magnitude more effective than UVA. (c) The product of action spectrum (b) with emission spectrum (a) gives a hazard spectrum. This shows that the small UVB content of sunlight is responsible for most of the erythema. Any sunscreen must give adequate protection over the hazard spectrum of the endpoint in question. This will vary with its action spectrum.

have been determined for human skin *in vivo* and the best characterized is that for erythema [6] as shown in Fig. 3.1(b). It is clear that UVB is several orders of magnitude more effective than UVA.

The generation of action spectra for the chronic effects of UVR on human skin is not possible for both logistical and ethical reasons. Thus, the only way to determine action spectra for skin cancer is in animal models. The most widely used of these is the hairless albino mouse. An action spectrum has been generated for squamous cell carcinoma (SCC) in the mouse model [7] and this is very similar to that for human erythema. The mouse photocarcinogenesis action spectrum has been used to calculate an action spectrum for SCC in humans, after taking differences in epidermal UVR transmission into account [7]. The conclusion from these calculations is that UVB is overwhelmingly the main cause of non-melanoma skin cancer.

At present, we lack action spectrum data for malignant melanoma in a mammalian model. Some spectral data for melanoma have been obtained from the South American opossum, *Monodelphis domestica*, in which it has been shown that UVA is relatively more effective at the induction of melanoma precursors than non-melanoma skin cancers [8]. However, a later study in the same animal model by the same author did not support a major role for UVA in the induction of melanoma [9]. More comprehensive data have been generated from a fish model [10]. These show that UVB is only about one order of magnitude more effective than UVA, and that melanoma can also be induced by visible radiation. Extrapolation of the fish action spectrum to humans would lead to the conclusion that 90% of malignant melanoma induction is caused by solar UVA and visible radiation [11]. Analysis of the relationship between latitude, UVA irradiance and melanoma incidence also lends support for a role for UVA in human melanoma induction [12]. However, it should be noted that xeroderma pigmentosum patients who specifically lack the ability to repair UVB-induced DNA damage are very prone to both melanoma and non-melanoma skin cancer [13]. Overall, it must be said that we do not know the action spectrum for human malignant melanoma.

Action spectra are crucial to the understanding of a given hazard from a given UVR emission spectrum such as sunlight. The product of a given action spectrum with a given emission spectrum results in an efficacy, or hazard, spectrum. For example, the small (≤5%) UVB component of solar radiation accounts for most of its erythemal efficacy in human skin as demonstrated in Fig. 3.1(c).

How do sunscreens work in sun protection?

Sunscreens are topical formulations that are designed to inhibit one acute effect of solar UVR exposure (sunburn). Their efficacy, determined under laboratory conditions, is expressed by their sun protection factor (SPF). This is a measure of the ability of a sunscreen to increase the time taken to achieve a minimal erythema dose (MED) where SPF = (MED with sunscreen)/(MED without sunscreen). The conditions for SPF assessment are tightly defined [14,15] and include a spectrally defined solar simulating radiation (SSR) source and a sunscreen application density of 2 mg/cm^2 skin. When a sunscreen is not used under these conditions the SPF will be different. For example, studies have shown that people usually apply 1 mg/cm^2 or less which will result in a very marked reduction of SPF [16,17]. The SPF may be misleading in terms of the percentage of erythemogenic radiation absorbed by the sunscreen as shown in Fig. 3.2. Increasing the SPF increases UVR attenuation in a non-linear fashion. Thus, only a 1% gain in UVR attenuation is achieved from increasing SPF from 20 to 25, or from 50 to 100. A true SPF of 15 is considered to be adequate for normal people under most conditions. However, there is a case for advocating higher SPFs, such as 20–30, to compensate for inadequate application density by the typical user.

The active ingredients of sunscreens are molecules that attenuate UVR in the solar region (~295–400 nm). These fall into two classes: (i) organic and (ii) inorganic. Organic molecules work by absorbing, and therefore attenuating UVR, whereas inorganic molecules work by scattering and absorbing UVR. Thus, sunscreen molecules may be regarded as exogenous chromophores applied to the skin, each with a characteristic absorption spectrum. There are about 50 sunscreen molecules that have been approved by regulatory authorities in different parts of the world and, of these, only two are inorganic. However, only nine sunscreen molecules as listed in Table 3.1 have met approval by all the major regulatory bodies. Typically, modern sunscreen formulations contain a mixture of organic and inorganic active molecules. Sunscreens have different category classifications in different parts of the world; they are drugs in the USA but cosmetics within the EU.

Sunscreens work by offering protection over the hazard spectrum of a given endpoint. The spectral properties of a sunscreen can be defined by their absorption profiles and *in vitro* assessments in which their monochromatic

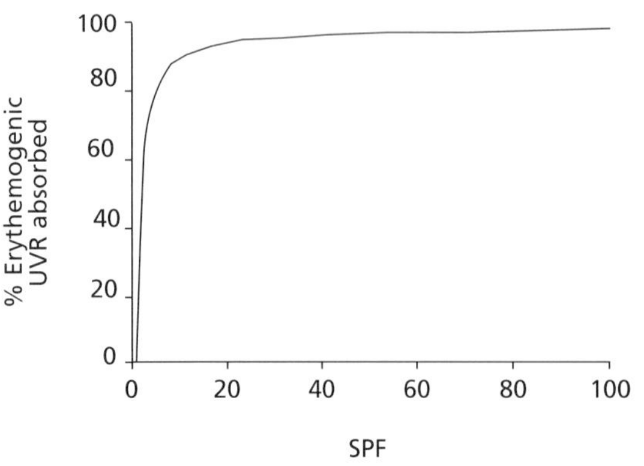

Fig. 3.2 The relationship between sun protection factor (SPF) and the amount of erythemogenic radiation that a sunscreen attenuates. The SPF is a ratio of (MED with sunscreen)/(MED without sunscreen). Sunscreen efficacy can also be expressed in absolute terms. Thus percentage transmission of erythemogenic UVR by a sunscreen is represented by $[(1/SPF) \times 100]$ and percentage attenuation of erythemogenic UVR by a sunscreen is represented by $\{[1-(1/SPF)] \times 100\}$.

Table 3.1 Sunscreens approved in the EU, USA, Japan and Australia. The spectral properties of the inorganic sunscreens depend on particle size

Molecule type	Molecule class	Name	Spectral category
Organic	Cinnamate	Octyl methoxycinnamate	UVB
	Salicylate	Homosalate	UVB
		Octyl salicylate	UVB
	PABA	PABA	UVB
		Octyl dimethyl PABA	UVB
	Benzophenone	Benzophenone-3	UVA
		Benzophenone-4	UVA
	Dibenzoylmethane	Butyl methoxydibenzoylmethane	UVA
Inorganic		Titanium dioxide	UVB + UVA
		Zinc oxide	UVB + UVA

Abbreviation: PABA, para-aminobenzoic acid.

protection factor (mPF) is plotted against wavelength. The hazard spectrum for erythema (Fig. 3.1c) shows that no sunscreen will work without attenuating UVB. Higher SPF sunscreens also require some attenuation of UVA. Since the 1990s there has been an increasing trend to formulate products with better UVA protection, resulting in products with a tendency towards flat absorption profiles, so-called neutral density filters. As yet there is no agreed standard for the assessment and representation of UVA protection. Various techniques have been proposed, some biological and others based on absorption profiles. Part of the problem of standardization lies in the fact that biological relevance of UVA is still uncertain. It is possible to have two sunscreen products, both with the same SPF but with quite different mPF profiles, as demonstrated in Fig. 3.3.

Does sunscreen use prevent skin cancer?

It is difficult to determine the role of sunscreens in the prevention of skin cancer. Human studies present ethical and logistical problems. Relevant biomarkers in humans may be used but the exact relationship between these, sunscreens and skin cancer is still unknown. Animal models may also be used but these too have limitations.

Biomarkers for skin cancer

Xeroderma pigmentosum patients, who show poor repair of di-pyrimidine DNA photolesions, such as cyclobutane pyrimidine dimers (CPD), have very high levels of all types of skin cancer including malignant melanoma [13]. Dipyrimidine DNA photolesions give rise to highly specific p53 mutations that

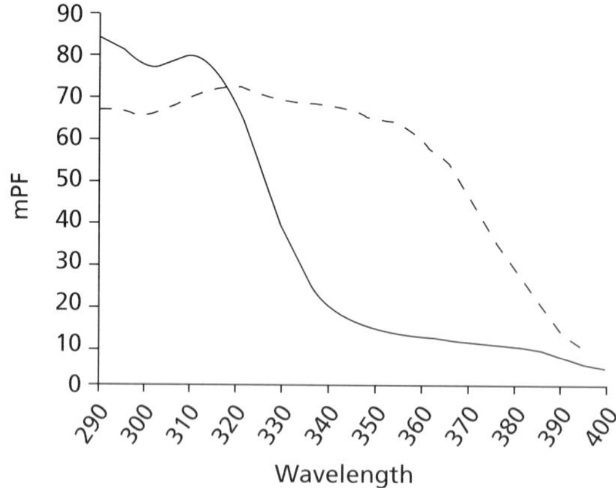

Fig. 3.3 Two sunscreens with SPF 60 have very different absorption profiles. This means that both products give comparable protection against sunburn. However, the broad-spectrum product would give much better protection from endpoints in which UVA had a greater role than for erythema. Given that we do not know the action spectra for malignant melanoma and other processes that may be important, such as immunosuppression, it may be prudent to use broad-spectrum formulations. The narrow-spectrum sunscreen is a water-in-oil emulsion (W/O) with 10% octyl methoxycinnamate, 3.1% titanium dioxide, 0.8% zinc oxide and 8.5% methylene bis-benzotriazolyl tetramethylbutylphenol. The broad-spectrum product is an oil-in-water emulsion (O/W) with 10% octocrylene, 2% terephthalylidene dicamphor sulphonic acid, 3% drometrizole trisiloxane and 5% titanium dioxide.

have an important role in non-melanoma skin cancer [18]. UVR readily induces CPD in human melanocytes *in situ* [19] and there can be little doubt that DNA photodamage is important in the pathogenesis of melanoma [13–20]. UVR-induced suppression of cell-mediated immunity is known to be important in photocarcinogenesis in the mouse [21] and a similar role is suspected in humans [22]. There is also evidence that immunosuppression is mediated via CPD [23]. This increasing understanding of the mechanistic aspects of skin cancer gives rise to the possibility of using different photobiological components of the disease process as biomarkers to assess sunscreen protection in skin cancer. Sunscreen protection against relevant biomarkers would not necessarily predict protection against skin cancer but failure to protect such biomarkers would suggest a lack of protection from skin cancer.

Erythema is the clinical endpoint against which sunscreen efficacy is judged. The use of a sunscreen that gave good protection from sunburn but poor protection against relevant biomarkers might unintentionally enhance skin cancer risk. For example, the use of an SPF 20 product that gave minimal protection from DNA photodamage would be a cause for concern. Thus, it is important to compare SPF with the relevant protection factor (RPF). Many, if not most studies have been designed to determine if a sunscreen protects against biomarkers without giving any indication of the RPF compared with the SPF. These studies are of limited benefit as they do not allow any assessment of risk in relation to erythema.

DNA photodamage and p53 mutation

There is evidence that DNA is a major chromophore for erythema [5] which would suggest that sunscreen protection from erythema should be associated with comparable levels of protection against DNA photodamage such as CPD. This has been demonstrated by Young *et al.* [24] with two sunscreens of the same SPF but with very different spectral profiles: one a UVB sunscreen and the other a broad-spectrum product. Furthermore, tanning has been associated with comparable levels of protection against erythema and DNA photodamage (CPD) in human skin [25]. Taken together, these data suggest that erythema is a good indicator of DNA photodamage and that prevention of sunburn by sunscreens is not associated with disproportionally high levels of DNA photodamage. However, it should be noted that DNA damage occurs with suberythemal exposure [5]. Sunscreens have been shown to inhibit UVR-induced p53 mutation in mouse skin [26,27]. There is also evidence that sunscreens inhibit UVR-induced p53 mutation in humans [28].

Suppression of cell-mediated immunity

There has been considerable controversy about the ability of sunscreens to afford protection against immunosuppression [29]. In some cases the observed lack of immunoprotection may be accounted for by poor experimental design [3]. Recent studies have shown that, even with good experimental design, the SPF may be higher than the immune protection factor (IPF) and that the relationship between IPF and SPF depends on the absorption spectrum of the sunscreen. In other words, there is indirect evidence that the action spectra for erythema and immunosuppression are different. Mouse [30] and human [31] studies suggest that protection from UVA may be more important for immunosuppression than for erythema and therefore erythema may not be a good indicator for immunosuppression. There is a need to confirm spectral conclusions from sunscreen studies with action spectra data for immunosuppression, but in the meantime it may be prudent to use broad-spectrum products to achieve good immunoprotection.

Animal photocarcinogenesis studies

Several studies have shown that topical application of sunscreens inhibits non-melanoma skin cancer by simulated solar radiation (SSR) in the hairless albino mouse model [32–34]. This would be expected if photocarcinogenesis is primarily caused by UVB as shown by action spectrum studies [7]. The IARC Working Group [3] evaluated all the published animal data and concluded: 'There is *sufficient evidence* that topical sunscreens have cancer-preventative activity in experimental animals. This evaluation is based on prevention by topical sunscreens of squamous cell carcinoma induction in the skin of mice by solar-simulated radiation.' However, studies to date have generally not assessed the degree of protection from skin cancer compared to the SPF of the product. An important limitation of mouse studies is that the effects of sunscreen application on UVR exposure behaviour are not taken into account. Animals with and without sunscreen spend the same amount of time under the UVR source, whereas humans may modify their behaviour when wearing a sunscreen.

Human non-melanoma skin cancer studies

Two randomized trials have shown that sunscreen use can inhibit actinic keratoses [35,36] that are considered to be a surrogate for risk of SCC. A long-term randomized trial in Australia has shown that sunscreen use significantly reduced the total number of SCCs in the sunscreen group, compared with the non-sunscreen group, but did not significantly reduce the number of people who developed new lesions [37]. No effect was seen with basal cell carcinoma, whether the data were analysed by total number of tumours or number of people with tumours. In the above studies, summarized in Table 3.2, the protective benefit of the sunscreens was relatively modest compared to the high SPF of the products used. Here it should be remembered that the mean ages of the study populations, in areas of high insolation, was ≥50 years. In these cases the benefits of sunscreen intervention, after genetic damage (e.g. p53 mutation) from several decades of UVR exposure, may be limited. At this stage, it is possible that sunscreens may act by inhibiting UVR-induced immunosuppression.

Melanocytic naevi and malignant melanoma

When considering the role of sunscreens in melanoma, it is important to consider that the pattern of solar exposure appears to be more important than cumulative exposure. Melanoma is associated with high-dose solar exposure (sunburn) in childhood and in adults [38]. Furthermore, it is more common in

Table 3.2 Summary of studies that have shown sunscreen protection from actinic keratoses and squamous cell carcinomas in humans. The protection factors are based on the ratios of the endpoints with and without sunscreen and are included to give some indication of efficacy

Study	Endpoint	Duration (years)	SPF	Result	PF	PF/SPF
Thompson *et al.* [35]	Mean change in AK	0.6	17	More remissions and fewer new lesions compared with vehicle	1.5	0.09
Naylor *et al.* [36]	Mean AK/year	2.0	29	Significant reduction compared with vehicle	2.1	0.07
Green *et al.* [37]	Total SCC	4.5	16	Significant reduction compared with no sunscreen	1.6	0.10

Abbreviations: AK, actinic keratosis; PF, protection factor; SCC, squamous cell carcinoma; SPF, sun protection factor.

people with indoor occupations who are exposed to sunlight in recreational activities [38]. One might assume that the use of sunscreens to prevent sunburn would confer a protective benefit. Furthermore, it is worth emphasizing that we do not know the action spectrum for human melanoma and that the sunscreens used in the epidemiological studies discussed below will have been primarily UVB-protecting products because good UVA protection was not common until the mid 1990s.

Naevi are accepted as risk indictors for malignant melanoma and can be legitimately used as surrogates to study the possible relationship between sunscreen use and malignant melanoma. Of several studies carried out in children, that of Autier *et al.* [39] is the most comprehensive. In this 2-year pan-European cross-sectional study of 631 children aged 6–7 years the sunscreen-associated relative risk (RR) for lesions ≥2 mm was 1.7 (95% CI = 1.1–2.6) and 1.5 (95% CI = 0.86–2.3) on the trunk and head/neck, respectively. The authors suggested that this may be caused by increased exposure time in the sun.

The results of 15 case–control studies on malignant melanomas are summarized in Table 3.3. A comprehensive account of these studies, and their possible flaws, has been published by IARC [3] and Weinstock [40] (12 studies). The data in Table 3.3 show a general trend for increased RR of malignant melanoma with sunscreen use. Five out of 15 (33%) studies show a RR of ≥2, 7/15 (47%) studies show a RR of 1.1–1.8 and 3/15 (20%) studies show a RR

Table 3.3 Summary of case–control studies that have addressed the relationship between sunscreen use and malignant melanoma. Relative risk (RR) adjusted for phenotypical and sun-related variables where possible except [44]. Study [49] in children only

Authors	Location	Study period	Cases/ controls	RR (95% CI)	Sunscreen trend
Klepp & Magnus [41]	Norway	1974–75	78/131	2.27 (1.3–4.1)	↑
Graham *et al.* [42]	USA	1974–80	404/521	2.2 (1.2–4.1)	↑
Herzfeld *et al.* [43]	USA	1977–79	324/415	2.58 (1.42–4.69)	↑
Beitner *et al.* [44]	Sweden	1978–83	523/505	1.8 (1.2–2.7)	↑
Elwoood & Gallagher [45]	Canada	1979–81	369/369	1.10 (0.75–1.62)	–
Holman *et al.* [46]	Australia	1980–81	507/507	1.1 (0.71–1.60)	–
Holly *et al.* [47]	USA	1981–86	452/930	0.62 (0.49–0.83)	↓
Osterlind *et al.* [48]	Denmark	1982–85	474/926	1.1 (0.8–1.5)	–
Whiteman *et al.* [49]	Australia	1987–94	50/156	2.2 (0.4–11.6)	↑
Westerdahl *et al.* [50]	Sweden	1988–00	400/640	1.8 (1.1–2.8)	↑
Rodenas *et al.* [51]	Spain	1989–93	105/138	0.2 (0.40–0.79)	↓
Espinosa Arranz *et al.* [52]	Spain	1990–94	116/235	0.48 (0.34–0.71)	↓
Autier *et al.* [53]	Europe	1991–92	418/438	1.50 (1.09–2.06)	↑
Wolf *et al.* [54]	Austria	1993–94	193/319	3.5 (1.8–6.6)	↑
Westerdal *et al.* [55]	Sweden	1995–97	571/913	1.8 (1.1–2.9)	↑

of <1. Thus it may be argued that about half the studies show no clear-cut effect of sunscreen use. Of the remaining eight studies, 63% show a positive correlation and 37% show a negative correlation.

At first inspection, it might appear that an overview of these studies shows, on balance, an association between sunscreen use and malignant melanoma. However, like other cancers, malignant melanoma has a long latent period the exact length of which is unknown. It must be stated that none of these studies was a randomized trial and all have been, less than ideal, case–control studies. This approach has inherent problems, especially when the use of sunscreens and their relationship with melanoma was not the main goal of most of the studies. Furthermore, these studies are highly susceptible to confounding. Having skin type I or II is a risk factor for malignant melanoma and these sun-sensitive skin types are also the most likely users of sunscreens, especially if they have a history of malignant melanoma or other skin cancers. An additional problem is the proper documentation of sunscreen use in relation to solar exposure. This includes the SPF (labelled and under actual conditions of use), product name, formulation, spectral profile and frequency of use. It is clear that recall on these matters is likely to be very poor. Furthermore, it is likely that different products with different SPF and spectral properties will have been used during the recall period. Overall, this means that existing studies on the benefits of sunscreen intervention are difficult to interpret.

Data from 11 of the case–control studies in Table 3.3 have been use for a meta-analysis of 9067 patients, published as an abstract [56]. This analysis showed no association between sunscreen use and malignant melanoma with RR of 1.11 (95% CI = 0.37–3.32) and 1.01 (95% CI = 0.46–2.28) when using hospital- and population-based studies combined or population-based studies alone, respectively. Thus, from this meta-analysis, one must conclude that there is no evidence that the use of sunscreens is associated with malignant melanoma. In fact, one might argue that sunscreens are protective if people have spent more time in the sun as a result of wearing a sunscreen [57].

What are the theoretical worries about sunscreens based upon how they work?

There is clearly much uncertainty about the role of sunscreens in the prevention of skin cancer. There are several reasons why sunscreens may not work as well as might be expected or even be associated with risk. These are discussed below.

Increased exposure time in the sun

The SPF is generally presented as a measure of how much longer one can spend in the sun to get a given level of sunburn rather than as a measure of erythemogenic dose reduction. This has resulted in some concern that sunscreens encourage people to spend longer in the sun. Autier *et al.* [57] reported that young Europeans who were given an unlabelled SPF 30 product stayed out in the sun for 25% longer than those given an unlabelled SPF 10 product. In a later study, Autier *et al.* [58] confirmed these findings and extended their observations by supplying volunteers with personal dosimeters. The dosimeters of SPF 30 group had a 17% higher median daily UVB exposure than those of the SPF 10 group. This increase was 26% if UVB dose was not assessed beyond late afternoon, but neither difference was significant ($P > 0.1$) and there was no difference in cumulative UVB exposure ($P = 0.4$) between the SPF 10 and SPF 30 groups. There was no evidence of any difference in UVA exposure in any of the defined exposure categories ($P > 0.3$).

All other things being equal, the important question here is not so much the time spent in the sun *per se*, but the UVR dose that has been received by the target chromophores [59]. Assuming correct usage, an SPF of 10 allows the wearer to spend 10 times longer in the sun to acquire the same level of erythema as unprotected skin. In such cases the erythemogenic dose would be no different with or without the sunscreen and no protection against erythema would have been obtained. The use of an SPF 10 sunscreen to spend five times longer in the sun compared with unprotected skin should result in a

50% reduction of the erythemogenic dose received, whatever the absorption profile of the sunscreen. In the case of a neutral density filter, there would be a 50% reduction at all wavelengths, making biological weighting redundant for other endpoints. However, in the case of a sunscreen that was not a neutral density filter, the degree of reduction would depend on the action spectrum of the endpoint in question.

However, all things may not be equal, and there is evidence for a failure of time–dose reciprocity for non-melanoma skin cancer in mice [60]. In other words, a given daily UVR dose may be more carcinogenic if delivered over an extended period. There was no evidence that the use of a high SPF sunscreen altered sun-exposure behaviour [61] in the large-scale Australian study to assess the role of sunscreens in the prevention of basal cell carcinoma (BCC) and SCC [37]. The Australian study population was much older than that of Autier *et al.* [57] and this may be a factor in sun-exposure behaviour, with younger people more inclined to be 'sun-seekers' in which sunburn might have been seen as a desirable biomarker for a tan [62].

Apart from a lower real-life SPF [16,17], studies have shown considerable variation in application thickness within areas of application [63]. This gives rise to the possibility of differential protection in different sites and the possibility of localized sunburn [64], a known risk factor for malignant melanoma [38].

Timing and location of maximum solar exposure

The standard advice given to minimize the risks of sunburn/skin cancer is to limit solar exposure between 10.00 a.m. and 4.00 p.m. and wear a sunscreen [1]. Implicit in this advice is the use of a sunscreen only during this period of high insolation. Assessments of UVR exposure are usually based on measurements made on horizontal surfaces. However, one study has shown a lack of correlation between solar UVR irradiance measurements made between horizontal and vertical surfaces and that the ratio of irradiance between such surfaces varies with time of day and wavelength [65]. When solar UVR irradiance was weighted with the action spectrum for erythema, horizontal surfaces—such as the shoulders and bridge of the nose—were at greatest risk at solar noon. However, vertical surfaces—such as the trunk/back and lower limbs—where melanoma is commonly found, were at greatest risk in mid-morning and mid-afternoon. This pattern correlated well with analysis of raw data at 300 nm. However, analysis of 400 nm data (to represent UVA) showed that peak exposure was in the early morning and late afternoon. These observations suggest that photoprotection advice may have to be reconsidered.

Spectral issues

In theory, the use of sunscreens that give good protection from erythema but less effective protection from endpoints relevant to skin cancer could enhance the risk of skin cancer. The level of sunscreen protection against skin cancer and relevant biomarkers will depend on a variety of factors including the action spectrum, and therefore hazard spectrum, of the endpoint in question and the absorption spectrum of the sunscreen. A neutral density sunscreen will screen all wavelengths equally, thus any differences in action spectra for different endpoints will have no effect on sunscreen efficacy. If the action spectrum is the same as that for erythema, one would predict comparable levels of protection, at least for acute endpoints, irrespective of the absorption spectrum of the sunscreen. However, protection factors would be expected to be different if the sunscreen is not a neutral density filter and the action spectrum for the endpoint in question was different than that for erythema. For example, an SPF 10 sunscreen that was primarily a UVB absorber would offer poor protection against an endpoint with an action spectrum that was primarily in the UVA region.

Relationship between SPF and protection from skin cancer

The cumulative effects of repeated low-dose exposure are likely to be important in skin cancer. For example, suberythemal exposure results in DNA damage to human melanocytes and keratinocytes *in situ* [19] and this damage is likely to accumulate with repeated UVR exposure if adequate DNA repair has not occurred [66]. Doses as low as 0.25 MED suppress cell-mediated immunity in skin types I/II but not in III/IV [67]. Thus cancer-relevant damage is likely to occur even when sunscreen use prevents erythema and the amount of repair between exposures is likely to be important.

The SPF is a measure of protection from a single UVR exposure. Repeated suberythemal doses—such as one might get with sunscreen use—results in the accumulation of erythema in sun-sensitive skin type II after a few days [68]. Under such conditions, depending on the UVR dose received through the sunscreen, its erythema protection factor might appear to be lower than its SPF. This means that the relationship between SPF and the level of protection from skin cancer is likely to be complex and may in fact never be known with any certainty in humans. All that one might be able to say is that sunscreens should be used to reduce solar UVR exposure dose.

Harmful effects of sunscreens

Vitamin D synthesis

The action spectrum for vitamin D synthesis is maximal in the UVB region [69] which raises the possibility that sunscreen use could be detrimental to this process. However, studies have shown that vitamin D synthesis is not unduly affected by sunscreen use [70], even in skin cancer prone xeroderma pigmentosum patients that take extreme photoprotection measures [71]. The reasons for this is that only relatively low doses of UVB over small areas of skin are necessary for the production of vitamin D.

Carcinogenic potential

There has been periodic concern that sunscreen molecules may have DNA damaging, mutagenic or photomutagenic properties that could result in carcinogenic potential [72–74]. It seems likely that some reports of adverse reports have resulted from contaminants in the test preparations [3]. To date all evidence for such concern has come from *in vitro* studies. One very common UVB sunscreen, octyl methoxycinnamate, has been studied for its ability to initiate skin cancer using the classical initiator–promoter chemical carcinogenesis model [32]. Mice were treated with the sunscreen followed by treatment with the tumour promoter TPA. There was no evidence for tumour initiation by the sunscreen.

Conclusions

There is no evidence that sunscreens *per se* cause skin cancer. Sunscreens clearly prevent non-melanoma skin cancer in animal models where behavioural factors play no part. There is evidence that sunscreens inhibit actinic keratoses. There is also evidence that they may inhibit squamous cell carcinoma in a long-term study that also suggested that there were no changes in sun-exposure behaviour. The most likely explanations for any correlation between sunscreen use and malignant melanoma are confounding factors and/or behavioural changes caused by sunscreen use. The true nature of the relationship between sunscreen use and malignant melanoma may not be known until a randomized long-term study is carried out.

Acknowledgements

I thank Dominique Moyal of L'Oréal Recherche, Paris for the data in Fig. 3.3 and Graham Harrison for preparing the figures.

References

1 Lim HW, Cooper K. The health impact of solar radiation and prevention strategies: report of the Environment Council, American Academy of Dermatology. *J Am Acad Dermatol* 1999; **41**: 81–99.

2 IARC. *Solar and Ultraviolet Radiation*, IARC Monographs on the Evaluation of Carcinogenic Risk to Humans, Vol. 55. Lyon: International Agency for Cancer Research, 1992.

3 IARC. *Sunscreens*, IARC Handbooks on Cancer Prevention, Vol. 5. Lyon: International Agency for Cancer Research, 2000.

4 Young AR. Chromophores in human skin. *Phys Med Biol* 1997; **42**: 789–802.

5 Young AR, Chadwick CA, Harrison GI, Nikaido N, Ramsden J, Potten CS. The similarity of action spectra for thymine dimers in human epidermis and erythema suggests that DNA is the chromophore for erythema. *J Invest Dermatol* 1998; **111**: 982–8.

6 McKinlay AF, Diffey BL. A reference action spectrum for ultraviolet radiation induced erythema in human skin. *CIE J* 1987; **6**: 17–22.

7 de Gruijl FR, van der Leun JC. Estimate of the wavelength dependency of ultraviolet carcinogenesis in humans and its relevance to the risk assessment of a stratospheric ozone depletion. *Health Phys* 1994; **67**: 319–25.

8 Ley RD. Ultraviolet radiation A-induced precursors to cutaneous melanoma in *Monodelphis domestica*. *Cancer Res* 1997; **57**: 3682–4.

9 Ley RD. Dose response for ultraviolet radiation A-induced focal melanocytic hyperplasia and nonmelanoma skin tumours in *Monodelphis domestica*. *Photochem Photobiol* 2001; **73**: 20–3.

10 Setlow RB, Grist E, Thompson K, Woodhead AD. Wavelengths effective in induction of malignant melanoma. *Proc Natl Acad Sci USA* 1993; **90**: 6666–70.

11 Setlow RB. Spectral regions contributing to melanoma: a personal view. I. Invest. *Dermatol Symp Proc* 1999; **4**: 46–9.

12 Moan J, Dahlback A, Setlow RB. Epidemiological support for an hypothesis for malignant melanoma indicating a role for UVA radiation. *Photochem Photobiol* 1999; **70**: 243–7.

13 Van Steeg H, Kraemer KH. Xeroderma pigmentosum and the role of UV-induced DNA damage in skin cancer. *Mol Med Today* 1999; **5**: 86–94.

14 European Cosmetic Toiletry and Perfumery Association, COLIPA: COLIPA Sun Protection Factor (SPF) Test Method. 1994. October ref 94/289.

15 FDA. Department of Health and Human Services Food and Drug Administration USA. Sunscreen drug products for over-the-counter human use: final monograph. *Federal Register* 1999; **64**: 27666–93.

16 Bech-Thomsen N, Wulf HC. Sunbathers' application of sunscreen is probably inadequate to obtain the sun protection factor assigned to the preparation. *Photodermatol Photoimmnol Photomed* 1992; **9**: 242–4.

17 Diffey BL, Grice J. The influence of sunscreen type on photoprotection. *Br J Dermatol* 1997; **137**: 103–5.

18 Ziegler A, Jonason AS, Lefell DJ, *et al.* Sunburn and p53 in the onset of skin cancer. *Nature* 1994; **372**: 773–6.

19 Young AR, Potten CS, Nikaido O, *et al.* Human melanocytes and keratinocytes exposed to UVB or UVA *in vivo* show comparable levels of thymine dimers. *J Invest Dermatol* 1998; **111**: 936–40.

20 Gilchrist BA, Eller MA, Geller AC, Yaar M. The pathogenesis of melanoma induced by ultraviolet radiation. *N Engl J Med* 1999; **340**: 1341–8.

21 Nishigori C, Yarosh DB, Donawho C, Kripke ML. The immune system in ultraviolet carcinogenesis. *J Invest Dermatol Symp Proc* 1996; **2**: 143–6.

22 Euvrard S, Kanitakis J, Pouteil-Noble C, Claudy A, Touraine JL. Skin cancers in organ transplant recipients. *Ann Transplant* 1997; **2**: 28–32.

23 Kripke ML, Cox PA, Alas LG, Yarosh DB. Pyrimidine dimers in DNA initiate systemic immunosuppression in UV-irradiated mice. *Proc Natl Acad Sci USA* 1992; **89**: 7516–20.

24 Young AR, Sheehan JM, Chadwick CA, Potten CS. Protection by ultraviolet A and B sunscreens against *in situ* dipyrimidine photolesions in human epidermis is comparable to protection against sunburn. *J Invest Dermatol* 2000; **115**: 37–41.

25 Sheehan JM, Cragg N, Potten CS, Young AR. Repeated UVR exposure offers the same protection against DNA photodamage and erythema in human skin types II and IV but is associated with faster repair in skin type IV. *J. Invest Dermatol* in press.

26 Ananthaswamy HN, Ullrich SE, Mascotto RE, *et al.* Sunlight and skin cancer: inhibition of p53 mutations in UV-irradiated mouse skin by sunscreens. *Nat Med* 1997; **3**: 510–2.

27 Ananthaswamy HN, Ullrich SE, Mascotto RE, *et al.* Inhibition of solar simulator induced p53 mutations and protection against skin cancer development in mice by sunscreens. *J Invest Dermatol* 1999; **112**: 763–8.

28 Rosentein BS, Phelps RG, Weinstock MA, *et al.* p53 Mutations in basal cell carcinoma arising in routine users of sunscreens. *Photochem Photobiol* 1999; **70**: 798–806.

29 Young AR, Walker SL. Photoprotection from UVR-induced immunosuppression. In: Krutmann J, Elmets CA, eds. *Photoimmunology*. Oxford: Blackwell Science, 1995: 285–97.

30 Fourtanier A, Gueniche A, Compan D, Walker SL, Young AR. Improved protection against solar-simulated radiation-induced immunosuppression by a sunscreen with enhanced ultraviolet A protection. *J Invest Dermatol* 2000; **114**: 620–7.

31 Kelly DA, Seed PT, Young AR, Walker SL. Sunscreen protection against ultraviolet radiation-induced immunosuppression is 50% lower than protection against sunburn in humans. Submitted.

32 Forbes PD, Davies RE, Sambuco CP, Urbach F. Inhibition of ultraviolet radiation induced tumors in hairless mice by topical application of the sunscreen 2-ethyl hexyl-p-methoxycinnamate. *J Toxicol Cut Ocular Toxicol* 1989; **8**: 209–26.

33 Young AR, Walker SL, Kinley JS, *et al.* Phototumorigenesis studies of 5-methoxypsoralen in bergamot oil: evaluation and modification of risk of human use in an albino mouse model. *J Photochem Photobiol B* 1990; **7**: 231–50.

34 Fourtanier A. Mexoryl SX protects against solar-simulated UVR-induced photocarcinogenesis in mice. *Photochem Photobiol* 1996; **64**: 688–93.

35 Thompson SC, Jolley D, Marks R. Reduction of solar keratoses by regular sunscreen use. *N Engl J Med* 1993; 1147–51.

36 Naylor MF, Boyd A, Smith DW, Cameron GS, Hubbard D, Neldner KH. High sun protection factor sunscreens in the suppression of actinic neoplasia. *Arch Dermatol* 1995; **131**: 170–5.

37 Green A, Williams G, Neale R, *et al.* Daily sunscreen application and betacarotene supplementation in prevention of basal cell and squamous cell carcinomas of the skin: a randomized controlled trial. *Lancet* 1999; **354**: 723–9.

38 Marks R. Epidemiology of melanoma. *Clin Exp Dermatol* 2000; **25**: 459–63.

39 Autier P, Doré JF, Cattaruzza MS, *et al.* Sunscreen use, wearing clothes, and number of nevi in 6- to 7-year-old European children. *J Natl Cancer Inst* 1998; **90**: 1873–80.

40 Weinstock MA. Do sunscreens increase or decrease melanoma risk: an epidemiologic evaluation. *J Invest Dermatol Symp Proc* 1999; **4**: 97–100.

41 Klepp O, Magnus K. Some environmental and bodily characteristics of melanoma patients: a case–control study. *Int J Cancer* 1979; **23**: 482–6.

42 Graham S, Marshall J, Haughey B, *et al.* An inquiry into the epidemiology of melanoma. *Am J Epidemiol* 1985; **122**: 606–19.

43 Herzfeld PM, Fiztgerald EF, Hwang S, Stark A. A case–control study of malignant melanoma of the trunk among white males in upstate New York. *Cancer Detect Prev* 1993; **17**: 601–8.

44 Beitner H, Norell SE, Ringborg U, Wennersten G, Mattson B. Malignant melanoma: aetiological importance of individual pigmentation and sun exposure. *Br J Dermatol* 1990; **122**: 43–51.

45 Elwood JM, Gallagher RP. More about: Sunscreen use, wearing clothes, and number of nevi in 6- to 7-year old European children. *J Natl Cancer Inst* 1999; **91**: 1164–6.

46 Holman CDJ, Armstrong BK, Heenan PJ. Relationship of cutaneous malignant melanoma to individual sunlight-

exposure habits. *J Natl Cancer Inst* 1986; **76**: 403–14.

47 Holly EA, Aston DA, Cress RD, Ahn DK, Kristiansen JJ. Cutaneous melanoma in women. I. Exposure to sunlight, ability to tan, and other risk factors related to ultraviolet light. *Am J Epidemiol* 1995; **141**: 923–33.

48 Osterlind A, Tucker MA, Stone BJ, Jensen OM. The Danish case–control study of cutaneous malignant melanoma II. Importance of UV-light exposure. *Int J Cancer* 1988; **42**: 319–24.

49 Whiteman DC, Valery P, McWhirter W, Green AC. Risk factors for childhood melanoma in Queensland, Australia. *Int J Cancer* 1997; **70**: 26–31.

50 Westerdahl J, Olsson H, Måsbåčk A, Ingvar C, Jonsson N. Is the use of sunscreens a risk factor for malignant melanoma? *Melanoma Res* 1995; **5**: 59–65.

51 Rodenas JM, Delgado-Rodriguez M, Herranz M, Tercedor J, Serrano S. Sun exposure, pigmentary traits, and risk of cutaneous malignant melanoma: a case–control study in a Mediterranean population. *Cancer Causes Control* 1996; **7**: 275–83.

52 Espinosa Arranz J, Sanchez Hernandez JJ, Bravo Fernandez P, *et al*. Cutaneous malignant melanoma and sun exposure in Spain. *Melanoma Res* 1999; **9**: 199–205.

53 Autier P, Doré JF, Schifflers E, *et al*. Melanoma and use of sunscreens: an EORTC case–control study in Germany, Belgium and France. *Int J Cancer* 1995; **61**: 749–55.

54 Wolf P, Quehenberger F, Mullegger R, Stranz B, Kerl H. Phenotypic markers, sunlight-related factors and sunscreen use in patients with cutaneous melanoma: an Austrian case–control study. *Melanoma Res* 1998; **8**: 370–8.

55 Westerdahl J, Ingvar C, Masback A, Olsson H. Sunscreen use and malignant melanoma. *Int J Cancer* 2000; **87**: 145–50.

56 Huncharek M, Kupelnick B. Use of topical sunscreens and risk of malignant melanoma: result of a meta-analysis of 9067 patients from 11 case control studies. *Am J Public Health* in press.

57 Autier P, Doré JF, Négrier S, *et al*. Sunscreen use and duration of sun exposure: a double-blind, randomized trial. *J Natl Cancer Inst* 1999; **91**: 1304–9.

58 Autier P, Doré JF, Grivegnée A, *et al*. Sunscreen use and intentional exposure to ultraviolet A and B radiation: a double blind randomised trial using personal dosimeters. *Br J Cancer* 2000; **83**: 1243–8.

59 Young AR. More about: Sunscreen use and duration of sun exposure: a double-blind, randomised trial. *J Natl Cancer Inst* 2000; **92**: 1532.

60 Kelfkens G, van Weeldon H, de Gruijl FR, van der Leun JC. The influence of dose rate on ultraviolet tumorigenesis. *J Photochem Photobiol B* 1991; **10**: 41–50.

61 Green A, Williams G, Neale R, Battistutta D. Betacarotene and sunscreen use. Author's Reply. *Lancet* 1999; **354**: 2163–4.

62 Autier P, Severi G, Boyle P, Doré JF. More about: Sunscreen use and duration of sun exposure: a double-blind, randomised trial. *J Natl Cancer Inst* 2000; **92**: 1532–3.

63 Rhodes LE, Diffey BL. Quantitative assessment of sunscreen application technique by *in vivo* fluorescence spectroscopy. *J Soc Cosmetic Chem* 1996; **47**: 109–15.

64 Diffey BL. Sunscreens, suntans, and skin cancer: people do not apply enough sunscreen for protection. *Br Med J* 1996; **313**: 942.

65 Webb AR, Weihs P, Blumthaler M. Spectral irradiance on vertical surfaces: a case study. *Photochem Photobiol* 1999; **69**: 464–70.

66 Young AR, Chadwick CA, Harrison GI, Hawk JLM, Nikaido O, Potten CS. The *in situ* repair kinetics of epidermal thymine dimers and 6–4 photoproducts in human skin types I and II. *J Invest Dermatol* 1996; **106**: 1307–13.

67 Kelly DA, Young AR, McGregor JM, Seed PT, Potten CS, Walker SL. Sensitivity to sunburn is associated with susceptibility to ultraviolet radiation-induced suppression of cutaneous cell-mediated immunity. *J Exp Med* 2000; **191**: 561–6.

68 Sheehan JM, Potten CS, Young AR. Tanning in human skin types II and III offers modest photoprotection against erythema. *Photochem Photobiol* 1998; **68**: 588–92.

69 Webb AR. Vitamin D synthesis under changing UV spectra. In: Young AR, Björn LO, Moan J, Nultsch W, eds. *Environmental UV Photobiology.* New York: Plenum Press, 1993: 185–202.

70 Marks R, Foley PA, Jolley D, Knight KR, Harrison J, Thompson SC. The effect of regular sunscreen use on vitamin D levels in an Australian population: results of a randomised controlled trial. *Arch Dermatol* 1995; **131**: 415–21.

71 Sollitto RB, Kraemer KH, DiGiovanna JJ. Normal vitamin D levels can be maintained despite rigorous photoprotection: six years' experience with xeroderma pigmentosum. *J Am Acad Dermatol* 1997; **37**: 942–7.

72 Knowland J, McKenzie EA, McHugh PJ, Cridland NA. Sunlight-induced mutagenicity of a common sunscreen ingredient. *FEBS Lett* 1993; **324**: 309–13.

73 Dunford R, Salinaro A, Cai L, *et al.* Chemical oxidation and DNA damage catalysed by inorganic sunscreen ingredients. *FEBS Lett* 1997; **418**: 87–90.

74 Stevenson C, Davies RJH. Photosensitisation of guanine-specific DNA damage by 2-phenylbenzimidazole and the sunscreen agent 2-phenyl-benzimidazole-5-sulfonic acid. *Chem Res Toxicol* 1999; **12**: 38–45.

4: Why are redheads so susceptible to melanoma?

Jonathan Rees

Introduction

The major covariants of most forms of skin cancer including melanoma are pigmentary phenotype and ambient ultraviolet radiation (UVR) [1–6]. In general, and ignoring recent human migrations, areas with ambient UVR load are inhabited by people with darker skin [7]. The major *genetic* risk factor for melanoma is therefore skin colour and, by association, hair colour; the major *environmental* risk factor is UVR. Differences in the degree and type of pigmentation account not just for differences in melanoma rates *between* broad groupings such as white or black people but also exist *within* these groups. For example, and relevant to the present chapter, it has been known for a long time that those with 'Celtic ancestry' are more susceptible to melanoma that those from southern Europe or even of 'Anglo-Saxon' stock [3,6,8–10].

This chapter reviews what we know of the genetics of the red hair phenotype, a phenotype known to be at increased risk of melanoma; what we know of the mechanisms linking allelic variation at the relevant genetic loci with different melanin pigments; and how these different pigments relate to differences in the cutaneous response to UVR. It is probably fair to say that whereas our understanding of pigment genetics is increasingly secure, our understanding of how differences in pigment physiology translate into disease susceptibility remains relatively murky.

What determines who has red hair?

Red hair is perhaps the most striking common variation of hair colour in people originating from Europe, and is of interest to all those interested in human genetics—professional and amateur. Indeed, hair colour is often used as an example in attempts to explain genetics to the lay public, yet it is only recently that we can claim even a rudimentary understanding of the genetic mechanisms operating. The medical, as compared with the biological, interest in red hair relates to the fact that it is a marker for a cutaneous phenotype characterized by sensitivity to the effects of UVR. This includes a tendency to burn rather than tan; a large number of freckles; the presence in later life of signs of sun damage, such as solar lentigos and solar elastosis; and an increased rate of melanoma and non-melanoma skin cancer. It is worth stating at the onset that this phenotype, however iconic, is poorly defined. For instance, there are many shades of red hair including strawberry blond, auburn and ginger; the epidemiology of the various red hair types has not been appropriately studied in depth; and, most important of all, whereas redheads usually tan poorly, some seem to tan well, and conversely not all persons with a poor ability to tan have red hair. None of these difficulties seem experimentally insurmountable, it is just that the subject remains neglected.

A number of studies early in the 20th century attempted to describe the pattern (mode) of inheritance of red hair [11–16]. Most favoured an autosomal recessive pattern, and some also postulated that red hair was hypostatic to black, but dominant to white. By today's standards these studies are not very robust. The major advance in our understanding of red hair genetics has come in the last few years and, like so many other aspects of biomedicine, owes much to the marriage of molecular genetics and the opportunities offered by the mouse mutant resource [17–19].

Cloning of the melanocortin 1 receptor (*MC1R*): a gene for red hair

The *MC1R* was cloned by two groups independently in 1992 and was shown to be a seven pass transmembrane (G-protein-coupled) receptor that signals via adenyl cyclase activation, leading to elevated intracellular cyclic adenosine monophosphate (cAMP) [20,21]. Whether the *MC1R* is involved in other signalling pathways remains undecided. Two physiological ligands (at least in mouse) are known to interact with the *MC1R*: α-melanocyte-stimulating hormone (αMSH), a tridecapeptide cleavage product of pro-opiomelanocortin (POMC) which acts so as to activate the receptor; and *agouti* which antagonizes the actions of αMSH [22–24]. Activation of the *MC1R* influences the relative amounts of eumelanin and phaeomelanin produced, with loss of activity being associated with red or yellow hair, depending on the animal [24]. Injection of αMSH or adrenocorticotrophin (ACTH)—which is also active at the *MC1R* but whose primary receptor is the melanocortin 2 receptor, (*MC2R*)—increases skin pigmentation although attempts to mimic the physiological or pharmacological context *in vitro* have proved uneven [25,26].

The critical experiments relating mutation at the *MC1R* with phenotype in the mouse were reported from Roger Cone's laboratory soon after the cloning of the *MC1R* [22]. They showed that various *extension* mutants in which the ratio of eumelanin to phaeomelanin (red/yellow melanin) was reduced (with a resulting yellow colour) were *MC1R* loss of function mutants. By contrast, dominant gain of function mutations of the *MC1R* resulted in black hair caused by increased eumelanin (blown/black melanin) biosynthesis. Subsequently, a similar pattern of mutants has been reported in a variety of other animals with loss of function leading to yellow or red hair and dominant mutations leading to black pigment [23,27–32].

The human *MC1R* located at 16q24.3 codes for a predicted 317 amino acid product and was originally thought like many G-coupled-receptors to be intronless [33]. Most early studies on the *MC1R* had assumed this to be the case. Recently, however, an intron at the 3′ end was described giving rise to two predicted RNA species, the functional significance of which is as yet unexplored [34]. The *MC1R* is expressed on a range of cell types including melanocytes, endothelial cells and keratinocytes [23,35–37]. The function of the *MC1R* in these various cell types apart from the melanocyte is unclear although there are those who argue that the *MC1R* may mediate some of the known effects of αMSH on a range of inflammatory and immune reactions [38,39]. Initial characterization of the human *MC1R* promoter has recently been published [40].

The first study ascribing a functional role to the *MC1R* in humans was a case–control study based on sequencing of the human *MC1R* in a small group of North European redheads and chose as controls individuals without red hair who tanned well rather than burned in response to UVR [41]. Allelic variants of the *MC1R* were common (>65%) and the frequency of variant alleles was higher in the redheaded group than the controls. However, there were a number of puzzling features. Many of the redheads had two allelic variants whereas others showed only one [42]. Furthermore, in some individuals more than one variant from wild type sequence was present on the same allele. It was not clear at this stage whether some variants may have been simple polymorphisms (with no phenotypic effect) and others mutations (the term variant is used so as to be neutral in respect of functional significance). A worrying feature of such allelic association studies—which of themselves do not provide functional evidence for equating a particular change on a allele with functional change—is that they may produce spurious results secondary to confounding brought about by hidden stratification of the populations studied. This is a particular concern where the case and control groups may have different genetic population histories.

Two subsequent studies partly clarified these issues—a twin study in Australia [43] and a population study in Ireland [44]—showing that the majority of redheads were homozygote for one of a limited number of alleles associated with red hair, including the Arg151Cys, Arg160Trp and Asp294His variants. Such alleles carried a risk ratio of red hair of >6 for one allele (heterozygote) and >20 for two alleles (compound heterozygote/homozygotes).

Subsequent functional studies using transient and stable transfections of the various putative mutant alleles showed that these three alleles were indeed loss of function mutants [45,46]. Most redheads are therefore compound heterozygotes for loss of function alleles of the *MC1R*. Family studies are in keeping with this, with a simple model of the inheritance of red hair as a recessive, allowing the guessing of the phenotype in more than 80% of individuals based on genotype. Subsequent studies also suggest that some of the other rarer alleles of the *MC1R* are also loss of function mutants [47].

What of individuals with red hair who are not compound heterozygote/homozygote mutants? Virtually all redheads (>95%) who are not compound heterozygotes (or homozygotes) are heterozygote for one of the above loss of function alleles. Mutations of the other allele may be present outside the coding region although searches have failed to identify any to date (unpublished data). However, the *MC1R* is not the only rate-limiting gene mutations which lead to red hair. Krude *et al.* [48] reported two siblings with bright red hair and a complicated endocrine phenotype who were subsequently shown to be compound heterozygotes for loss of function mutations of POMC. The endocrine phenotype was predictable on the basis of the known physiology of POMC, but the red hair confirms that in humans POMC is the precursor for the ligand that is physiologically active at the *MC1R*. By contrast, there are occasional individuals who possess compound heterozygote/homozygote mutations of the *MC1R* but do not have red hair. The explanation for this is at present unclear.

In summary, the majority of redheads are compound heterozygotes/homozygotes for a limited number of loss of function mutations of the *MC1R*. Perhaps one-quarter of redheads are 'just' heterozygotes, and there are occasional persons with red hair without any known mutations of the *MC1R* locus. There are also occasional persons who harbour two *MC1R* mutations but who do not have red hair.

How are the different patterns of melanogenesis related to sunburn?

If the genetics of red hair is becoming clearer, then the biochemistry linking the genes with the physiology of the UVR response remains difficult.

When activated, the *MC1R* elevates intracellular cAMP [23]. This signalling cascade then influences the amounts or, more particularly, the ratio of the two main sorts of melanin produced: eumelanin (black/brown) and phaeomelanin (red/yellow) [23]. However, the steps linking cAMP and melanogenesis are poorly understood, as is the involvement of other signalling pathways [49,50]. Much of the difficulty lies with the problems of working with melanin. Although convenient for usage, as has been the case so far in the present chapter, melanin is not a single chemical entity, rather it is a complex mixture of polymer products that is very unfriendly to chemical analysis [51–53]. It has been likened to plastic—there are lots of different sorts [54,55]! There is therefore no single chemical formula for melanin or the various melanins. Add to this the fact that the optical properties of melanin depend on the macromolecular structure in which melanin is packaged, rather than just the chemistry, then it is possible to appreciate the technical difficulties those interested in pigment biology face [54,55]. Thus, whereas the term phaeomelanin describes a class of compounds that share a common pathway of melanogenesis involving incorporation of cysteine, it is difficult to be more precise than this. For the present, examination at the gross level may be more meaningful: mutations at the *MC1R* result in yellow hair (in mouse and some other animals) or red hair (humans and some animals). The reasons for the species differences in hair colour (red or yellow), however homologous, are still unclear.

Relating the type and amount of melanin to UVR susceptibility

Despite assertions to the contrary [56], melanin effectively protects against the effects of UVR [57]. The evidence for this comes from the ecological associations between skin cancer and pigmentation, the grossly elevated rates of skin tumours seen in albinos, and the obvious example of patients focally deficient in melanin or melanocytes (vitiligo) who only burn in response to UVR in areas of skin without melanin [6,57,58]. Again, despite statements to the contrary, melanin is not a neutral density filter but rather shows peak absorption at the shorted wavelengths where UVR is most hazardous to cellular macromolecules [55].

However, the different types or classes of melanin do differ—obviously because they are different colours—in respect of their optical qualities [51,52]. Here again the most convincing data relates to physiology rather than to direct biochemical analyses of the various melanins. The issue still undecided in the literature is whether the sensitivity of the redheaded phenotype is caused by deficiency of eumelanin *per se* or rather the presence of more phaeomelanin (or an increased ratio of phaeomelanin : eumelanin) [52,53,59–62]. The author's view is that this issue is still experimentally unresolved. A number of experiments have been reported showing that phaeomelanin is a less effective 'sun-block' than eumelanin and that when irradiated it generates more harmful free radicals [56,63,64]. However, the physiological relevance of the models used seems highly debatable. By contrast, if the redheaded phenotype is sun-sensitive because of deficiencies in eumelanin rather than the presence of pheomelanin, then one could predict no difference between blond individuals with pale skin and redheads with pale skin, both who would have little eumelanin. As an extreme case, one could ask whether melanoma is underrepresented (over what one might expect based on non-melanoma skin rates) in albinos given their complete absence of pigment. There is some evidence that albinos are comparatively resistant to melanoma—certainly in comparison with non-melanoma skin cancer—and it is possible to argue that the absence of melanin might be safer than the presence of small amounts of phaeomelanin [65,66]. Interesting though these speculations are, they suffer from a lack of robust experimental data. Our understanding at present therefore remains that it is uncertain whether the increased risk of melanoma in redheads is as a result of decreased eumelanin or an increased ratio of phaeomelanin : eumelanin; or, put another way, whether the elevated risk is as a result of a reduced amount of a natural sun-block or the presence of a sun-block that is in reality harmful when irradiated.

MC1R, red hair and melanoma susceptibility

There are a large number of epidemiological studies relating pigmentary phenotypes and melanoma incidence [1–4]. In interpreting them it is useful to spell out what are the likely causal relations between red hair and cutaneous sensitivity.

Most people with red hair tend to burn rather than tan in response to the sunshine. An individual with red hair if exposed to a set dose of UVR on unexposed skin, such as the buttock, may show slightly more erythema than non-red-haired individuals but the difference is not large. However, if a typical redhead receives repeated doses of UVR then, unlike a 'normal' non-red-haired individual, tanning does not occur, and there is therefore a failure of adaption to the effects of UVR that occurs in persons able to tan. The difference therefore between the redhead and non-redhead relate predominantly to the degree to which photoadaptation occurs.

The relation between red hair and the cutaneous phenotype is also worth exploring. As stated above, most people with red hair are sun-sensitive, and this most likely relates to the increased ratio of phaeomelanin : eumelanin in their skin. However, there are also individuals who have a similar cutaneous phenotype to those with red hair but have, say, black hair. The explanation for this is unclear but one suggestion that has received recent support is that these individuals are heterozygote mutants at the *MC1R* [67]. While there are going to be many loci that are important determinants of skin type, a heterozygote effect at the *MC1R* has recently been shown to be one of them [67].

To understand studies relating red hair and other pigmentary phenotypes to melanoma, the interrelation between various markers of the red hair phenotype must be understood. If you statistically adjust the data for, say, skin type, you may well be effectively overmatching (to use the epidemiological term) and removing or diminishing a genuine causal relation. Similarly, freckling results from UVR exposure in the context of a particular genotype and so again may result in overmatching if 'adjusted' for in the analysis. Finally, any relation with red hair and UVR may actually underestimate the biological strength of relation between phenotype and melanoma. This is because individuals who know themselves to be sun-sensitive will often, if not usually, behave differently from those who do not burn easily. The dose of UVR they receive may therefore be smaller. Such selection may also confound studies relating occupational factors or pattern of exposure to UVR. There may well be a degree of conscious selection against outdoor occupations in those with red hair in areas with high ambient UVR. It is not impossible that such factors might bias attempts to explain the higher rate of melanoma in those with indoor occupations in comparison with those with outdoor occupations.

Studies of the *MC1R* and melanoma

Few studies have been published, and even fewer are methodologically sound [37,68–70]. The first published study showed [70] an association between mutations at the *MC1R*, in particular the Asp84Glu variant, and melanoma. However, a subsequent study by the same group failed to confirm this association, suggesting that the original report was a chance finding of testing of a large number of possible alleles [37]. Other published studies are also open to criticism in that only some of the alleles associated with red hair were tested and that the functional status of many pseudo-wild type alleles were classified as wild type [68,71].

The most thorough and largest study of melanoma and the *MC1R* was reported recently from Australia [69]. This study showed a clear association between the *MC1R* mutation, red hair and melanoma, with a risk ratio of around 2 for each of three red-hair associated alleles when present in the heterozygote state and 4 when homozygote or compound heterozygote. Interestingly, the effect of mutant alleles persisted even in those without red hair and with skin types 3 and 4 (using the Fitzpatrick classification). What are the possible explanations for this? While red hair approximates to an autosomal recessive, as mentioned above, there is a heterozygote effect on skin type so it is not too surprising that an *MC1R* effect is seen outside the redheaded group [72]. Does the MC1R mediate effects on melanoma through other means than just effects on skin type? This question, although mooted in an earlier study [70], was more comprehensively examined in the study from Sturm *et al.* [69]. In this (latter) study adjusting for skin type did not completely remove the effects of *MC1R* on melanoma risk. There is some evidence that αMSH, presumably acting through the *MC1R*, may influence melanocyte growth and such an effect may therefore be relevant to melanoma [62]. On the contrary, skin typing as performed in many studies, and perhaps inherently [73], is remarkably lacking in robustness and, in the author's view, the evidence does not convincingly argue for effects of the *MC1R* beyond the cutaneous response to UVR. Future studies will need to be large, ideally based in different genetic backgrounds or populations, and use explicit models of the effects of the various alleles.

Relevance of the mouse?

Murine genetics has provided a powerful way to identify genes involved in melanocyte development and melanogenesis [18,19]. Murine models of non-melanoma skin cancer have also informed opinion on the hazards of UVR for human non-melanoma skin cancer [74]. However, the value of murine models in connection with red hair and melanoma appears limited for a number of reasons. Mouse melanocytes are predominantly follicular rather than interfollicular and current (murine) models of melanoma are limited. These limitations may be surmountable. Engineering of melanocyte position within the epidermal compartment in the mouse is feasible, and such systems would provide interesting approaches to study the relation between melanogenic intermediaries and phototoxicity—something that is very hard if not impossible to achieve in humans. Complementing these sort of approaches, however, is an urgent need to improve our knowledge of pigmentary phenotypes in humans, and our understanding of how persons with different genetic backgrounds differ in response to UVR.

Conclusions

The genetic basis of red hair is rapidly being resolved as the necessary technical tools are in hand. The role of the *MC1R* in determining skin type is less advanced and may require new experimental methods of treating the interaction between *MC1R* allelic variation and the cutaneous skins response to UVR as a quantitative trait. Further human genetic epidemiological studies of the *MC1R* and melanoma are required and far greater attention to the quality of the phenotypic assessment may be important if we are to understand the physiological pathways linking genotype to phenotype.

References

1 Gallagher RP, Ho X, Ho VC. Environmental and host risk factors. In: Grob JJ, Stern RS, MacKie RM, Weinstock MA, eds. *Epidemiology, Causes and Prevention of Skin Diseases*. Oxford: Blackwell, 1998: 235–42.

2 Weinstock MA. Epidemiology of ultraviolet radiation. In: Grob JJ, Stern RS, MacKie RM, Weinstock MA, eds. *Epidemiology, Causes and Prevention of Skin Diseases*. Oxford: Blackwell, 1998: 121–8.

3 Bliss JM, Ford D, Swerdlow AJ *et al.* Risk of cutaneous melanoma associated with pigmentation characteristics and freckling: systematic overview of 10 case–control studies. The International Melanoma Analysis Group (IMAGE). *Int J Cancer* 1995; **62**: 367–76.

4 Elwood JM, Jopson J. Melanoma and sun exposure: an overview of published studies. *Int J Cancer* 1997; **73**: 198–203.

5 Urbach F, Rose DB, Bonnem RDH, Bonnem M. Genetic and environmental interactions in skin carcinogenesis. In: Urbach F, Rose DB, Bonnem RDH, Bonnem M, eds. *Genetic and Environmenatal Carcinogenesis*. Baltimore: Williams & Wilkins, 1972: 355–71.

6 Urbach F. The cumulative effects of ultraviolet radiation on the skin: photocarcinogenesis. In: Hawk JLM, ed. *Photodermatology*. London: Arnold, 1999: 89–102.

7 Bodmer WF, Cavalli-Sforza LL. *Genetics, Evolution and Man*. San Fransisco: W.H. Freeman, 1976.

8 Gallagher RP, Hill GB, Bajdik CD *et al.* Sunlight exposure, pigmentation factors, and risk of nonmelanocytic skin cancer. II. Squamous cell carcinoma. *Arch Dermatol* 1995; **131**: 164–9.

9 Lock-Andersen J, Drzewiecki KT, Wulf HC. The measurement of constitutive and facultative skin pigmentation and estimation of sun exposure in caucasians with basal cell carcinoma and cutaneous malignant melanoma. *Br J Dermatol* 1998; **139**: 610–17.

10 Lock-Andersen J, Drzewiecki KT, Wulf HC. Eye and hair colour, skin type and constitutive skin pigmentation as risk factors for basal cell carcinoma and cutaneous malignant melanoma: a Danish case–control study. *Acta Derm Venereol* 1999; **79**: 74–80.

11 Neel JV. Concerning the inheritance of red hair. *J Hered* 1943; **34**: 93–6.

12 Reed TE. Red hair colour as a genetical character. *Ann Eugen* 1952; **17**: 115–39.

13 Sunderland E. Hair-colour variation in the United Kingdom. *Hum Genet* 1956; **20**, 312–30.

14 Singleton WR, Ellis B. Inheritance of red hair for six generations. *J Hered* 1964; **55**: 261.

15 Rife DC. The inheritance of red hair. *Acta Genet Med Gemellol (Roma)* 1967; **16** (4): 342–9.

16 Nicholls EM. The genetics of red hair. *Hum Hered* 1969; **19**: 36–42.

17 Jackson IJ. Molecular and developmental genetics of mouse coat color. *Ann Rev Genet* 1994; **28**: 189–217.

18 Barsh GS. The genetics of pigmentation: from fancy genes to complex traits. *Trends Genet* 1996; **12** (8): 299–305.

19 Jackson IJ. Homologous pigmentation mutations in human, mouse and other model organisms. *Hum Mol Genet* 1997; **6**: 1613–24.

20 Chhajlani V, Wikberg JE. Molecular cloning and expression of the human melanocyte stimulating hormone receptor cDNA. *FEBS Lett* 1992; **309**: 417–20.

21 Mountjoy KG, Robbins LS, Mortrud MT, Cone RD. The cloning of a family of genes that encode the melanocortin receptors. *Science* 1992; **257**: 1248–51.

22 Cone RD, Mountjoy KG, Robbins LS *et al.* Cloning and functional characterization of a family of receptors for the melanotropic peptides. *Ann N Y Acad Sci* 1993; **680**: 342–63.

23 Cone RD, Lu D, Koppula S *et al.* The melanocortin receptors: agonists, antagonists, and the hormonal control of pigmentation. *Recent Prog Horm Res* 1996; **51**: 287–317.

24 Lu D, Chen W, Cone RD. Regulation of melanogenesis by the MSH receptor. In: Nordlund JJ, Boissy RE, Hearing VJ, King RA, Ortonne JP, eds. *The Pigmentary System: Physiology and Pathophysiology*. New York: Oxford University Press, 1998: 183–98.

25 Friedmann PS, Wren F, Buffey J, MacNeil S. Alpha-MSH causes a small rise in cAMP but has no effect on basal or ultraviolet-stimulated melanogenesis in human melanocytes. *Br J Dermatol* 1990; **123**: 145–51.

26 Lerner AB. The discovery of the melanotropins. *Ann N Y Acad Sci* 1993; **680**: 1–12.

27 Joerg H, Fries HR, Meijerink E, Stranzinger GF. Red coat color in Holstein cattle is associated with a deletion in the MSHR gene. *Mamm Genome* 1996; **7**: 317–18.

28 Klungland H, Vage DI, Gomez-Raya L, Adalsteinsson S, Lien S. The role of melanocyte-stimulating hormone (MSH)

receptor in bovine coat color determination. *Mamm Genome* 1995; **6**: 636–9.

29 Takeuchi S, Suzuki S, Hirose S *et al.* Molecular cloning and sequence analysis of the chick melanocortin 1-receptor gene. *Biochim Biophys Acta* 1996b; **1306**: 122–6.

30 Våge DI, Lu DS, Klungland H, Lien S, Adalsteinsson S, Cone RD. A non-epistatic interaction of *agouti* and *extension* in the fox, *Vulpes vulpes*. *Nat Genet* 1997; **15**: 311–15.

31 Våge DI, Klungland H, Lu D, Cone RD. Molecular and pharmacological characterization of dominant black coat color in sheep. *Mamm Genome* 1999; **10**: 39–43.

32 Marklund L, Moller MJ, Sandberg K, Andersson L. A missense mutation in the gene for melanocyte-stimulating hormone receptor (MC1R) is associated with the chestnut coat color in horses. *Mamm Genome* 1996; **7**: 895–9.

33 Gantz I, Yamada T, Tashiro T *et al.* Mapping of the gene encoding the melanocortin-1 (alpha-melanocyte stimulating hormone) receptor (MC1R) to human chromosome 16q24.3 by fluorescence *in situ* hybridization. *Genomics* 1994; **19**: 394–5.

34 Tan CP, McKee KK, Weinberg DH *et al.* Molecular analysis of a new splice variant of the human melanocortin-1 receptor. *FEBS Lett* 1999; **451**: 137–41.

35 Chakraborty AK, Funasaka Y, Pawelek JM, Nagahama M, Ito A, Ichihashi M. Enhanced expression of melanocortin-1 receptor (MC1-R) in normal human keratinocytes during differentiation: evidence for increased expression of POMC peptides near suprabasal layer of epidermis. *J Invest Dermatol* 1999; **112**: 853–60.

36 Hartmeyer M, Scholzen T, Becher E, Bhardwaj RS, Schwarz T, Luger TA. Human dermal microvascular endothelial cells express the melanocortin receptor type 1 and produce increased levels of IL-8 upon stimulation with α-melanocyte-stimulating hormone. *J Immunol* 1997; **159**: 1930–7.

37 Healy E, Todd C, Jackson IJ, Birch-Machin M, Rees JL. Skin type, melanoma, and melanocortin 1 receptor variants. *J Invest Dermatol* 1999; **112**: 512–13.

38 Bhardwaj RS, Luger TA. Pro-opiomelanocortin production by epidermal cells: evidence for an immune neuroendocrine network in the epidermis. *Arch Dermatol Res* 1994; **287**: 85–90.

39 Scholzen T, Armstrong CA, Bunnett N, Luger TA, Olerud J, Ansel JC. Neuropeptides in the skin: interactions between the neuroendocrine and the skin immune systems. *Exp Dermatol* 1998; **7**: 81–96.

40 Moro O, Ideta R, Ifuku O. Characterization of the promoter region of the human melanocortin-1 receptor (*MC1R*) gene. *Biochem Biophys Res Commun* 1999; **262**: 452–60.

41 Valverde P, Healy E, Jackson I, Rees JL, Thody AJ. Variants of the melanocyte-stimulating hormone receptor gene are associated with red hair and fair skin in humans. *Nat Genet* 1995; **11**: 328–30.

42 Spritz RA. A study in scarlet [news; comment]. *Nat Genet* 1995; **11**: 225–6.

43 Box NF, Wyeth JR, O'Gorman LE, Martin NG, Sturm RA. Characterization of melanocyte stimulating hormone receptor variant alleles in twins with red hair. *Hum Mol Genet* 1997; **6**: 1891–7.

44 Smith R, Healy E, Siddiqui S *et al.* Melanocortin 1 receptor variants in an Irish population. *J Invest Dermatol* 1998; **111**: 119–22.

45 Frändberg PA, Doufexis M, Kapas S, Chhajlani V. Human pigmentation phenotype: a point mutation generates nonfunctional MSH receptor. *Biochem Biophys Res Commun* 1998; **245**: 490–2.

46 Schioth HB, Phillips S, Rudzish R, Birch-Machin M, Wikberg J, Rees JL. Loss of function mutations of the human melanocortin 1 receptor are common and associated with red hair. *Biochem Biophys Res Commun* 1999; **260**: 488–91.

47 Rees JL, Birch-Machin M, Flanagan N, Healy E, Phillips S, Todd C. Genetic studies of the human melanocortin 1 receptor (*MC1R*). *Ann N Y Acad Sci* 1999; **885**: 134–42.

48 Krude H, Biebermann H, Luck W, Horn R, Brabant G, Grüters A. Severe early-onset obesity, adrenal insufficiency and red hair pigmentation caused by *POMC* mutations in humans. *Nat Genet* 1998; **19**: 155–7.

49 Ao Y, Park HY, Olaizola-Horn S,

Gilchrest BA. Activation of cAMP-dependent protein kinase is required for optimal α-melanocyte-stimulating hormone-induced pigmentation. *Exp Cell Res* 1998; **244**: 117–24.

50 Furumura M, Sakai C, Potterf SB, Vieira WD, Barsh GS, Hearing VJ. Characterization of genes modulated during pheomelanogenesis using differential display. *Proc Natl Acad Sci USA* 1998; **95**: 7374–8.

51 Ito S. Advances in chemical analysis of melanins. In: Nordlund JJ, Boissy RE, Hearing VJ, King RA, Ortonne JP, eds. *The Pigmentary System: Physiology and Pathophysiology*. New York: Oxford University Press, 1998: 439–50.

52 Prota G. *Melanins and Melanogenesis*. San Diego: Academic Press, 1992.

53 Prota G, Misuraca G. Melanins and related metabolites in skin photoprotection. In: Altmeyer P, Hoffman K, Stücker M, eds. *Skin Cancer, UV Radiation*. Berlin: Springer-Verlag, 1997: 148–57.

54 Chedekel MR. Photophysics and photochemistry of melanin. In: Zeise L, Chedekel MR, Fitzpatrick TB, eds. *Melanin: its Role in Human Photoprotection*. Overland Park: Valdenmar, 1995: 11–22.

55 Kollias N, Sayre RM, Zeise L, Chedekel MR. Photoprotection by melanin [Review]. *J Photochem Photobiol B* 1991; 9: 135–60.

56 Hill HZ. The function of melanin or six blind people examine an elephant. *Bioessays* 1992; **14** (1), 49–56.

57 Pathak MA, Fitzpatrick TB. The role of natural photprotective agents in human skin. In: Fitzpatrick TB, Pathak MA, Harber LC, Seiji M, Kukita A, eds. *Sunlight and Man*. Tokyo: Univeristy of Tokyo Press, 1974: 725–50.

58 Gilchrest BA, Eller MS, Geller AC, Yaar M. The pathogenesis of melanoma induced by ultraviolet radiation. *N Engl J Med* 1999; **340**: 1341–8.

59 Barker D, Dixon K, Medrano EE *et al.* Comparison of the responses of human melanocytes with different melanin contents to ultraviolet B irradiation. *Cancer Res* 1995; **55**: 4041–6.

60 Memoli S, Napolitano A, d'Ischia M, Misuraca G, Palumbo A, Prota G. Diffusible melanin-related metabolites are potent inhibitors of lipid peroxidation. *Biochim Biophys Acta* 1997; **1346**: 61–8.

61 Vincensi MR, d'Ischia M, Napolitano A *et al.* Phaeomelanin versus eumelanin as a chemical indicator of ultraviolet sensitvity in fair skinned subjects at high risk for melanoma: a pilot study. *Melanoma Res* 1998; **8**: 53–8.

62 Thody AJ, Graham A. Does α-MSH have a role in regulating skin pigmentation in humans. *Pigment Cell Res* 1998; **11**: 265–74.

63 Menon IA, Persad S, Ranadive NS, Haberman HF. Effects of ultraviolet-visible irradiation in the presence of melanin isolated from human black or red hair upon Ehrlich ascites carcinoma cells. *Cancer Res* 1983; **43**: 3165–9.

64 Persad S, Menon IA, Haberman HF. Comparison of the effects of UV-visible irradiation of melanins and melanin-hematoporphyrin complexes from human black and red hair. *Photochem Photobiol* 1983; **37**: 63–8.

65 Diffey BL, Healy E, Thody AJ, Rees JL. Melanin, melanocytes, and melanoma. *Lancet* 1995; **346**: 1713.

66 Lookingbill DP, Lookingbill GL, Leppard B. Actinic damage and skin cancer in albinos in northern Tanzania: findings in 164 patients enrolled in an outreach skin care program. *J Am Acad Dermatol* 1995; **32**: 653–8.

67 Healy E, Birch-Machin MA, Rees JL. The human Melanocortin-1 receptor. In: Cone RD, ed. *The Melanocortin Receptors*. New Jersey: Humana Press, 2000: 341–60.

68 Ichii-Jones F, Lear JT, Heagerty AHM *et al.* Susceptibility to melanoma: influence of skin type and polymorphism in the melanocyte stimulating hormone receptor gene. *J Invest Dermatol* 1998; **111**: 218–21.

69 Palmer JS, Duffy DL, Box NF *et al.* Melanocortin-1 receptor polymorphisms and risk of melanoma: is the association explained solely by pigmentation phenotype? *Am J Hum Genet* 2000; **66**: 176–86.

70 Valverde P, Healy E, Sikkink S *et al.* The Asp84Glu variant of the melanocortin 1 receptor (MC1R) is associated with melanoma. *Hum Mol Genet* 1996; **5**: 1663–6.

71 Strange RC, Ichii-Jones F, Lear JT,

Hutchinson PE, Fryer AA. Skin type, melanoma and melanocortin 1 receptor variants: reply. *J Invest Dermatol* 1999; **112**: 513.

72 Healy E, Flanagan N, Ray AJ *et al.* Melanocortin-1-receptor gene and sun sensitivity in individuals without red hair. *Lancet* 2000; **335**: 1072–3.

73 Rampen FH, Fleuren BA, de Boo TM, Lemmens WA. Unreliability of self-reported burning tendency and tanning ability. *Arch Dermatol* 1988; **124**: 885–8.

74 de Gruijl FR, Forbes PD. UV-induced skin cancer in a hairless mouse model [Review]. *Bioessays* 1995; **17**: 651–60.

5: The management of patients with atypical naevi

Julia A. Newton Bishop

Introduction

The management of patients with an atypical naevus phenotype, and even the presence of one or two atypical naevi often causes concern, not least because there is commonly uncertainty in the mind of the clinician as to the risk of melanoma implied. The management of affected patients can, however, be approached in a straightforward manner, based upon published data.

What are atypical moles?

Atypical moles are usually defined as moles with a diameter of 5 mm or larger, with an irregular shape and variable pigmentation (Fig. 5.1). Although such moles have a characteristic histological appearance, the diagnosis is a clinical one: the risk associated with such naevi has been calculated using clinical appearance, not histological characteristics.

Most moles grow in diameter with age but usually to a maximal diameter of 2 mm or so. At this stage most lesions will show a loss of junctional activity histologically: melanocytes disappear from the dermoepidermal junction and the dermal cells differentiate towards a rather neural appearance. Lever likens them to Schwann cells [1]. Thus, a junctional naevus matures via a compound naevus to a dermal cellular naevus. It seems appropriate to speculate that the melanocytes have senesced.

Atypical moles appear to behave in a different way. Junctional proliferation of melanocytes continues longer so that the lesion increases in diameter and dermalization takes longer to occur. Indeed, the naevus may continue to increase in diameter to an excess of 10 mm. Naevi such as this are less numerous in the elderly and the assumption is that in the majority of cases even large atypical naevi will mature and disappear. Indeed, that is the author's experience in the pigmented lesion clinic, and cross-sectional data on naevi suggest that naevi disappear with age [2].

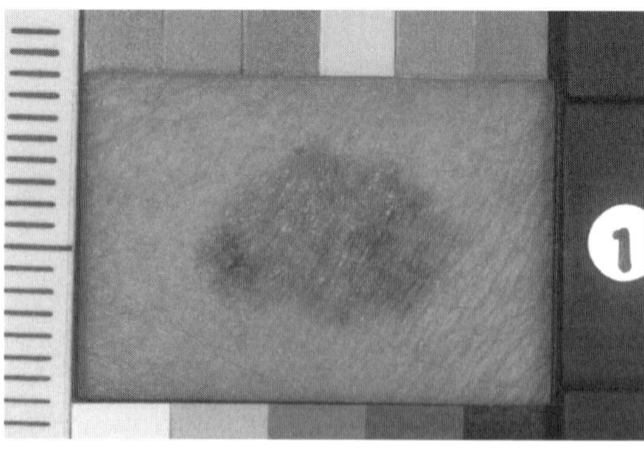

Fig. 5.1 An atypical naevus showing the characteristic features of size ≥ 5 mm in diameter, irregular pigmentation and an irregular edge.

The atypical naevus phenotype

It is common to have one or two clinically atypical naevi. In our UK case–control study performed in the south of England, 3.5% of the adult control population had one atypical naevus, and 2.8% had two or more. Most of these individuals were under the age of 50 years. In the city of Leeds where the author runs a pigmented lesion clinic, then there must, by extrapolation, be at least 30 000 such patients. For an individual with no family history of melanoma, and without an excess of naevi in total, the risk of melanoma arising in such a naevus is very low but difficult to quantify.

However, a small proportion of the general population have a more markedly unusual naevus phenotype, the so-called atypical naevus syndrome phenotype (AMS). This was first described in the 19th century in the context of familial susceptibility to melanoma [3] but was first properly explored by Wallace Clark and was given the name the B-K mole syndrome and then the dysplastic naevus syndrome [4]. The same phenotype was recognized by Wilma Bergman in Dutch families prone to melanoma and was named the familial atypical multiple mole and melanoma (FAMMM) syndrome [5] . The term 'dysplastic naevus' attracted a good deal of controversy some years ago, largely related to concerns about the implications of the word 'dysplastic' to histopathologists [6–9] and hence forth many have chosen to use the term 'atypical mole syndrome phenotype' instead (AMS). This is the author's preferred name.

The AMS is characterized by the presence of large numbers of naevi, clinically atypical naevi and an abnormal distribution of naevi such that affected patients often have naevi in sites where they are less common in the general population. These sites include the ears, the scalp, the buttocks and the dorsae of the feet. Rona MacKie described the phenotype as being consistent with 'an activated and expanded population of melanocytes' [10], and indeed that is what the phenotype suggests clinically. The patients with this phenotype have

Table 5.1 The AMS scoring system used in studies by our group and in the clinic

	Score	
100 or more naevi 2 mm or bigger (50 or more if under 20 or over 50 years)	1 point	AMS 1
Two or more atypical naevi	1 point	AMS 2
One or more naevi in the anterior scalp	1 point	AMS 3
One naevus on buttocks or two or more on dorsae of feet	1 point	AMS 4
One or more iris naevi	1 point	AMS 5

Patients are considered to have the 'AMS phenotype' if the total score is 3 or more.

an increased tendency to naevi such that they develop increased numbers of them and naevi in uncommon sites, even in the iris [11].

Some patients have very large numbers of naevi, more than 400, 2 mm or more in diameter, yet have few or no clinically atypical naevi. Others have large numbers of atypical naevi although their total overall naevus count is small. The differences between patients may cause confusion and concern. What particular phenotype is associated with the greatest risk and how should we define the AMS?

There have been several definitions used to define the AMS. We use a scoring system based upon dichotomous variables. The maximum score is 5 and we consider someone to have the AMS if their score is 3 or more (Table 5.1). Our use of this scoring system in data from the NE Thames case–control study showed that a score of 3 or more is seen in 2% of the general population and 15% of melanoma patients giving an odds ratio of 10 for a score of 3 or more compared with a score of 0 [12]. We have created here a discontinuous phenotype out of what is clearly a continuous one, as was recognized by Professor Happle and Dr Traupe years ago [13], but the scoring system works in practice. It is a reproducible robust system which can be taught in a relatively short period [14]. It is easy to use in clinic and defines a population of people who are at increased risk of melanoma, which is quantifiable, albeit imperfectly. Furthermore, it takes into account the variations in the phenotype between individuals, as described above.

What does the presence of the AMS mean?

Although the AMS phenotype was described in the context of familial melanoma, its relationship to familial susceptibility remains unclear. It is common to see the same phenotype in patients with no family history of melanoma. In the UK, 2% of the general population have the AMS as we have defined it [12,14,15]. It is true that families at increased risk of melanoma commonly also have the AMS, but the AMS is not diagnostic of familial susceptibility. All we can say at the moment is that it defines a population at increased risk of melanoma.

The complicated relationship between the AMS and familial susceptibility to melanoma is illustrated by some genotype–phenotype studies we carried out in fine families carrying germline mutations in the *CDKN2A* gene which predisposes to melanoma [16,5]. The family members were examined prior to discovery of *CDKN2A* and the naevus phenotype was subsequently correlated with mutation status. Mutation carriers were significantly more likely to have two or more atypical naevi ($P=0.03$), naevi on the buttocks ($P=0.005$), naevi on the dorsum of the feet ($P=0.002$) and a larger number of naevi ($P=0.002$) than their family members with wild type or normal *CDKN2A*. However, the overlap between relatives with mutations and those without was considerable, such that it became clear that the AMS cannot be used in families to predict who is a gene carrier and who is not: the studies produced some evidence that *CDKN2A* is naevogenic but that the relationship between *CDKN2A* and naevi is complex.

Much work is currently taking place to dissect the relationship between the AMS and melanoma risk. Meanwhile, the bottom line is that family history is the major determinant of risk and individuals with a strong family history of melanoma should be regarded as at risk, whether they have the AMS or not. Patients with the AMS and no family history have an increased risk, but that risk is much more moderate. Estimates of relative risk in the UK population are given in Table 5.2. The risk estimates given in Table 5.2 are based upon a large case–control study [12] and there should be some caution in applying them to clinical practice in absolute terms; however, they can be used to order the risk.

Table 5.2 Estimates of increased risk of melanoma in the UK

Risk factor	Odds ratio with 95% CI
Red hair (with reference to dark brown hair)	2.5 (1.5–4.2)
Fitzpatrick skin type I relative to type IV	9.2 (3.8–21.6)
AMS score 3 or more with no family history*	10.2
1 atypical naevus	3.9 (2.1–7.3)
2–3 atypical naevi	5.3 (2.3–12.1)
4 or more atypical naevi	28.7 (8.6–95.6)
25–49 naevi 2 mm or more in diameter†	1.6 (0.9–3.0)
50–99 naevi	2.2 (1.2–4.2)
100 or more naevi	3.1 (1.4–6.7)
CDKN2A mutation carrier status [18]	50‡

* Relative to a score of 0.

† Adjusted for atypical naevi.

‡ Based upon work in progress (Bishop, Goldstein and Desmenais on behalf of the Melanoma Genetics Consortium) [12].

Carrying a germline mutation in *CDKN2A* is associated with the greatest risk [17], followed by a strong family history of melanoma, then the AMS and, finally, phenotypic characteristics indicative of sun sensitivity, such as red hair and a reported tendency to burn in the sun. The only more specific statistic that I find useful in clinical practice is the following. In our hands the AMS is associated with an odds ratio for melanoma of around 10. As the lifetime risk for melanoma in the UK is around 1 in 200 this produces an approximate lifetime risk for an AMS patient with no family history of about 1 in 20. As the general population do not all have an AMS score of O, this estimate $1/_{20}$ is probably a little high. However, many AMS carriers have increased now due to the presence of fair skin or freckles and $1/_{20}$ therefore is a good 'working' estimate in the clinic. This is significant, but lower than the risk of breast cancer for any woman in the UK. The table of relative risk shows some evidence that large numbers of clinically atypical naevi are associated with a greater risk, so that in clinical practice these patients should probably receive extra care. It seems unwise to attach more specific risk estimates pending results of ongoing further research. Finally, these risk estimates are multiplicative: a *CDKN2A* gene carrier with red hair is likely to have a higher risk than a gene carrier with olive skin.

What is the biological explanation for the AMS?

It is not yet clear what underlies the AMS but its association with familial susceptibility and *CDKN2A* mutation carrier status suggests that it is genetically determined.

Studies of normal moles in twins provide strong evidence that the variation between individuals in their naevus phenotype is largely genetically controlled [18–21]. There is some effect of ultraviolet (UV) light exposure on expression of those genes [21], but genes are the major determinants of variation. There remains much that is not known about the precise relationship between putative naevus genes and UV but there are data to suggest that UV exposure may have an effect on the rate of emergence of naevi [22,23] and some to suggest that sunlight may have a particular effect on the development of clinically atypical naevi [24].

Our hypothesis is that the atypical naevus phenotype is under genetic control but that its expression is probably influenced by UV exposure. Furthermore the genes which control the naevus phenotype are melanoma susceptibility genes. We have some evidence that these genes are moderate to low penetrance susceptibility genes, but this is not yet clear and forms the focus of the current research in the Genetic Epidemiology Division of the Imperial Cancer Research Fund (ICRF) Clinical Centre in Leeds, UK.

It is likely that putative melanoma–naevus susceptibility genes interact with low-penetrance susceptibility genes, such as *MC1R*. Human pigmentation is, in part, determined by the ratio of eumelanin in the skin (brown/black pigment) to phaeomelanin (red pigmentation). This is partly determined by the action of α-melanocyte-stimulating hormone (MSH) on its type 1 receptor (*MC1R*). Genetic variants in *MC1R* are common in white-skinned populations and have been shown to 'explain' a very large proportion of red hair and, presumably, sun sensitivity [25]. The variants also appear to be related to the risk of skin cancer even in people with darker hair [26,27].

How should dermatologists manage patients with the AMS?

1 Estimation of risk.

Does the patient have the AMS? The AMS scoring system is useful to define this.

Is there a family history of melanoma and, if so, how distant were the relatives?

Does the patient have a sun-sensitive phenotype: red hair, freckles and type 1 skin?

2 If there is a family history, construct a pedigree and seek the advice of a clinical geneticist or a specialist pigmented lesion clinic, if there are either:

- three or more cases of melanoma; or
- two cases and one had multiple primaries or the AMS phenotype.

3 Regardless of the need to seek expert genetics help in families, patients with the AMS need to be taught how to monitor their own naevi. I find it helpful to teach the patient and whoever has the responsibility for keeping an eye on their back together. The two need to know which moles (the clinically atypical) need to be watched and, most importantly, they need to see good colour photographs of melanomas: they need to know what they are looking for. I take two colour polaroids of the atypical naevi, one for the hospital notes, one for the patient. The family takes these home with a colour leaflet bearing photographs of melanomas with which they can compare their own naevi. Once a month the skin should be examined in a good light. Families need time and a few visits to the clinic to feel in control. Some never feel entirely comfortable and these patients may need long-term follow-up. The clinical trial evidence that self-examination works is lacking, but in clinical practice it certainly seems to. The critical factor is to spend time with your patient in teaching, to tailor the teaching to the patient and to have an open door to your clinic for the worried.

4 The diagnosis of the AMS, as discussed above, is clinical and therefore there is no point in biopsy unless there is concern that a naevus is evolving into a melanoma. When faced with a patient with atypical naevi, the aim should be to monitor lesions safely without unnecessary surgery. The dermatoscope and photography are very useful here, as discussed in Chapter 8.

5 It is my practice to offer open screening to family members in the presence of a family history of melanoma. Undiagnosed melanomas occasionally appear and the intent is to inform and educate.

6 Clear advice about limiting sun exposure should be given. Patients should be advised to avoid the midday sun, keep their clothes on and never get burnt. Because of recent anxieties that over-reliance on sunscreens could actually increase sun exposure, patients must be convinced that they cannot rely upon 'Factor 30'.

7 The length of follow-up will vary:

- *AMS and no family history.* Until the doctor and the patient are happy that the naevi are stable and the patient is confident and knows what he or she is looking for. Some patients, who are anxious or who cannot be persuaded to self-examine, may need long-term follow-up but most patients will require only two or three visits. Some authors recommend particular surveillance at a time when naevi are prone to change, such as around puberty or in pregnancy. Some patients have particularly unusual naevi and I would keep such patients under long-term surveillance whatever their family history.
- *AMS and one case of melanoma in the family.* As above.
- *AMS and two or more cases of melanoma in the family.* Long-term surveillance.
- *Two or more cases in the family and one with multiple primaries, or three or more cases of melanoma in the family, whatever their naevus phenotype.* Long-term follow-up. Whether this equates to lifelong follow-up in a hospital will depend on the patient, the health care system and whether gene testing eventually becomes routine.
- *AMS and a personal history of melanoma.* Lifelong follow-up.

What do I do about patients with one or two atypical naevi only?

It is my practice to remove lesions which appear to be changing, or which have atypical dermatoscopic features. The overwhelming majority of such lesions which present in the clinic, however, have neither of these features. I will then take a Polaroid photograph and review in 4 months. If at 4 months the lesion is clearly unchanged I discharge the patient with their own copy of the photograph, with an open appointment to return if there is a change.

A considerable proportion of the population have such naevi and the absolute risk of any one such lesion evolving into a melanoma is tiny, although unquantified. My experience in the pigmented lesion clinic suggests that melanoma *in situ* (MIN) may remain stable for years before becoming invasive. A policy of removal of lesions clinically suggestive of atypical naevi only if they are changing may therefore theoretically result, rarely, in failure to remove an *in situ* lesion. The critical issue then is to have a sufficiently low threshold for excision and here dermatoscopy is of value. A banal appearance down the dermatoscope increases the likelihood that the lesion really is benign. These issues are discussed in Chapter 8.

References

1 Lever W, Schaumburg-Lever G. Melanocytic nevus. In: *Histopathology of the Skin*. Philadelphia: Lippincott and Co., 1990: 756–805.

2 MacKie RM, *et al.* The number and distribution of benign pigmented moles (melanocytic naevi) in a healthy British population. *Br J Dermatol* 1985: **113**; 167–74.

3 Norris W. A case of fungoid disease. *Edinb Med Surg J* 1820: **16**; 562–5.

4 Clark W, *et al.* Origin of familial malignant melanoma from hereditable melanocytic lesions: the B-K mole syndrome. *Arch Dermatol* 1978: **114**; 732.

5 Bergman W, Palan A, Went LN. Clinical and genetic studies in six Dutch kindreds with the Dysplastic Naevus Syndrome. *Ann Hum Genet* 1986: **50**; 249–58.

6 Piepkorn M, *et al.* The dysplastic melanocytic nevus: a prevalent lesion that correlates poorly with clinical phenotype. *J Am Acad Dermatol* 1989: **20**; 407–15.

7 Shapiro PE. Making sense of the dysplastic nevus controversy. *Am J Dermatopathol* 1992; **14** (4): 350–6.

8 Happle R. Dysplastic nevus 'syndrome': the emergence and decline of an erroneous concept. *J Eur Acad Dermatol* 1993: **2**; 275–80.

9 Ackerman AB, Milde P. Naming acquired melanocytic nevi: common and dysplastic, normal and atypical or Unna, Miescher, Spitz and Clark. *Am J Dermatopathol* 1992; **14** (5): 447–53.

10 MacKie RM. Multiple melanoma and atypical melanocytic naevi: evidence of an activated and expanded melanocytic system. *Br J Dermatol* 1982: **107**; 621–9.

11 Rodriguez-Sains RS. Ocular findings in patients with dysplastic nevus syndrome. *An update. Dermatol Clinics* 1991: **9** (4); 723–8.

12 Bataille V, *et al.* Risk of cutaneous melanoma in relation to the numbers,types and sites of naevi: a case–control study. *Br J Cancer* 1996: **73**; 1605–11.

13 Traupe H, Happle R. Reply: The dysplastic nevus 'syndrome' is not a dichotomic, but a continuous phenotype. *Am J Med Genet* 1990: **35**; 295–6.

14 Newton JA, *et al.* How common is the atypical mole syndrome phenotype in apparently sporadic melanoma? *J Am Acad Dermatol* 1993: **29**; 989–96.

15 Newton Bishop J, *et al.* Teaching non-specialist health care professionals how to identify the atypical mole syndrome phenotype: a multi-national study. *Br J Dermatol* 2000: **142**; 331–7.

16 Wachsmuth R, Harland M, Newton Bishop J. The atypical mole syndrome and predisposition to melanoma. *New Engl J Med* 1998: **339**; 348–9.

17 Bishop D, Goldstein A, Demenais F. Geographical variation in CNKN2A penetrance for melanoma. *Am J Hum Genet* 2000: **67** (4); 16.

18 Easton D, *et al.* Genetic susceptibility to naevi: a twin study. *Br J Cancer* 1991: **64**; 1164–7.

19 Zhu G, *et al.* A major quantitative-trait locus for mole density is linked to the familial melanoma gene CDKN2A: a maximum-likelihood combined linkage and association analysis in twins and their sibs. *Am J Hum Genet* 1999: **65**; 483–92.

20 Bataille V, *et al.* Genetics of risk factors for melanoma: an adult twin study of nevi and freckles. *J Natl Cancer Inst* 2000: **92**; pp 457–63.

21 Wachsmuth RC, *et al.* A twin study of the effect of environmental exposures (ultraviolet light) on genes determining variation in nevus density. *J Invest Dermatol* 2001: **4**, in press.

22 Harrison SL, MacKie RM, MacLennan R. Development of melanocytic nevi in the first three years of life. *J Natl Cancer Inst* 2000: **92** (17); 1436–8.

23 Kelly J, *et al.* Sunlight: a major factor associated with the development of melanocytic nevi in Australian schoolchildren. *J Am Acad Dermatol* 1994: **30**; 40–8.

24 Bataille V, *et al.* The association between naevi and melanoma in populations with different levels of sun exposure: a joint case–control study of melanoma in the UK and Australia. *Br J Cancer* 1998: **77**; 505–10.

25 Valverde P, *et al.* Variants of the melanocyte stimulating hormone receptor gene are associated with red hair and fair skin in humans. *Nat Genet* 1995: **11**; 328–30.

26 Box NF, *et al.* Melanocortin-1 receptor genotype is a risk factor for basal and squamous cell carcinoma. *J Invest Dermatol* 2001: **116** (2); 224–9.

27 Palmer JS, *et al.* Melanocortin-1 receptor polymorphisms and risk of melanoma: is the association explained solely by pigmentation phenotype? *Am J Hum Genet* 2000: **66** (1); 176–86.

6: Guidelines for the management of those at high risk for developing cutaneous melanoma

Richard F. Kefford

Introduction

Cutaneous melanoma, like other cancers, is the result of the convergence of genetically determined constitutional factors and environmental DNA damaging factors. Melanoma is unique because the environmental agent, ultraviolet radiation, is clearly defined, and at least some of the factors determining genetic predisposition have been identified. Current international research is directed at a precise analysis of the interaction between environment and constitution in determining causation. The continuing refinement of our understanding of this interaction will continue to guide public health and clinical measures in melanoma prevention, screening and early detection. The ability to define high-risk groups will allow for a higher degree of precision and cost effectiveness in directed programmes of this type.

Risk factors for cutaneous melanoma

Those at highest risk for developing cutaneous melanoma are members of particularly melanoma-prone families. Typically, these families are characterized by the presence of three or more affected members in two or more generations, on the same side of the family. A typical pedigree is shown in Fig. 6.1. Members of such families have an approximate relative risk of 35–70 for the development of cutaneous melanoma [1]. Some, but not all, of these families also display inheritance of the phenotype of multiple atypical naevi. It is important to note that not all patients reporting the presence of a family history of melanoma are at such high risk. First, there is a false-positive rate as high as 40% in patient reporting of melanoma in their relatives [2]. Secondly, the mere presence of a positive family history, defined as 'one or more affected first-degree relatives' confers an approximate relative risk of 2–3 [3].

The presence of multiple benign naevi is a strong marker for melanoma risk across all continents [4]. In an Australian study, the risk of melanoma was raised 12 times in those with more than 100 naevi compared with those with

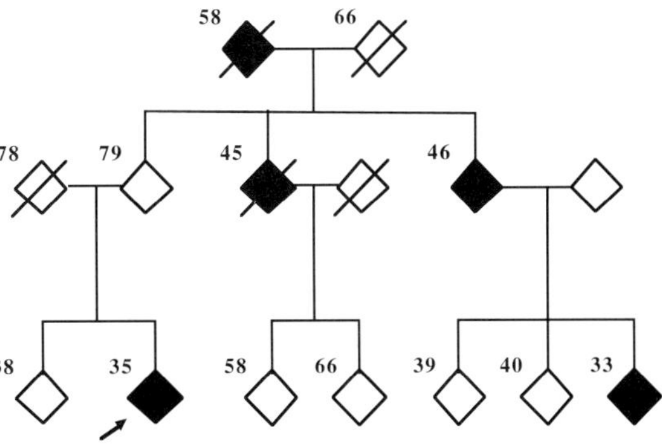

Fig. 6.1 Typical pedigree of melanoma-prone kindred showing the age of onset of melanoma. Gender has been scrambled to preserve confidentiality. Opaque diamonds indicate a melanoma case. The arrow indicates the proband.

less than 10 [5]. The atypical mole syndrome (AMS)/dysplastic naevus syndrome (DNS) phenotype confers potent risk, carrying in the UK, for example, a relative risk of around 10 for melanoma in the general population [6,7]. There is evidence for both a genetic [6] and an environmental [8–10] component in determining 'moliness'. It seems that genetic predisposition to melanoma is in part expressed as an ultraviolet-vulnerable skin type and/or 'moliness', and that this predisposition also interacts strongly with sun exposure.

Other important risk factors for cutaneous melanoma are the presence of a history of previous primary cutaneous melanoma (relative risk 8.5) [10], skin that burns readily and fails to tan (relative risk 1.4) [11], freckling (relative risk 2–3) [11,12], blue eyes (relative risk 1.6) [11,12], red hair (relative risk 2.4–4) [11,12] and personal history of blistering sunburn (relative risk 2–3) [11,12]. Many of these risk factors relate to sun sensitivity, and are compounded for those individuals living in locations of high ambient ultraviolet radiation.

Genetic basis of melanoma

Constitutional mutations have been found in two genes that confer a high risk for the development of melanoma. These are the genes CDKN2A on chromosome 9p (coding for the cyclin-dependent kinase inhibitor, p16^{INK4A}), and the cyclin-dependent kinase, CDK4. Both genes play a critical part in the regulation of the cell cycle. The proportion of all cutaneous melanomas that is attributable to the inheritance of autosomal dominantly inherited mutations in melanoma susceptibility genes is unknown, but is estimated by to be < 1–2% [13].

Approximately one-third of those hereditary melanoma families containing three or more affected first- or second-degree relatives show inheritance of mutations in the CDKN2A gene [14]. Mutations occur throughout the gene [15], frustrating the ability to perform simple targeted analyses for 'hot-spot' mutations. Because current information on each mutation is limited and confined to data from large specifically ascertained families, the confidence limits on current estimates of the penetrance of mutations in the CDKN2A gene are very wide. There are few data on the prevalence of CDKN2A mutations in the population. In a large population-based study in Queensland, the prevalence of CDKN2A mutations was 9/87 (10.3%) in the subgroup of kindreds exhibiting the strongest familial clustering, and the overall prevalence in the population was estimated to be 0.2% [16].

Two families in the USA and one in France have mutations in the CDK4 gene on chromosome 12q, which inhibits binding of its inhibitor, $p16^{INK4A}$ [17,18]. The genetic basis for the remaining 60–80% of families, in which highly penetrant genes may be operating, is the subject of active research by the International Melanoma Genetics Consortium [13].

Genetic testing for melanoma

It is possible to identify certain pointers to the presence of constitutional mutations in melanoma susceptibility genes within an individual. The best predictor at present is the presence in a melanoma-affected person of a strong family history of melanoma [14]. Other pointers include a history of multiple primary melanomas [19,20], and an early age of onset of first melanoma [21].

Despite these known correlations with genetic susceptibility, at present predictive genetic testing for melanoma susceptibility in unaffected individuals should only be performed very rarely outside of a research setting [13]. The reasons for this are as follow.

- Only approximately one-third of multiple-affected-member melanoma kindreds are accounted for by currently known melanoma susceptibility genes [13,22]. While the hunt for other genes continues, DNA testing in the majority of such families will be uninformative.
- Even where a defined mutation in a known melanoma susceptibility gene has been identified in one affected family member, this information is frequently of little value to other family members because of a lack of knowledge about the penetrance of such mutations. In the case of the CDKN2A gene, penetrance appears to be partially influenced by exposure to sunlight [23]. It is therefore not possible to offer even near-accurate estimates of the lifetime risk of melanoma in individuals carrying a constitutional mutation in a melanoma susceptibility gene such as CDKN2A. In certain cases, for example, gene carriers have survived to advanced years without developing melanoma [24]. Such lack of precision confounds attempts at accurate predictive DNA testing even within the context of such relatively rare multiple-case families.

- While certain CDKN2A mutations have a clear and demonstrable functional effect on the p16^{INK4A} protein [25], others do not, and may represent population polymorphisms of no predictive value with respect to melanoma occurrence.
- It is not uncommon to find atypical naevi and even melanoma in *non*-mutation carriers in high-risk melanoma kindreds [22,26,27]. This may be because of common environmental exposure by family members, or to the common inheritance of less highly penetrant melanoma susceptibility genes, or modifier genes. Whatever the reason, the practical clinical result is that *all* members of such families should be subjected to the same protocol of prevention and surveillance.
- There is currently only limited data on the efficacy of prevention and surveillance strategies for melanoma [28].

Advice for those at risk

Given current gaps in knowledge about the expression of melanoma susceptibility genes in the population, DNA testing cannot be used as a guide to clinical practice of prevention and surveillance. All individuals deemed to be at high risk of melanoma should be managed with the same attention to the following measures, as outlined for those at high risk of melanoma [29,30]. In the absence of randomized controlled clinical trial-based data, the evidence for each of these measures is Level IV, (a consensus view).

- Education of all family members about the need for sun protection is essential. Parents in particular should be educated about sun-protective measures during infancy and childhood [29,31,32] including the use of sun-protective clothing, hats and sunglasses, broad-spectrum UVA- and UVB-protective sunscreens [33,34], avoidance of peak ultraviolet conditions and absolute avoidance of sunburns.
- From the age of 10 years, family members should have a baseline skin examination with characterization of moles. Overview photographs of the entire skin surface and close-up photographs of atypical naevi are useful.
- Individuals should be taught about routine self-examination in the hope that this will prompt earlier diagnosis and removal of melanomas. Patients may be given their own copy of photographs and shown how to use these in self-examination. The significance of change in size or shape of pigmented lesions should be understood and the ABCD rules are often helpful in this regard [35]. Colour photographs of early melanomas and atypical moles may be given to the patient as an aid.
- Self-examination should be supplemented where possible with examination by a similarly trained parent, partner or family member.
- An appropriately trained health care provider should carry out 6-monthly

skin examinations until the naevi are stable and the patient is judged competent in self-surveillance. Subsequently, the individual should be seen annually or have prompt access to that health care provider as necessary. During puberty or pregnancy, when the naevi may be unstable, more frequent health care provider examinations may be indicated. Examination should include adequate examination of the scalp and genitalia. Skin surface microscopy (epiluminescence microscopy) [36,37] may be helpful in a surveillance programme.

- The indication for surgical removal of a pigmented lesion is the same as in the general population; that is, suspicion of malignant change. There is no justification for prophylactic excision of moles because the probability of a single naevus becoming melanoma is low and, with time, most naevi will mature and disappear. Furthermore, melanomas may occur on previously entirely normal skin [38] so that 'prophylactic' excision of all moles would not change guidelines on surveillance by the patient or the health care provider.
- Screening and surveillance guidelines for other cancers should be carried out as in the general population. Rarely, melanoma occurs in the context of the Li–Fraumeni syndrome. The hallmark for the Li–Fraumeni syndrome is the presence of sarcomas and other early onset cancers, particularly breast cancer, in the pedigree. Screening should be conducted in accordance with guidelines for this condition. Certain hereditary melanoma families carrying CDKN2A mutations have an increased incidence of pancreatic adenocarcinoma [39,40]. Even within this minority of families, the occurrence of pancreatic cancer is a rare event. At present there is no reliable screening method for early operable pancreatic carcinoma and survival is poor even with optimal treatment of early disease [41].
- Where cases of ocular melanoma have occurred in the family, annual fundoscopy is recommended, although it is of unproved efficacy in screening or early detection. The risk in any individual of developing this tumour is likely to be low.

Conclusions

The discovery of mutations in the melanoma susceptibility genes CDKN2A and CDK4 in families showing an inherited pattern of cutaneous melanoma has led to the possibility of genetic testing for this disease. However, it is currently premature to offer predicative DNA testing for melanoma outside of defined research protocols because of the low likelihood of finding mutations; current uncertainties about the functionality and penetrance of mutations, even if found; and the lack of proved efficacy of prevention and surveillance strategies, even for mutation carriers. Rather than singling out those deemed to be at high risk because of family history, all patients carrying risk factors for melanoma should be subject to stringent programmes of sun protection and skin surveillance.

Acknowledgements

The Melanoma Genetics Programme at Westmead Institute for Cancer Research is jointly supported by the Melanoma and Skin Cancer Research Institute, University of Sydney. This programme is funded by the National Health and Medical Research Council, the New South Wales Cancer Council, the Melanoma Foundation, the University of Sydney Cancer Research Fund, the Millennium Foundation and the Leo and Jenny Cancer Research Foundation.

References

1 Goldstein AM, Tucker MA. Genetic epidemiology of familial melanoma. *Dermatol Clin* 1995; **13**: 605–12.

2 Aitken JF, Youl P, Green A, *et al.* Accuracy of case-reported family history of melanoma in Queensland, Australia. *Melanoma Res* 1996; **6**: 313–7.

3 Ford D, Bliss JM, Swerdlow AJ, *et al.* Risk of cutaneous melanoma associated with a family history of the disease. The International Melanoma Analysis Group (IMAGE). *Int J Cancer* 1995; **62**: 377–81.

4 Berwick M, Halpern A. Melanoma epidemiology. *Curr Opin Oncol* 1997; **9**: 178–82.

5 Grulich AE, Bataille V, Swerdlow AJ, *et al.* Naevi and pigmentary characteristics as risk factors for melanoma in a high-risk population: a case–control study in New South Wales. *Int J Cancer*, 1996; **67**: 485–91.

6 Newton JA, Bataille V, Griffiths K, *et al.* How common is the atypical mole syndrome phenotype in apparently sporadic melanoma? *J Am Acad Dermatol* 1993; **29**: 989–96.

7 Bataille V, Bishop JA, Sasieni P, *et al.* Risk of cutaneous melanoma in relation to the numbers, types and sites of naevi: a case–control study. *Br J Cancer* 1996; **73**: 1605–11.

8 Harrison SL, MacLennan R, Speare R, *et al.* Sun exposure and melanocytic naevi in young Australian children. *Lancet* 1994; **344**: 1529–32.

9 Green A, Siskind V, Green L. The incidence of melanocytic naevi in adolescent children in Queensland, Australia. *Melanoma Res*, 1995; **5**: 155–60.

10 Tucker MA, Boice JD Jr, Hoffman DA. Second cancer following cutaneous melanoma and cancers of the brain, thyroid, connective tissue, bone, and eye in Connecticut, 1935–82. *Natl Cancer Inst Monogr* 1985; **68**: 161–89.

11 Marrett LD, King WD, Walter SD, *et al.* Use of host factors to identify people at high risk for cutaneous malignant melanoma. *Can Med Assoc J* 1992; **147**: 445–53. [Published erratum appears in *Can Med Assoc J* 1992; **147** (12): 1764, see comments.]

12 Bliss JM, Ford D, Swerdlow AJ, *et al.* Risk of cutaneous melanoma associated with pigmentation characteristics and freckling: systematic overview of 10 case–control studies. The International Melanoma Analysis Group (IMAGE). *Int J Cancer* 1995; **62**: 367–76.

13 Kefford RF, Newton Bishop JA, Bergman W, *et al.* Counseling and DNA testing for individuals perceived to be genetically predisposed to melanoma: a consensus statement of the Melanoma Genetics Consortium. *J Clin Oncol* 1999; **17**: 3245–51.

14 Goldstein AM, Tucker MA. Screening for CDKN2A mutations in hereditary

melanoma [editorial; comment]. *J Natl Cancer Inst* 1997; **89**: 676–8.

15 Hayward NK. The current situation with regard to human melanoma and genetic inferences. *Curr Opin Oncol* 1996; **8**: 136–42.

16 Aitken J, Welch J, Duffy D, *et al.* CDKN2A variants in a population-based sample of Queensland families with melanoma. *J Natl Cancer Inst* 1999; **91**: 446–52.

17 Zuo L, Weger J, Yang Q, *et al.* Germline mutations in the p16INK4a binding domain of CDK4 in familial melanoma. *Nat Genet* 1996; **12**: 97–9.

18 Soufir N, Avril MF, Chompret A, *et al.* Prevalence of p16 and CDK4 germline mutations in 48 melanoma-prone families in France. *Hum Mol Genet* 1998; **7**: 209–16.

19 Monzon J, Liu L, Brill H, *et al.* CDKN2A mutations in multiple primary melanomas. *N Engl J Med* 1998; **338**: 879–87.

20 Burden AD, Newell J, Andrew N, *et al.* Genetic and environmental influences in the development of multiple primary melanoma [see comments]. *Arch Dermatol* 1999; **135**: 261–5.

21 Goldstein AM, Fraser MC, Clark WH Jr, *et al.* Age at diagnosis and transmission of invasive melanoma in 23 families with cutaneous malignant melanoma/dysplastic nevi. *J Natl Cancer Inst* 1994; **86**: 1385–90.

22 Goldstein AM, Falk RT, Fraser MC, *et al.* Sun-related risk factors in melanoma-prone families with CDKN2A mutations. *J Natl Cancer Inst* 1998; **90**: 709–11.

23 Cannon-Albright LA, Meyer LJ, Goldgar DE, *et al.* Penetrance and expressivity of the chromosome 9p melanoma susceptibility locus (MLM). *Cancer Res* 1994; **54**: 6041–4.

24 Holland EA, Beaton SC, Becker TM, *et al.* Analysis of the p16 gene, CDKN2, in 17 Australian melanoma kindreds. *Oncogene* 1995; **11**: 2289–94.

25 Ranade K, Hussussian CJ, Sirkosi RS, *et al.* Mutations associated with familial melanoma impair p16INK4 function. *Nat Genet* 1995; **10**: 114–16.

26 Wachsmuth RC, Harland M, Bishop JA. The atypical-mole syndrome and predisposition to melanoma [letter]. *N Engl J Med* 1998; **339**: 348–9.

27 Gruis NA, Sandkuijl LA, van der Velden PA, *et al.* CDKN2 explains part of the clinical phenotype in Dutch familial atypical multiple-mole melanoma (FAMMM) syndrome families. *Melanoma Res* 1995; **5**: 169–77.

28 Tucker MA, Fraser MC, Goldstein AM, *et al.* The risk of melanoma and other cancers in melanoma-prone families. *J Invest Dermatol* 1993; **100**: 350S–355S.

29 National Institutes of Health Consensus Development Conference Statement on Diagnosis and Treatment of Early Melanoma, January 27–29, 1992 [see comments]. *Am J Dermatopathol* 1993; **15**: 34–43, discussion 46–51.

30 Slade J, Marghoob AA, Salopek TG, *et al.* Atypical mole syndrome: risk factor for cutaneous malignant melanoma and implications for management. *J Am Acad Dermatol* 1995; **32**: 479–94.

31 Ferrini RL, Perlman M, Hill L. American College of Preventive Medicine practice policy statement: skin protection from ultraviolet light exposure. *Am J Prev Med* 1998; **14**: 83–6.

32 Gasparro FP, Mitchnick M, Nash JF. A review of sunscreen safety and efficacy. *Photochem Photobiol* 1998; **68**: 243–56.

33 Setlow RB, Grist E, Thompson K, *et al.* Wavelengths effective in induction of malignant melanoma. *Proc Natl Acad Sci USA* 1993; **90**: 6666–70.

34 Krien PM, Moyal D. Sunscreens with broad-spectrum absorption decrease the *trans* to *cis* photoisomerization of urocanic acid in the human stratum corneum after multiple UV light exposures. *Photochem Photobiol* 1994; **60**: 280–7.

35 McGovern TW, Litaker MS. Clinical predictors of malignant pigmented lesions: a comparison of the Glasgow seven-point checklist and the American Cancer Society's ABCDs of pigmented lesions. *J Dermatol Surg Oncol* 1992; **18**: 22–6.

36 Kenet RO, Kang S, Kenet BJ, *et al.* Clinical diagnosis of pigmented lesions using digital epiluminescence microscopy: grading protocol and atlas. *Arch Dermatol* 1993; **129**: 157–74.

37 Menzies SW, Ingvar C, McCarthy WH. A sensitivity and specificity analysis of the surface microscopy features of invasive melanoma. *Melanoma Res* 1996; **6**: 55–62.

38 Kelly JW, Yeatman JM, Regalia C, *et al.* A high incidence of melanoma found in patients with multiple dysplastic naevi by photographic surveillance. *Med J Aust* 1997; **167**: 191–4.
39 Goldstein AM, Fraser MC, Struewing JP, *et al.* Increased risk of pancreatic cancer in melanoma-prone kindreds with p16INK4 mutations. *N Engl J Med* 1995; **333**: 970–4.
40 Hille ET, van Duijn E, Gruis NA, *et al.* Excess cancer mortality in six Dutch pedigrees with the familial atypical multiple mole–melanoma syndrome from 1830 to 1994. *J Invest Dermatol* 1998; **110**: 788–92.
41 Nitecki SS, Sarr MG, Colby TV, *et al.* Long-term survival after resection for ductal adenocarcinoma of the pancreas: is it really improving? *Ann Surg* 1995; **221**: 59–66.

7: Borderline melanocytic lesions

Nigel Kirkham

Are *in situ* melanomas real melanomas?

Because effective treatments for malignant melanoma have proved so elusive there has been an emphasis on looking for the early lesion. It is possible to diagnose malignant melanoma both clinically and histologically at an early stage when the lesion is small, flat and confined to the epidermis. This is what is meant by the term '*in situ* melanoma'. Simple excision of an *in situ* melanoma has the potential to produce a cure. The tumour is prevented from evolving into a larger tumour with a greater potential for metastasis [1]. This begs the question of whether *in situ* melanomas are real melanomas.

It has been proposed that primary malignant melanomas evolve from melanocytic precursor lesions and this evolution goes through stages described as radial and vertical growth phases. The radial growth phase includes *in situ* melanoma, but also includes microinvasive tumours and describes tumours that are not tumourigenic: they lack the capacity for metastasis. The prognosis in radial growth phase is excellent, irrespective of tumour thickness or other prognostic variables [2].

The biological behaviour of the intraepidermal component of radial growth phase or superficial spreading melanoma has significantly different properties to the cells in a vertical growth phase melanoma. The main debate has been about the criteria for diagnosing *in situ* melanoma and whether there exists a group of atypical *in situ* melanocytic lesions that are neither melanomas nor naevi. This debate has not usually been informed by many relevant data [3,4].

Underdiagnosis of malignancy

The underdiagnosis of malignancy is not a large problem in terms of absolute numbers, as most histopathologists will not make this sort of mistake very often. When it does happen it can become a very real problem for the pathologist as well as for the patient. For the patient, the development of metastatic disease some time after being told that the mole that they were so worried about and had had excised was benign is obviously unsettling to say the least. For the pathologist, there is a blow to professional pride but also a very real possibility of being sued by the patient or the patient's dependants.

When a patient develops metastatic disease and the biopsy had originally been diagnosed as benign then there are questions that need to be answered. It is often the case that the diagnosis of malignancy has been missed. The application of the retrospectoscope to the sections in the file will usually show that the lesion was a melanoma.

Overdiagnosis of malignancy

The overdiagnosis of malignancy is a slightly different problem to that of underdiagnosis. Instead of the patient who turns up with unexpected metastases we have the patient who 'fails to die'. The cynic would say that this is not a problem at all; by overdiagnosing malignancy the pathologist can never be wrong. When the lesion really is malignant then nobody is surprised. When the lesion was actually benign but was called malignant, then the pathologist can sit back and reflect that the patient 'has done very well' or that 'the treatment must have worked'. So, to take an extreme example, if every appendix or gall-bladder was called malignant, the pathologist would never 'be wrong' and the vast majority of the patients 'would do very well'. The skill comes in riding along the border and assigning lesions into the appropriate categories of benign or malignant. The perfect diagnostician would never have a lesion diagnosed as benign show subsequent evidence of metastasis and would not label many patients with a malignant diagnosis that was not warranted. We can all strive to achieve perfection but how often it is attained is another matter.

The main issues here relate to the differentiation of benign and dysplastic naevi from melanomas and there is the subsidiary problem of dividing

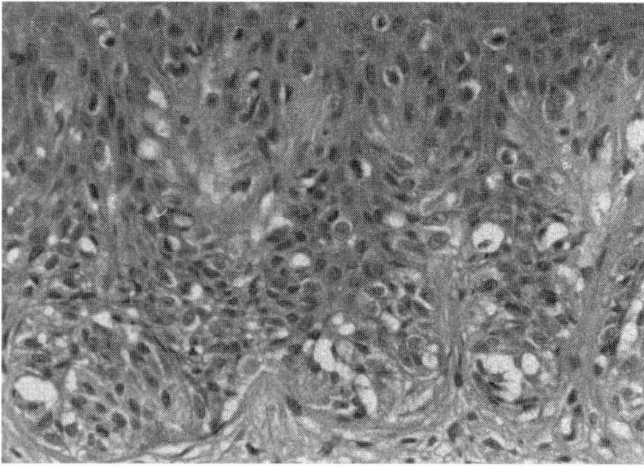

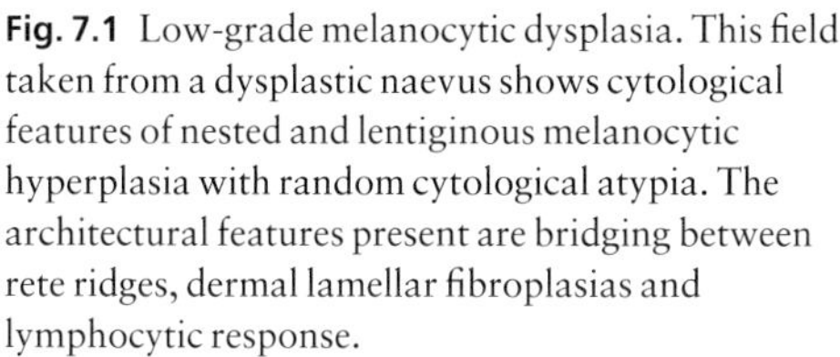

Fig. 7.1 Low-grade melanocytic dysplasia. This field taken from a dysplastic naevus shows cytological features of nested and lentiginous melanocytic hyperplasia with random cytological atypia. The architectural features present are bridging between rete ridges, dermal lamellar fibroplasias and lymphocytic response.

melanomas into those with and those without the potential for metastasis. This has caused a lot of heart searching in recent years, but the clouds that have lain over the area are starting to clear away and the issues are becoming more easily defined.

There is really little substantial difference between these problems and those seen with tumours in other organ systems. For instance, the distinction between actinic keratosis and squamous cutaneous carcinoma is a problem of attempting to distinguish between a tumour that can be cured by local removal and a tumour that has the potential for distant metastasis. In the uterine cervix the subclassification of cervical intraepithelial neoplasia (CIN) and the debate about microinvasive disease is really a debate about how to spot those lesions that will cured by local removal or ablation and to distinguish them from those tumours that have the potential for metastasis. Similar problems are encountered in the endometrium in the distinction between endometrial hyperplasia, dysplasia and carcinoma. There are other examples that come to mind, but all have in common the recognition that some tumours have the ability to metastasize while others, similar in other ways, do not.

There is probably more room for manoeuvre than has been generally appreciated. The late Dr Vincent McGovern of Sydney, Australia, is reported to have said that if a melanocytic lesion 'is difficult then it is benign'. There is some justice in this remark. Most melanomas with a real potential for metastasis are relatively straightforward to diagnose. Many of the borderline lesions, where the pathologist is not sure of the correct diagnosis, have little or even no potential for metastasis.

So there is room for overdiagnosis of malignancy aplenty here. The debate about dysplastic naevi that has taken place in recent years is largely empty, because whatever you choose to call those lesions they have in common a signal lack of ability to metastasize. Similarly, the distinction between a dysplastic naevus and a 'melanoma *in situ*', whatever its merits, is nothing to do with recognizing a tumour with the potential for metastasis. Even the distinction between a Level I and II melanoma does not necessarily do this either. The definition of melanoma in radial growth phase includes both 'melanoma *in situ*' and 'superficial spreading melanoma'. The important distinction to make is between radial and vertical growth phase, on the basis that the radial growth phase melanoma is the melanocytic equivalent of 'CIN' or an 'epithelioma'; a tumour that may recur locally if it is not excised completely, but will not metastasize. The vertical growth phase melanoma has the potential for metastasis but even this is not absolute. Several prognostic models have been produced showing a variation in the probability of regional or distant metastasis that is determined by a number of variables, including tumour thickness, but emphasizes that not all melanomas are equally malignant. Therefore there is room for manoeuvre at all points.

In situ melanomas are real melanomas but they have not progressed to the stage of vertical growth phase at which they might be expected to metastasize. They are part of the spectrum of radial growth phase melanoma. In practice it can often be difficult to distinguish between Level I and II melanomas. True *in situ* melanomas are clinically benign if completely excised; if not, they have the potential to progress to vertical growth phase.

Melanocytic intraepidermal neoplasia

The distinction between possible diagnostic categories of naevus, atypical melanocytic lesion, *in situ* melanoma, microinvasive melanoma and invasive malignant melanoma lies at the centre of the pathological debate. This has been studied in relation to lentigo maligna [5]. These authors hypothesized that in the case of lesions described as lentigo maligna, two categories could be defined: a precursor lesion and *in situ* melanoma. The criteria used for *in situ* melanoma were pagetoid spread, confluence and nesting of atypical melanocytes. In the study, 42 consecutive cases of invasive lentigo maligna melanoma were reviewed to determine the nature of the intraepidermal component overlying the invasive tumour, on the basis that this would be representative of the epidermal changes in the preinvasive tumour. In all cases the epidermal component fulfilled the criteria for *in situ* melanoma. The authors conclude that this is strong evidence for *in situ* melanoma being a step in tumour progression that lies between atypical melanocytic hyperplasia (lentigo maligna) and invasive malignant melanoma. Their findings support the case for a distinction to be made between these three entities.

Pagetoid spread does appear to be a reliable criterion for *in situ* melanoma. Its presence is inversely correlated with tumour thickness, level of invasion, growth phase and mitotic count, and positive correlation with the presence and severity of regression. Thus, pagetoid infiltration of the epidermis is most

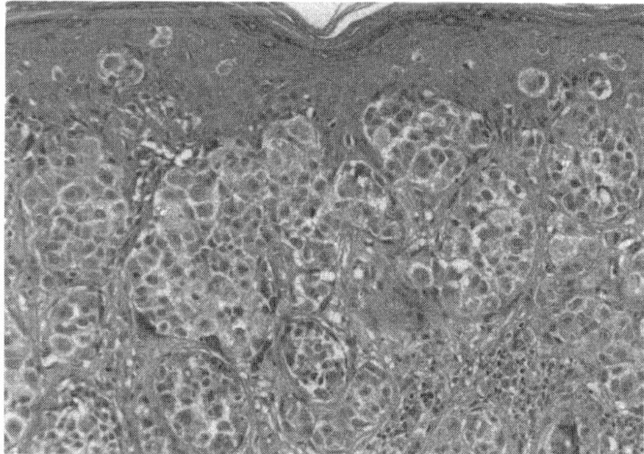

Fig. 7.2 *In situ* melanoma/radial growth phase melanoma/high-grade melanocytic dysplasia/MIN with microinvasion. This field taken from a radial growth phase melanoma shows cytological features of severe cytological atypia and pagetoid spread. The architectural features asymmetry, expansile nests of melanocytes and probable microinvasion of the dermis.

common in *in situ* or thin radial growth phase melanomas, and may be absent in thicker primary tumours [6]. In another study of the diagnosis of thin melanoma pagetoid spread, severe cytological atypia and asymmetry of the lesion were each found in over 80% of lesions, while lesser features were present less often [7].

One of the main problems is that of diagnostic consistency. A study using four experienced pathologists found considerable disagreement amongst them on the diagnosis of melanoma vs. other pigmented lesions [8]. Tumour thickness and presence of ulceration were the most reproducible histological features of cutaneous melanoma between these four pathologists.

In a study performed in England and Scotland eight pathologists evaluated consistency in the use of histopathological terms for features of diagnostic and prognostic importance for cutaneous malignant melanoma, especially in borderline lesions [9]. It was found that overall levels of interobserver agreement were much better when the group worked together to discuss and define the terms that were being used in diagnosis. These included architectural and nuclear atypia, pagetoid infiltration and radial and vertical growth phases. A high level of agreement was achieved for an overall benign or malignant diagnosis ($\kappa=0.77$) but use of more specific terms, such as benign naevi with atypia and melanoma ≤ 0.76 mm thickness, was associated with only an intermediate level of agreement. The poor concordance in distinguishing severe dysplasia in the junctional component of melanocytic proliferations from melanoma *in situ* and superficial dermal invasion improved only modestly despite intensive efforts.

As melanoma *in situ* and severe dysplasia could not be distinguished by objective measurements and because their clinical management is the same, it was suggested that attempts to separate them in diagnostic reports should be discontinued and they could both be referred to as melanocytic intraepidermal neoplasia (MIN). It was also suggested that dermal invasion without a vertical growth component can be managed identically to MIN, and so this invasive radial phase may be appropriately referred to as microinvasion and linked to MIN for the purposes of clinical management.

In a further study, a random sample of 148 UK histopathologists participated in two circulations, the first with 20 slides and the second with 25 slides [10]. The results were compared with those for the panel in the first study, consisting of seven histopathologists and one dermatopathologist, which had developed and evaluated diagnostic criteria. In the first circulation, when no standardized diagnostic criteria were used, a fair level of agreement was achieved for an overall diagnosis using the categories benign naevi with no atypia, benign naevi with atypia and melanoma ($\kappa=0.45$). This was low compared with the agreement of the panel that had used agreed criteria ($\kappa=0.75$). Moreover, participants in the nationwide survey were more likely to diagnose melanoma and less likely to diagnose benign naevi without atypia than the panel. In the second circulation, when diagnostic criteria and diagrams were used, there was a higher level of agreement for overall diagnosis using the categories benign MIN with or without microinvasion and melanoma with vertical growth phase, which was the same as that achieved by the panel using the same criteria ($\kappa=0.68$). It was concluded that it was important that standardized diagnostic criteria be used to ensure accurate reporting of thin melanomas [10].

The value of agreed criteria in improving levels of interobserver agreement has been studied elsewhere. In one such study a stratified random sample of 112 melanocytic tumours was chosen [11]. The original diagnoses included typical and dysplastic melanocytic naevi and melanomas. A single representative slide for each case was interpreted independently by each of the five panel dermatopathologists and two melanoma specialists. They had no prior knowledge of the original diagnosis or the diagnoses of the other panel members. Each case was graded on a five-point scale from no dysplasia to melanoma and correlation among the panel members was 0.67 (95% CI= 0.59–0.73). The Pearson correlations of each of the five panel dermatopathologists with the mean of the two melanoma specialists ranged from 0.67 to 0.84, and the correlations of the mean of the panel with the two melanoma specialists were 0.79 and 0.82; the mean reading of the melanoma specialists correlated 0.89 with the mean panel reading. It was concluded that the level of agreement was substantial to excellent for the histopathological diagnosis of 112 melanocytic tumours by dermatopathologists. Using predetermined criteria, melanocytic dysplasia can be reproducibly graded among diverse general dermatopathologists [11].

In summary, the proponents of MIN suggested, first, that severe intraepidermal melanocytic dysplasia and *in situ* melanoma could not be distinguished and could be described by the same term; and, secondly, that microinvasive melanoma could be included within this description. This in effect is a restatement of part of the concept of tumour progression proposed by others, including Clark *et al.* [12]. The term MIN (with or without microinvasion) is a synonym for radial growth phase melanoma.

Treatment of *in situ* melanoma/melanocytic intraepidermal neoplasia

Although wide surgical excision has in the past been the accepted treatment for thin malignant melanomas, there is reason to believe that narrower margins may be adequate. It is clear that the form of local treatment has no influence on the presence or absence of subsequent metastasis. The purpose of local excision is twofold: first, to remove the tumour at an early stage before it has developed the capacity for metastasis; and, secondly, to ensure local clearance of disease so as to avoid local recurrence of tumour.

Some authors have suggested that with excision margins of 0.5–1 cm, local recurrence has not been a problem [13]. In a randomized prospective study to assess the efficacy of narrow excision (excision with 1-cm margins) for primary melanomas no thicker than 2 mm, narrow excision was performed in 305 patients, and wide excision (margins of 3 cm or more) was performed in 307 patients.

The major prognostic criteria were well balanced between the two groups. The mean thickness of melanomas was 0.99 mm in the narrow-excision group and 1.02 mm in the wide-excision group. The subsequent development of metastatic disease involving regional nodes and distant organs was not different in the two groups (4.6 and 2.3%, respectively, in the narrow-excision group, compared with 6.5 and 2.6% in the wide-excision group). Disease-free survival rates and overall survival rates (mean follow-up period, 55 months) were also similar in the two groups. Only three patients had a local recurrence as a first relapse. All had undergone narrow excision, and each had a primary melanoma with a thickness of 1 mm or more. The absence of local recurrence in the group of patients with a primary melanoma thinner than 1 mm and the very low rate of local recurrences indicate that narrow excision is a safe and effective procedure for such patients [14].

In situ melanoma should be treated by complete histological excision with a maximum surgical margin of 1.0 cm. The excision specimen should then be examined in detail by an experienced pathologist to rule out the presence of a vertical growth phase in the tumour [4]. In practice this may often be a two-stage procedure, with an initial excision biopsy being performed with a 2-mm clinical margin, followed by a second re-excision procedure to achieve a further 5–8 mm radius around the biopsy scar. The re-excision specimen should be examined to look for any residual disease, although if the initial excision was complete it is unlikely that any will be found. In the case of an initial complete excision with no macroscopic pigmentation in the sliced re-excision specimen, a single block from the centre of the specimen is all that need be taken [15,16].

What should we tell patients about *in situ* melanomas?

Patients with thin primary melanomas (≤ 1 mm) generally have an excellent prognosis, especially if the tumour is unequivocally *in situ* or radial growth phase. Nevertheless, there is a small subset of patients with thin malignant melanomas who do develop metastases [17]. Features that may help differentiate higher and lower risk lesions in this thickness range include the patient's age and sex, anatomical site and diameter of the primary lesion, Clark level of invasion, development of a vertical growth phase, the mitotic index, ulceration, regression and cellular aneuploidy. However, of these, the presence of a vertical growth phase is probably the feature that is most likely to have an adverse effect on survival rate.

It is not always clear that a vertical growth phase component is present when the tumour is first reported. For instance, in an audit of 66 cases of *in situ* melanoma randomly selected from the files at the Royal Brisbane Hospital, Australia, when multiple deeper sections were cut from the paraffin blocks, an invasive component (Level II) was found in eight cases [18]. The tumours with an invasive component had a Breslow thickness ranging from 0.19 to 0.45 mm. No recurrences or metastases had developed after at least 5 years. Focal areas of regression were present in the initial sections in all but one of these eight cases. The presence of regression is probably a feature that should preclude a diagnosis of *in situ* melanoma, because it implies that a vertical growth phase component is likely to have been present. Similarly, the presence of increased dermal vascularity is an indicator that some degree of angiogenesis has taken place. This angiogenesis is likely to be associated with the presence of a vertical growth phase [19].

It must be remembered that the rate of the subsequent development of metastatic disease involving regional nodes and distant organs is low. In the WHO study Veronesi *et al.* [14] reported rates of 4.6–6.5% for regional node involvement and 2.3–2.6% for distant metastasis for T1 melanomas.

The development of sentinel node biopsy as a staging procedure offers the prospect of an answer in difficult cases, on the basis that the presence of a nodal metastasis precludes a diagnosis of *in situ* or radial growth phase melanoma in which nodal involvement and metastasis would not be expected.

In one study of 235 patients with clinically localized cutaneous melanomas who underwent successful sentinel lymph node biopsy, 71 had lesions 1 mm or smaller, with a vertical growth phase identified on the primary lesion [20]. The rate of occurrence of sentinel lymph node metastasis was 15.2% in patients with melanomas >1 mm thick and 5.6% in patients with thin melanomas <1 mm thick. Three patients with thin melanomas and a positive sentinel lymph node had low-risk lesions, based on a highly accurate six-variable multivariate logistic regression model for predicting 8-year survival in stage I/II melanomas. The fourth patient had a low-to-intermediate-risk lesion based on this model. At the time of the lymphadenectomy, one patient had two additional nodes with metastasis.

Sentinel node biopsy therefore appears to be a sensitive staging procedure for distinguishing *in situ* and radial growth phase melanomas from those with a vertical growth phase. Furthermore it is tailored to the individual and so is likely to be more accurate than the use of a multivariate logistic regression model that incorporates thickness, mitotic rate, regression, tumour-infiltrating lymphocytes, sex and anatomical site. At the present time there are no effective adjuvant therapies but patients do have the possibility of entering trials of adjuvant therapy when stage III disease is found [20].

Patients with *in situ* melanoma can be told that they have probably been cured by complete local excision, but that they have a statistical possibility of a 4.6–6.5% chance of regional node involvement and a 2.3–2.6% chance of distant metastasis [14].

References

1 Ackerman AB. Malignant melanoma *in situ*: the flat, curable stage of malignant melanoma. *Pathology* 1985; **17**: 298–300.
2 Elder D. Tumor progression, early diagnosis and prognosis of melanoma. *Acta Oncol* 1999; **38**: 535–47.
3 Flotte TJ. Malignant melanoma *in situ*. *Hum Pathol* 1990; **21**: 1199–201.
4 Kirkham N. Optimal handling and criteria for melanoma diagnosis. *Histopathology* 2000; **37**: 467–9.
5 Tannous ZS, Lerner LH, Duncan LM, Mihm MC Jr, Flotte TJ. Progression to invasive melanoma from malignant melanoma *in situ*, lentigo maligna type. *Hum Pathol* 2000; **31**: 705–8.
6 Fallowfield ME, Cook MG. Pagetoid infiltration in primary cutaneous melanoma. *Histopathology* 1992; **20**: 417–20.
7 Stolz W, Schmoeckel C, Welkovich B, Braun-Falco O. Semiquantitative analysis of histologic criteria in thin malignant melanomas. *J Am Acad Dermatol* 1989; **20**: 1115–20.
8 Corona R, Mele A, Amini M, *et al.* Interobserver variability on the histopathologic diagnosis of cutaneous melanoma and other pigmented skin lesions. *J Clin Oncol* 1996; **14**: 1218–23.
9 Cook MG, Clarke TJ, Humphreys S, *et al.* The evaluation of diagnostic and prognostic criteria and the terminology of thin cutaneous malignant melanoma by the CRC Melanoma Pathology Panel. *Histopathology* 1996; **28**: 497–512.
10 CRC Melanoma Pathology Panel. A nationwide survey of observer variation in the diagnosis of thin cutaneous malignant melanoma including the MIN terminology. *J Clin Pathol* 1997; **50**: 202–5.
11 Weinstock MA, Barnhill RL, Rhodes AR, Brodsky GL. Reliability of the histopathologic diagnosis of melanocytic dysplasia. The Dysplastic Nevus Panel. *Arch Dermatol* 1997; **133**: 953–8.
12 Clark WH Jr, Elder DE, Guerry D, Epstein MN, Greene MH, Van Horn M. A study of tumor progression: the precursor lesions of superficial spreading and nodular melanoma. *Hum Pathol* 1984; **15**: 1147–65.
13 Alper JC, Bogaars H, Sober AJ, Schoenfeld E. The surgical management of *in situ* melanoma. *J Dermatol Surg Oncol* 1982; **8**: 771–3.
14 Veronesi U, Cascinelli N, Adamus J, *et al.* Thin stage I primary cutaneous malignant melanoma: comparison of excision with margins of 1 or 3 cm. *N Engl J Med* 1988; **318**: 1159–62.
15 Martin HM, Birkin AJ, Theaker JM. Malignant melanoma re-excision specimens: how many blocks? *Histopathology* 1998; **32**: 362–7.
16 Kirkham N. What is there to find in malignant melanoma re-excision specimens? *Histopathology* 1998; **32**: 566–7.
17 Salman SM, Rogers GS. Prognostic factors in thin cutaneous malignant melanoma. *J Dermatol Surg Oncol* 1990; **16**: 413–18.
18 Weedon D. A reappraisal of melanoma *in situ*. *J Dermatol Surg Oncol* 1982; **8**: 774–5.
19 Barnhill RL, Levy MA. Regressing thin cutaneous malignant melanomas (≤ 1.0 mm) are associated with angiogenesis. *Am J Pathol* 1993; **143**: 99–104.
20 Bedrosian I, Faries MB, Guerry D, *et al.* Incidence of sentinel node metastasis in patients with thin primary melanoma (≤ 1 mm) with vertical growth phase. *Ann Surg Oncol* 2000; **7**: 262–7.

Part 2: Diagnosis, Screening and Prevention

8: How can we improve the early diagnosis of melanoma?

Wilma Bergman

Tools to improve early diagnosis of melanoma

The prognosis of malignant cutaneous melanoma is directly related to the tumour thickness at presentation. In order to facilitate early diagnosis of melanoma many tools have been mentioned in the literature, from the use of simple ABCD rules to the use of artificial neural networks.

This chapter deals with tools to improve the process of recognition of early melanoma once the patient has come to see the doctor. Patient education and the subject of screening (Chapter 9) are also approaches to early diagnosis but at a different level: primary and secondary prevention. However, the most important approach to improve early diagnosis is the management of individuals and families with the atypical mole syndrome, as this is the most important high-risk category for melanoma. Chapters 5 and 6 deal with this subject.

Table 8.1 summarizes the many tools that are available for the early detection of melanoma, some of which will be discussed in more detail.

Risk profile

In clinical practice it is of utmost importance to establish the risk profile of an individual patient by counting his or her risk factors, even before seeing the lesion in question. Has the patient atypical moles, relatives with melanoma or is he or she a redhead? Has the patient noticed any symptoms from the mole? In the author's experience the sum of these risk factors may be of more importance than the actual aspect of the specific lesion in deciding about removal of a lesion so it is possible, especially within the context of familial melanoma, to decide on excision of a certain lesion before even having seen the mole. Symptoms such as itch or stinging from a pigmented lesion should be considered relevant to the early diagnosis of melanoma. However, a very innocent and common lesion, occurring in the same age group as melanoma (40–60 years of age) usually causes complaints of mild itch: the seborrhoeic wart.

Table 8.1 Approaches to the early detection of melanoma

1	Primary prevention by education of the population about ultraviolet protection
2	Patient education on early warning signs
	personal risk charts
	self-examination
3	Population-screening
4	Screening of selected high-risk phenotypes
5	Training of primary care workers
	seven-point check list
	ABCDs of the American Cancer Society
6	Set-up of pigmented lesion clinics
	quick referral type
	superspecialist type
7	Epiluminescence microscopy/dermatoscopy
8	Teledermatology
9	Digital image analysis systems

In the author's opinion, symptoms such as itch or stinging or even an almost instinctive distrust are especially relevant for patients recognizing the development of their second or next primary melanoma. In the context of familial melanoma, patients continue to develop primary melanomas; up to 10 or even more. I remember patients coming directly to my surgery clinic and saying: 'I feel I have another one, so I made the appointment for excision right away.' An important warning sign of early melanoma is change, be it change in size, shape or colour [1]. Behaviour of a pigmented lesion over time is believed to be more important than its immediate appearance at time of presentation.

Table 8.2 summarizes established risk factors for the development of melanoma. More than one risk factor can be present in a patient and they should be constructed into a total risk profile. Table 8.2 also gives an elegant mnemonic for increased melanoma risk awareness. Each letter represents one of the major risk factors for cutaneous melanoma. This MMRISK mnemonic was first presented by Professor Thomas B. Fitzpatrick, Dublin, Ireland in 1997.

Patients with high-risk profiles should be referred to pigmented lesion clinics (PLCs) for regular follow-up and photodocumentation. When a newly diagnosed melanoma patient has other family members with cutaneous melanoma, this family should be registered by the National Cancer Family Registry or referred to the Centre for Human Genetics. In the Netherlands there is the Netherlands Foundation for the Detection of Hereditary Tumours, where families with cancer are registered and (presymptomatic) screening is facilitated and monitored.

Patients with atypical moles are at significantly increased risk of

Table 8.2 Summary of risk factors for the development of melanoma

Changing or symptomatic mole in adult patient
Melanoma in patient history
Presence of atypical moles in patient
Melanoma in first-degree relative(s)
Large numbers of normal moles
Skin type I, freckles and red hair
Xeroderma pigmentosum
Immunocompromised patient
Sunburn(s) before the age of 15
(Giant) congenital naevi
MMRISK*
A mnemonic for increasing melanoma risk awareness among patients and physicians. Each letter represents one of the major risk factors for cutaneous melanoma
M Moles: atypical moles (> 10)
M Moles: common moles (numerous)
R Red hair and freckling
I Inability to tan: skin phototypes 1–2
S Sunburn: severe sunburn before age 14
K Kindred: family history of melanoma

* By Professor Thomas B. Fitzpatrick, Dublin, September 1997.

Table 8.3 Strategy for early diagnosis of melanoma in primary care

1	Make an inventory of the patient's risk factors
2	Investigate the mole in question and all the skin of the patient, trying to find more risk factors
3	When in doubt use a dermatoscope if available
4	When still in doubt refer the patient to a dermatologist or remove the lesion *in toto* with 2 mm margins for histological investigation
5	Does the patient (because of a high-risk profile) need regular follow-up? If so, refer to pigmented lesion clinic

melanoma. The incidence of melanoma in European countries is still too low, however, to refer each individual with one or a few atypical moles to a dermatologist or a PLC, especially with a negative family history of melanoma. The patient's absolute risk of melanoma remains low. Therefore, in the author's opinion, these patients can be followed-up in primary health care, provided they get an appropriate amount of patient education on the early warning signs of melanoma. Table 8.3 gives a strategy for the early detection of melanoma in primary health care.

It must be appreciated that legal aspects, which play an important part in the USA, might alter medical strategies concerning patients with relatively low cancer risks. In other countries, such as Australia and New Zealand, melanoma risk of the population might be sufficiently high to warrant more strict referral strategies. On the other hand, in these non-densely populated countries early diagnosis of melanoma might be facilitated by teledermatology, as this may be an efficient option in providing dermatological care in medically underserved areas.

Early warning signs: assessing the individual lesion

It is important to have sufficient lighting in the investigation room and this should be of daylight type as yellow or pink hues in the light are very distracting when judging the spectrum of colours of the pigmentation. Bluish, grey or blue–pink shades should especially not be missed, as these are suspicious for melanoma. Two mnemonics have been developed to help remember the features of early melanoma: the seven-point checklist and the ABCD rules.

Seven-point checklist

A seven-point scoring system was adopted by the Cancer Research Campaign in Scotland in the 1980s to help non-dermatologists recognize (early) melanoma. The seven points of this score were the following:

1 minor itch;
2 over 1 cm diameter;
3 recent growth;
4 irregular edge;
5 irregular pigmentation;
6 inflammation; and
7 bleeding or weeping.

Each feature scored 1, thus the maximum score was 7 [2]. The Scottish group suggested that lesions with scores of 3 or more should be referred for specialist opinion and that where the score is 4 or more, 90% are melanomas.

Later, others reported the score to be less useful so another Scottish group reviewed it, especially in the light of increasing referral of patients with pigmented lesions [3]. It was found that the seven-point checklist was too inclusive; substantial percentages of benign lesions, especially seborrhoeic warts, scored 3 or more, whereas two melanomas scored only 2. A logistic regression analysis showed that the single feature required to give the best discrimination between melanoma and not melanoma was the assessment of marginal irregularity (point 4) as recognized by the doctor. However, this feature was too difficult for the public or the patient to recognize.

Although this seven-point checklist used as a screening test seems inaccurate, it is important to appreciate that the list has been designed by very experienced clinicians and also, in the author's opinion, all seven points are worth considering when investigating patients with pigmented lesions.

The seven-point checklist was later modified by its draftsmen into major and minor signs, emphasizing a history of change. Major signs are changes in size, shape or colour. Minor signs are inflammation, crusting or bleeding, sensory change (e.g. itch) and a diameter of 5 mm or more.

ABCD of pigmented lesions

The American Cancer Society advertises its ABCD of pigmented lesions to help recognize and seek early medical evaluation of suspicious pigmented lesions. The four features are as follow:

A Asymmetry
B Border irregularity
C Colour irregularity
D Diameter > 6 mm.

This mnemonic is more specifically directed to the public than the seven-point checklist, which was designed for non-dermatological medical personnel. The ABCD system is widely used in public education; many leaflets are dedicated to this simple aid to memory and it is clear that all four features are also part of the seven-point checklist.

A comparison of the ABCD system and the original seven-point checklist has been carried out [4]. The investigators concluded that the simpler ABCD score had a better sensitivity and an equal specificity to the seven-point checklist, therefore these authors preferred the ABCD system.

Many of the signs and symptoms of early melanoma are also common features of benign lesions. Public education campaigns encouraging people to seek advice for any change in a pigmented lesion will cause a huge workload for GPs, who should be able to provide the necessary reassurance.

When the lesion in question cannot be judged to be benign with certainty with the naked eye, a magnifying lens or dermatoscope can be used to aid diagnosis. If still in doubt, a primary care physician should refer the patient to a dermatologist or remove the lesion *in toto*, with a small margin of 2–3 mm of surrounding normal skin to facilitate the pathologist's diagnosis and assessment of the extent of the excision. When the histological diagnosis is available, one should then act as appropriate according to the national consensus on the treatment of melanoma. The histological diagnosis should also be used as a feedback tool for the primary care physician's diagnostic accuracy, which only works by mentioning the diagnosis of preference to the pathologist or at least writing it down in the patient's record.

In the absence of a single test for melanoma, diagnostic criteria have been recommended for use by patients and GPs to identify (most) melanomas, yet exclude benign lesions. Grin *et al.* [5] have studied the accuracy of the clinical diagnosis of (early) melanoma. The diagnosis of melanoma was made in

Table 8.4 Pigmented skin lesions to be differentiated from melanoma

Non-melanocytic lesions
Seborrhoeic wart
Dermatofibroma
Basal cell carcinoma (pigmented type)
Haemangioma (especially thrombosed)
Pyogenic granuloma
Melanocytic lesions
Atypical naevus
Solar/senile lentigines
Congenital naevus
Blue naevus
Spitz naevus (epithelioid and spindle cell naevi)

84.5% of the histologically proved cases of melanoma, reflecting a high degree of diagnostic accuracy. The results of a recent study from Sweden also reflected a clinical detection rate of 85% [6]. Thus it seems appropriate to presuppose a diagnostic accuracy among experienced dermatologists of over 80%. For the early detection of melanomas it is more relevant that GPs and the public know the signs and symptoms of melanoma. All pre-existing moles exhibiting changes in adults are worth a visit to a doctor and this is an important part of the message to the public. Again, this early warning sign will bring in many patients with seborrhoeic warts.

Table 8.4 summarizes the most commonly occurring pigmented lesions that must be differentiated from melanoma. In many instances the use of the dermatoscope will be very helpful, especially in differentiating between melanocytic lesions and non-melanocytic lesions. Many of the lesions mentioned in Table 8.4 do not pose a problem for diagnosis when showing typical features, furthermore they have different clinical characteristics such as a different preferential age category (Spitz naevus, pyogenic granuloma) or a different medical history (congenital naevus). But patients with these diagnoses can sometimes be seen with very uncharacteristic signs and symptoms which are more difficult to differentiate from melanoma.

Pigmented lesion clinics

A pigmented lesion clinic (PLC) can be established to deal with the referrals generated by publicity campaigns, patient self-referral or GP referral (quick referral PLC) or can also be viewed as a superspecialist clinic for the follow-up of individuals with a high-risk profile for melanoma.

In Leiden, the Netherlands, a PLC of the latter type was established in 1982, facilitating the regular follow-up of members of melanoma-prone families (familial dysplastic naevus syndrome/familial atypical multiple mole–melanoma syndrome) and patients with sporadic atypical mole syndrome. Other patients at increased risk of melanoma, such as those with giant congenital naevi and xeroderma pigmentosum, also attend this clinic on a regular basis. This type of PLC does not allow for self-referrals or even GP referrals. This concentration of high-risk patients facilitates expertise to be built up and the training of dermatology residents and primary care physicians.

Furthermore, a PLC generates the possibility of clinical research. The commitment of research nurses, psychologists, medical photographers or other auxiliaries can be realized by concentrating high-risk patients in a PLC. A superspecialist PLC for the regular follow-up of selected high-risk individuals results in thinner melanomas being diagnosed, as concluded from a Dutch study on high-risk patients from melanoma-prone families who were under surveillance in such a PLC [7].

What is the rationale for the open or rapid referral PLC? The intention is to provide rapid screening of lesions by clinicians with high diagnostic accuracy, thereby providing early diagnosis cost effectively. The clinical accuracy of the diagnosis of cutaneous melanoma by dermatologists was determined by the group running the university hospital PLC in Glasgow, Scotland [8]. The diagnostic accuracy for melanoma by experienced dermatologists from this PLC was very high, when compared to training dermatologists or dermatologists seeing less than 10 melanomas per year. It is concluded that pigmented lesions of virtually all types can be diagnosed and treated within dermatology departments, making dermatologists the appropriate first point of referral for suspected early melanoma.

The value of PLCs for the early detection of melanoma has been questioned. Osborne *et al.* [9] have examined the effect of the availability of a PLC on the referral interval between patients with suspicious moles presenting to their GP and their attendance at hospital. They found that in 1994 only 48% of melanomas in their district were referred to a PLC established in 1986. These authors conclude that PLCs are of value in early diagnosis of melanoma, but only if they are appropriately utilized by GPs. Mallet *et al.* [10] assessed the effect of a quick referral PLC on referral patterns and thickness of melanoma by comparing the yield of a public awareness campaign in two districts: one without a PLC and one served by a PLC. They concluded that a quick referral PLC conferred no obvious benefit other than satisfying a demand from both GPs and patients and providing a centralized base for the collection of data. Almost the same conclusions were reached by Bataille *et al.* [11] from the PLC at St George's Hospital, London. They concluded that the role of PLCs in reducing mortality caused by melanoma remains to be established, although it is likely that these clinics have an important role in terms of public health education regarding sun avoidance and early warning signs of skin cancer. A Dutch study by Rampen *et al.* [12] studied the workload after a regional screening campaign. In the week immediately after the campaign, GPs noticed a small increase in the number of consultations for suspected skin cancer. Thereafter the number of consultations decreased to precampaign levels in 6 weeks. These findings might discourage the set-up of quick referral PLCs but stress the need to train GPs in recognizing early melanoma.

Kirkpatrick *et al.* [13] have reported the results of the first year of their quick referral PLC in terms of numbers of patients, numbers of excisions and the mean Breslow thickness of melanomas. They did not find thinner melanomas; however, they viewed the advantages of their PLC to be the bypassing of the waiting list for regular dermatology clinics and herewith reducing anxiety to patients and their families.

A quick referral PLC appears to be a more efficient service for the patient than a tool for early diagnosis of melanoma.

Epiluminescence microscopy

Epiluminescence microscopy (ELM) is a non-invasive clinical examination technique that can improve the differential diagnosis of pigmented lesions (Table 8.5). ELM is also known as dermatoscopy or dermascopy.

The technique consists of placing a thin layer of mineral oil on the skin and inspecting pigmented structures below the skin surface with a hand-held 10× magnifying lighted scope. ELM has been developed by the Vienna Department of Dermatology, Austria. Initially—almost 20 years ago—a large, very sophisticated machine was used which almost completely filled the investigation room. However, nowadays almost every dermatologist uses a simple and inexpensive dermatoscope, Delta 10, developed by Heine Optotechnik (Herrsching, Germany) with the help of the Vienna group. Several other groups (Naples and Florence, Italy; Boston and New York, USA) have now published papers on the use of ELM and this technique is now widely used in dermatology departments.

Table 8.5 Application of epiluminescence microscopy in clinical practice

Differentiation of non-melanocytic lesions (absence of pigment network)	
Seborrhoeic warts	
Haemangiomas	
Blue naevi	
Identifying high- and low-risk melanocytic lesions (pigment network present)	
High	ELM features of early melanoma
Medium	Atypical naevi
Low	Benign naevi

The literature on ELM is profuse and in choosing publications to be included in the references I selected the most recent ones, as well as several classical papers and reviews. Several atlases on ELM are also available with clear colour instructions on the various ELM features. The first one was printed in 1993 in German and the first English version was released in 1994 [14]. These types of atlases should be consulted if ELM is being seriously considered. This chapter only gives an overview of the possibilities and briefly mentions the features that are relevant for ELM.

It is important to realize that more can be seen by using a dermatoscope; a new dimension of epidermal structures—not visible to the naked eye—can be visualized during ELM examination and more features are available to aid a more specific clinical diagnosis so this device yields a pure profit to dermatology. ELM can be used to differentiate melanocytic lesions from non-melanocytic lesions and this is the most important gain, especially for non-dermatologists or training dermatologists (Figs 8.1–8.5). Non-melanocytic lesions usually lack a reticular pigment network pattern. Thrombosed haemangiomas or blue naevi can be identified with more accuracy with the help of ELM. In seborrhoeic keratosis ELM is helpful, although sometimes a pigment network can be present in one small region. ELM can also be used to identify high- and low-risk melanocytic lesions and thus reach a sharper

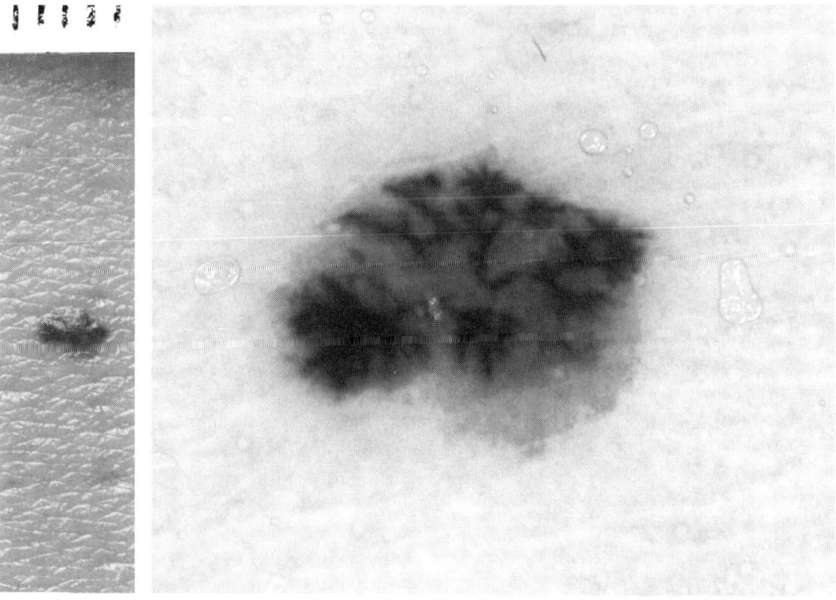

Fig. 8.1 This very dark, small naevus showed much more detail by dermatoscopy. The pigment network is very coarse with abrupt stops and branched streaks at the periphery. The centre of the lesion seems slightly veiled. Diagnosis: dysplastic naevus, severe atypia.

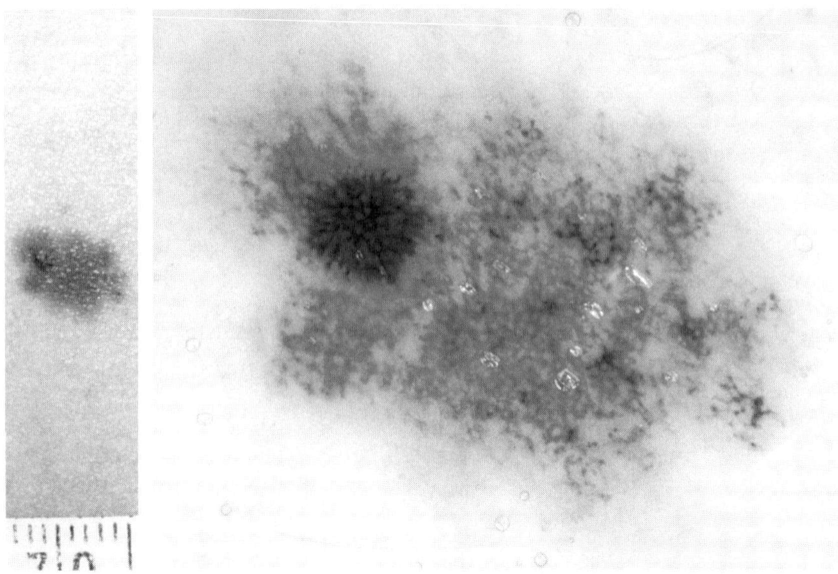

Fig. 8.2 The presence of a pigment network confirms this lesion as melanocytic. The pigment network is (slightly) irregular. The darkest region is at the periphery. Diagnosis: dysplastic naevus, mild atypia.

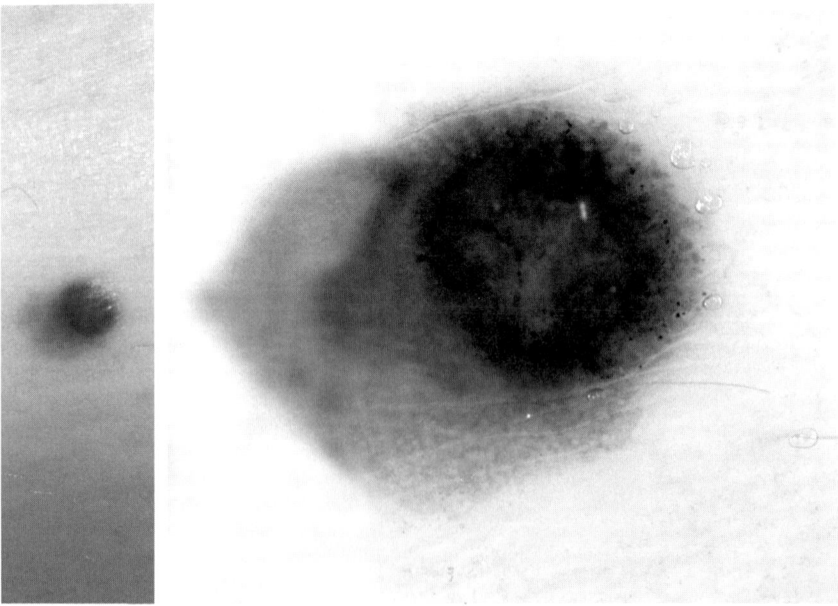

Fig. 8.3 This small nodule on the ankle of a young woman grew progressively for 5 months, in a pre-existing mole. Blue–grey areas, branched streaks and globules at the periphery could be detected by dermatoscopy. Diagnosis: malignant melanoma, tumour thickness 0.8 mm.

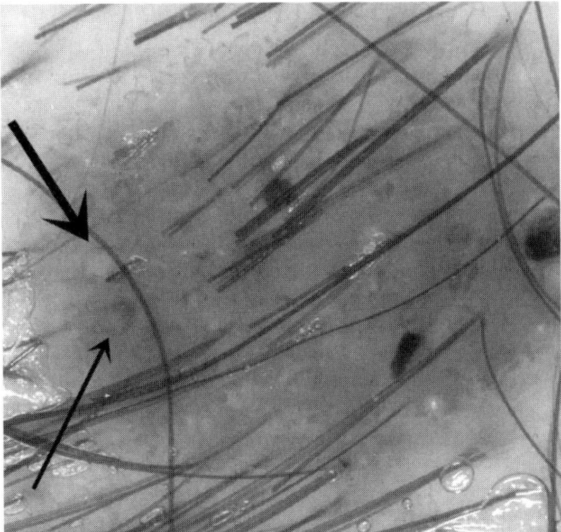

Fig. 8.4 In this lesion a pigment network is lacking and pseudofollicular openings (→) and horny pseudocysts (→) are indications of the diagnosis. Diagnosis: seborrhoeic keratosis.

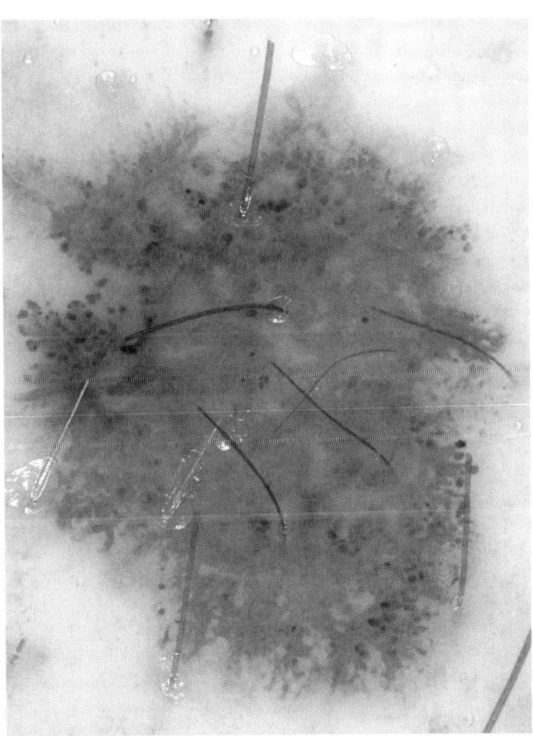

Fig. 8.5 In this melanocytic lesion (diameter 7 mm) many pigmented globules and dots are located at the periphery. The centre of the lesions shows whitish veiled and structureless areas. Diagnosis: malignant melanoma, tumour thickness 0.5 mm.

indication for removal of pigmented lesions. This second area of use is more subtle and specifically experienced dermatologists will benefit from this application of ELM.

Binder *et al.* [15] have investigated the intraobserver and interobserver agreement between experienced ELM dermatologists and dermatologists without ELM experience. ELM was found to increase sensitivity in formally trained dermatologists, but to decrease diagnostic ability in dermatologists not formally trained in the ELM technique. These authors suggest that training in ELM should be offered to dermatologists. Dermatologists not used to applying ELM techniques should not include it in their clinical management of pigmented lesions before having studied an ELM atlas or before having trained in a PLC.

Although ELM offers additional criteria for the identification of high-risk pigmented lesions, I have never yet dared to wait and see what happened to a lesion that appeared as an early melanoma to the naked eye although showing quite reassuring ELM features. After consideration, I think I apply ELM especially to:

1 support my 'already made up' clinical impression in low- to medium-risk naevi to help in the decision to wait and see; or

2 to investigate darkly pigmented lesions, where the naked eye is not able to discriminate the architecture of the pigment network pattern.

ELM features: the ABCD rule and seven-point checklist again?

With experience ELM improves diagnostic accuracy. As for clinical diagnosis, various attempts have been made to improve the diagnostic accuracy, particularly for learners. The ABCD rule of dermatoscopy was reported to be of high prognostic value in the diagnosis of doubtful melanocytic skin lesions by the Vienna group [16]. This ABCD rule for dermatoscopy provides an approach to the interpretation of ELM images on the basis of:

A Asymmetry
B Border
C Colour
D Differential structure.

A semiquantitative scoring system has been developed with maximum scores for A being 2, 8 for B, 6 for C and 5 for D. This scoring system (the total dermatoscopy score) has been validated for the differentiation between benign and malignant melanocytic lesions, with specificity and sensitivity both over 90%. In this investigation the score was determined directly using a dermatoscope, just as in clinical practice.

As the ABCD rule for dermatoscopy does not provide 100% diagnostic accuracy, Lorentzen *et al.* [17] have tested it by applying an intricate statistical method on photo-slides. They found that only 85% of melanomas had a higher total dermatoscopy score than non-melanoma skin lesions. The observers in this study also provided their own overall dermatoscopy diagnosis based on clinical experience and this diagnosis appeared to be higher in sensitivity as compared to the ABCD rules. Kittler *et al.* [18] have recently developed an extension of the ABCD rule in considering change of the lesion as an additional feature. They found that information about the morphological changes of pigmented lesions as reported by the patient add to the diagnostic accuracy. This finding is not surprising, as in clinical practice too it is of vital importance to be informed about recent symptoms such as change in pigmented lesions.

Argenziano *et al.* [19] have conducted a comparison of the ABCD rule of dermatoscopy and a new seven-point checklist based on pattern analysis. The seven points these authors selected were the following: atypical pigment network; grey–blue areas; atypical vascular pattern; radial streaming; irregular diffuse pigmentation (blotches); irregular dots and globules; and a regression pattern. These seven features have been selected as they have relevant histological correlates. The ELM seven-point checklist in the hands of experienced observers gave the highest sensitivity, especially in the subgroup of early melanoma, as compared to the ABCD rule. The specificity of the seven-point method was lower comparing these two ELM scoring methods, because of the tendency to overclassify atypical moles as melanomas.

In the American literature on ELM, the system of pattern analysis has been advocated, which has been extensively explained in pictures in the publication of Kenet *et al.* [20]. These authors—after a consensus meeting—suggest a three-step approach:

1 global ELM features;
2 local ELM features; and
3 network features.

Table 8.6 gives a systematic approach of the ELM investigation of a melanocytic lesion with the American system as a guideline. This table has been simplified by the author from Table 1 of Kenet *et al.* [20]. Furthermore, the features of ELM in Table 8.6 have been assigned a degree of risk with regard to a diagnosis of early melanoma or severe atypia. These degrees of risk have been estimated from the literature on ELM but have not been tested by logistic regression analysis. Each feature is non-specific for melanoma, only suggesting the possibility of melanoma, especially in the presence of one or more other risk features. As always, nodular melanoma and amelanotic melanoma can be very difficult to recognize, even with the help of ELM. A large-scale evaluation of the role of ELM in the differential diagnosis of pigmented lesions was conducted by Ascierto *et al.* [21]. Almost 500 lesions were removed and histologically examined. In this study the pattern analysis system

Table 8.6 Systematic approach of ELM investigation for melanocytic lesions

Step	Feature	Degree of risk*
1 Global ELM features	Multicomponent pattern	+++
	Darkest region at periphery	+
	Erythema	+
2 Local ELM features	Whitish veil	+++
	Blue–grey areas	+++
	Pseudopods/radial streaming/branched streaks at periphery	+++
	Dots/globules at periphery	++
3 Network features	Prominent/irregular network	+
	Pigment network fading at periphery	0

* Degrees of risk modified in numbers of crosses by the author.

of ELM from Kenet & Fitzpatrick [22] was used for evaluating ELM. Sensitivity and specificity of ELM in the analysis of melanocytic lesions were both very high (92.3 and 91.2%, respectively).

Unfortunately, no system of ELM shows 100% sensitivity in diagnosing (early) melanoma and therefore ELM should always be integrated with data from both the history and clinical evaluation, as has been suggested already in Table 8.3.

Digital photography in dermatology

Digital imaging systems are currently being used to teach medical students and physicians-in-training about skin diseases directly or with the help of telecommunications (teledermatology) This technology is being used increasingly to enhance clinical record-keeping in dermatological practices. The resolution of digital imaging is now considered to be sufficiently high enough for use in clinical dermatology and several dermatology textbooks are now available on CD-ROM.

A recent review advises on the selection of digital cameras and hardware requirements [23]. This paper also includes Internet resources that may be helpful in selecting the components of a digital imaging system.

Digital technology and melanoma

Digital imaging systems are currently available to assist in diagnosing malignant melanoma. Most digital imaging analysis systems for early diagnosis of melanoma use a combination of ELM and computerized measurements of size, shape and colour of images. By assembling a database of the ELM features of malignant and atypical pigmented lesions, computer systems are being formulated to identify melanomas simply by scanning an image of the lesion and evaluating its characteristics [24]. My PLC has recently acquired such a commercial machine.

The results of these analyses can be interpreted by the dermatologist or by an artificial neural network [25]. Computer diagnosis has legal drawbacks in Europe, although computer-assisted diagnosis (in which the dermatologist has to make the final decision, aided by arguments presented by the computer) is permitted.

Early diagnosis of melanoma by digital technology is especially useful in following high-risk patients with clinically atypical lesions over time. It is my personal view that PLCs would benefit from the purchase of such a machine. The images of the past visits are readily available and can be compared with the new images without any difficulty. The image can also be sent to an expert for a teledermatological consultation. However, it is important to realize that the inclusion of one patient with atypical moles will take half an hour, and the follow-up visit will also take more time than thorough inspection of the skin with the naked eye only. The help of a (research) nurse is indispensable. Furthermore, taking into consideration the high costs of these sophisticated systems, although they are useful, I doubt whether they are really needed in most clinical practices. Experienced dermatologists can recognize most melanomas very early and in the worst case some unnecessary biopsies will be performed [8]. Moreover, the best computerized image analysis still does not yield 100% diagnostic accuracy and in inexperienced hands might even be harmful. The technical procedure of mole checks by computers may induce a false feeling of safety in the patient, when an alert attitude is needed, especially for members of melanoma-prone families.

Telediagnosis of early melanoma

In the last 2 years, several studies have been performed demonstrating that teledermatology represents a useful diagnostic tool, especially to support underserved communities with respect to dermatological services.

Provost *et al.* [26] reported a high clinical and dermatoscopic concordance in the diagnosis of atypical melanocytic naevi and early melanoma when comparing conventional slides with digital images. Piccolo *et al.* [27] studied digital photographs of pigmented lesions and compared face-to-face diagnosis vs. telediagnosis via e-mail. The diagnostic concordance was 91%, the level obtained by telediagnosis being only a little lower than clinical diagnosis.

It is very plausible that teledermatology, including expert consultation of pigmented lesions via the Internet, will be common practice by the year 2005.

References

1 MacKie RM. Clinical recognition of early invasive malignant melanoma. *Br Med J* 1990; **301**: 1005–6.
2 Mackie RM. Edenburgh. *An Illustrated Guide to the Recognition of Early Malignant Melanoma*. Blackwood, Pillans and Wilson, 1986.
3 Keefe M, Dick DC, Wakeel RA. A study of the value of the seven-point checklist in distinguishing benign pigmented lesions from melanoma. *Clin Exp Dermatol* 1990; **15**: 167–71.
4 McGovern TW, Litaker MS. Clinical predictor of malignant lesions: a comparison of the Glasgow seven-point checklist and the American Cancer Society's ABCDs of pigmented lesions. *J Dermatol Surg Oncol* 1992; **18**: 22–6.
5 Grin CM, Kopf AW, Welkovich B, Bart RS, Levenstein MJ. Accuracy in the clinical diagnosis of malignant melanoma. *Arch Dermatol* 1990; **126**: 763–6.
6 Lindelöf B, Hedblad MA, Sigurgeirsson B. Melanocytic naevus or malignant melanoma? A large-scale epidermiological study of diagnostic accuracy. *Acta Derm Venereol* 1998; **78**: 284–8.
7 Vasen HFA, Bergman W, van Haeringen A, Scheffer E, van Sloten EA. The familial dysplastic nevus syndrome: the natural history and the impact of screening on the prognosis. *Eur J Cancer Clin Oncol* 1989; **25**: 337–41.
8 Morton CA, Mackie RM. Clinical accuracy of the diagnosis of cutaneous malignant melanoma. *Br J Dermatol* 1998; **138**: 283–7.
9 Osborne JE, Bourke JF, Holder J, Colloby P, Graham-Brown RAC. The effect of the introduction of a pigmented lesion clinic on the interval between referral by family practitioner and attendance at hospital. *Br J Dermatol* 1998; **138**: 418–21.
10 Mallett RB, Fallowfield ME, Cook MG, Landells WN, Holden CA, Marsden RA. Are pigmented lesion clinics worthwhile? *Br J Dermatol* 1993; **129**: 689–93.
11 Bataille V, Sasieni P, Curley RK, Cook MG, Marsdens RA. Melanoma yield, number of biopsies and missed melanomas in a British teaching hospital pigmented lesion clinic: a 9-year retrospective study. *Br J Dermatol* 1990; **140**: 243–8.
12 Rampen FHJ, Berretty PJM, van Huystee BEWL, Kiemeny LALM, Nijs CHHM. General practitioners' workload after skin cancer/melanoma screening clinics in the Netherlands. *Dermatology* 1993; **186**: 258–60.
13 Kirkpatrick JJR, Taggart I, Rigby HS, Townsend PLG. A pigmented lesion clinic: analysis of the first year's 1055 patients. *Br J Plast Surg* 1995; **48**: 247–51.
14 Stolz W, Braun-Falco O, Bilek P, Landthaler M, Cognelta AB. *Colour Atlas of Dermatoscopy*. Oxford: Blackwell Science, 1994.
15 Binder M, Schwarz M, Winkler A, *et al.* Epiluminescence microscopy: a useful tool for the diagnosis of pigmented skin lesions for formally trained dermatologists. *Arch Dermatol* 1995; **131**: 286–91.
16 Nachbar F, Stolz W, Merkle T, *et al.* The ABCD rule of dermatoscopy: high prospective value in the diagnosis of doubtful melanocytic skin lesions. *J Am Acad Dermatol* 1994; **30**: 551–9.
17 Lorentzen H, Weismann K, Secher L, Petersen CS, Larsen FG. Dermatoscopic ABCD rule does not improve diagnostic accuracy malignant melanoma. *Acta Derm Venereol* 1999; **79**: 469–72.
18 Kittler H, Seltenheim M, Dawid M, Pehamberger H, Wolff K, Binder M. Morphologic changes of pigmented skin lesions: a useful extension of the ABCD rule for dermatoscopy. *J Am Acad Dermatol* 1999; **40**: 558–62.
19 Argenziano G, Fabrocini G, Carli P, De Giorgi L, Sammarco E, Delfino M. Epiluminescence microscopy for the diagnosis of doubtful melanocytic skin lesions. *Arch Dermatol* 1998; **134**: 1563–70.
20 Kenet RO, Kang S, Kenet BJ, Fitzpatrick TB, Sober AJ, Barnhill RL. Clinical diagnosis of pigmented lesions using digital epiluminescence microscopy. *Arch Dermatol* 1993; **129**: 157–74.
21 Ascierto PA, Satriano RA, Palmieri G, Parasole R, Bosco L, Castello G. Epiluminescence microscopy as a useful approach in the early diagosis of cutaneous malignant melanoma. *Melanoma Res* 1998; **8**: 529–37.
22 Kenet RO, Fitzpatrick TB. Reducing mortality and morbidity of cutaneous

melanoma: a six year plan. (B) Identifying high and low risk pigmented lesions using epiluminescence microscopy. *J Dermatol* 1994; **21**: 881–4.

23 Ratner D, Thomas CO, Bickers D. The uses of digital photography in dermatology. *J Am Acad Dermatol* 1999; **41**: 749–56.

24 Andreassi L, Perotti R, Rubegni P, *et al.* Digital dermoscopy analysis for the differentiation of atypical nevi and early melanoma. *Arch Dermatol* 1999; **135**: 1459–65.

25 Binder M, Kittler H, Seeber A, Steiner A, Pehamberger H, Wolff K. Epiluminescence microscopy-based classification of pigmented skin lesions using computerized image analysis and an artificial neural network. *Melanoma Res* 1998; **8**: 261–6.

26 Provost N, Kopf AW, Rabinovitz HS, *et al.* Comparison of conventional photographs and telephonically transmitted compressed digitized images of melanomas and dysplastic nevis. *Dermatology* 1998; **196**: 299–304.

27 Piccolo D, Smolle J, Wolf IH, *et al.* Face-to-face diagnosis vs. telediagnosis of pigmented skin tumors. *Arch Dermatol* 1999; **135**: 1467–71.

9: What are the prospects for population screening for melanoma?

Mark Elwood

Introduction

Melanoma is one of the most common cancers in European origin populations living in sunny countries, such as Australia, New Zealand, Hawaii and California; and even in moderate incidence areas, such as North America and Europe, it is an important disease. However, in higher incidence countries, the survival rate tends to be higher. It is the mortality rate rather than the total incidence which assesses the potential value of screening. The improved survival rate in higher incidence countries is likely to be because of both increased public awareness of the disease and more effective management, particularly in initial diagnosis. In most countries, at least until recently, the trend in incidence and mortality rates has been upwards [1]. In Australia and the USA mortality rates are stabilizing or beginning to fall in younger age groups, but they continue to increase in older subjects [2,3].

Depth distribution of melanoma

The main determinant of mortality risk is the tumour histological (Breslow) depth distribution. In high incidence countries, such as Australia and New Zealand, the depth distribution of melanoma is more favourable than in lower incidence areas, such as the UK, and survival rates are correspondingly greater. In South Australia, the proportion of melanoma >1.5 mm thick declined from 35% in 1981–83 to 21% in 1990–92 [4]. The 10-year survival for lesions <0.76 mm is over 95%, compared to <50% for lesions 3 mm or thicker [5,6].

Purpose of screening

The purpose of screening for melanoma is to reduce mortality and morbidity. This will happen only if intervention at an earlier stage in the natural history results in a better outcome for the patient. This cannot be assumed to be always true. Early intervention for a lesion which is not progressive will not be beneficial. There is substantial evidence that a proportion of thin melanomas may not progress or progress only very slowly [7–9]. Also, if the normal process of diagnosis gives an excellent result, as the survival figures for very thin lesions show, then an earlier diagnosis may confer no extra benefit.

It would be expected that a reduction in mortality would be seen only several years after the introduction of an effective early diagnosis campaign. The more immediate effect is a shift in the proportion of thin lesions, because of an increase in the incidence rate of thin lesions and, within a few years, a decrease in the incidence rate of thick lesions. Using only the proportional distribution by thickness is misleading as an indicator of the benefits of screening. The incidence rate of thick melanomas should be a good predictor of the mortality rate from melanoma, but such information is only available over a substantial time period in very few countries.

Any campaign of education or screening is likely to produce a short-term increase in the total incidence of melanoma. If the programme is successful and is continued, this short-term increase in incidence should fall away, being replaced by a similar constant incidence rate as before, but with a thinner depth distribution. However, if increased surveillance is causing the diagnosis of non-progressive lesions, then this later stable incidence rate will be higher than that occurring before screening.

Two other effects of a screening programme are more difficult to assess. Education and skin surveillance programmes will lead to the diagnosis of basal cell and squamous cell cancers, lentigo maligna lesions, and a wide range of other skin lesions. The earlier diagnosis is unlikely to be of great benefit, as these lesions have excellent outcomes even if diagnosed in normal clinical practice.

If screening does produce reduced mortality or morbidity, the relevant questions then relate to the comparison of the extent of these benefits with the costs and detrimental effects, such as false-positives, of screening. This comparison will be more favourable in populations with a higher mortality rate and a higher incidence rate of deeply invasive melanoma.

Options for early diagnosis programmes

Screening is only one method of achieving earlier diagnosis (Table 9.1). Programmes for the early diagnosis of melanoma include several options:

1 media-based education to the general public about the early signs of melanoma;

2 open access clinics, offering skin checks or a spot check, often without charge and in an informal setting such as a community hall or on the beach, and often by volunteer doctors;

1	Mass media education
2	Open access clinics
3	Case finding in primary care
4	Active promotion of self-screening
5	Active invitation and screening in primary care
6	Active invitation and screening as a new service

Table 9.1 Six approaches to the earlier diagnosis of melanoma, in (approximately) increasing order by the resources needed

3 case finding as a component of routine primary care;
4 active promotion of self-screening;
5 specific invitation-based screening programmes based in routine primary care; and
6 specific invitation-based screening programmes as a new service additional to current services.

Part of the difficulty of assessing options for the early detection of melanoma is that the separation between normal practice and a new programme may not be very clear, in contrast to screening programmes using a new technology, such as mammography.

Public education

Public education is concerned with both the earlier recognition of a suspicious skin lesion, and with obtaining a medical opinion more quickly once a suspicious skin lesion is recognized. It is difficult to disentangle these two features. One of the British campaigns [10] showed a substantial increase in melanomas diagnosed, but in most the abnormal signs had been present for many months; so the campaign had precipitated action rather than early recognition.

Media education has been assessed carefully in Scotland, with a programme of public education in 1985 about the early signs of melanoma, backed by educational efforts to GPs in dealing with pigmented lesions. This was followed by reductions in the incidence rate of thick melanoma and in melanoma mortality through the next 5 years, but only in women; no beneficial trend was seen in men [11–14]. These trends were seen in data for the whole of Scotland, although the programme was carried out only in western Scotland, and no useful control data are available. After a similar campaign in south-eastern Scotland, the proportion of thin melanomas rose, but the frequency of thick melanomas did not decrease [15]. Programmes in several other areas of the UK have been followed by increases in the incidence of thin melanomas, without any decrease in thick melanoma [16]. An educational campaign in Austria showed a temporary fall in the proportion of thick lesions, but campaigns in France and Switzerland showed no significant effect on depth distribution [17,18]. There is no clear evidence from controlled studies showing a reduction in deep melanomas or in mortality. Educational campaigns may have substantial effects on the demand for referral services [10,19]. In Queensland, a descriptive analysis by time period in one city looked at the effect of two public education campaigns, showing a 24% increase in the total number of melanocytic skin lesions excised in relationship to the campaigns [20]. The authors question the effectiveness of such campaigns, as they found no evidence for a change in thickness of melanoma or an increased detection rate.

Free access skin checks

These range from beach patrols and informal skin screening sessions in community halls, to a process by which GPs or specialists will open their premises on occasions specifically to offer free skin checks. This approach has been used considerably in several countries, and large numbers of subjects have participated [21–23]. Open access clinics have been assessed in the USA by the American Academy of Dermatology (AAD) [24–27], in the Netherlands [28–31] and in Western Australia [32]. The participation rates in these clinics on a population basis are usually low, despite the large number of attenders. For example, the US total of some 282 000 subjects screened in 1992–94 [27] translates to only about 2% of the at-risk population, if that is defined as white-skinned adults over the age of 30. This compares to participation rates of over 70% for many cervical smear and mammography screening programmes. The detection rate of melanoma in that programme was 1.3 per 1000 screened, 90% being *in situ* or less than 0.76 mm deep.

The positivity rate is a central issue, both in its amount and its definition. Defining this as the proportion of subjects given a label of suspected melanoma or somcthing similar, gives modest positivity rates of between 1 and 4%, and the predictive value (the proportion of such patients who are subsequently found to have melanoma) is substantially high. The AAD programme, for example, defined 1.6% of participants as having suspected melanoma, and this was confirmed in 8.2% [27]. Even in the AAD programme, around 20% who screened positive apparently received no follow-up assessment or treatment. This may be acceptable as long as the service is seen as an extra voluntary effort, but is unlikely to be unacceptable for an established programme. Failure to ensure follow-up in screening programmes for breast or cervical cancer has raised medicolegal issues, and screening for hypertension without follow-up has been shown to have detrimental effects [33].

Although the proportions identified as having suspect melanoma are modest, the proportions of subjects who have a positive screening result (in management terms they are recommended to take further action) are much higher, being 10–12% in the Netherlands [28,31], 31% in the early Massachusetts

AAD programme [24] (reduced later) and 17% in Western Australia [32]. Any population screening programme with more than 10% of subjects being referred for further assessment creates a large requirement for follow-up services; in comparison, in breast and colorectal screening, the expected positivity rates would be closer to 5%. Most of the subjects referred were clinically labelled as having suspected basal cell carcinomas, squamous cell carcinomas, or a range of other conditions including dysplastic naevi; all these conditions have such good outcomes in normal clinical practice that any improvement from screening is unlikely.

Melanoma screening programmes would be much more manageable and cost effective if only subjects with clinically suspected melanomas were referred. However, this requires clinical and medicolegal assurance that this is acceptable. If only those with clinically suspected melanomas are followed up, some melanomas will be missed; more selective referral accepts a reduction in sensitivity for a substantial gain in specificity. In the Geraldton (Australia) survey [34], six out of 20 melanomas diagnosed were clinically labelled basal cell carcinoma, and would have been missed by a selective referral process.

Examination of the entire skin has been recommended to avoid missing lesions not noticed by the patient; in a US study, 13 of 14 melanomas found from an open access clinic were on body sites normally covered [35]. In the Netherlands, in a voluntary self-referral clinic in which participants were asked to indicate whether they wanted one or a few specific lesions assessed or a complete skin check, there was a small increase in clinically suspicious lesions after the additional skin examination, and no change in confirmed melanomas. The authors question the value of offering full skin examination [36].

There are several studies of inter- and intraobserver agreement in skin cancer or skin lesion assessment carried out after referral of patients to hospitals or clinics, but relatively few in a community setting. In one such study in the USA, kappa (κ) values for interobserver agreement between dermatologists ranged from 0.38 for squamous cell cancer, based on only a very few cases, to 0.78 for squamous keratoses [37]. However, agreement on the simple management issue of whether to refer or excise or not would be more valuable. The performance of nurses who had been given special training has been assessed [38,39]. In Western Australia [39], nurses showed a sensitivity of 95% and a specificity of 84% compared to a surgeon's clinical assessment, showing that they could be more cost effective. Nurses as screeners have also been assessed in Sweden [40] where nurses referred some 10% of subjects as having suspicious lesions, compared to 3.5% referred for biopsy by doctors.

The benefits of open access clinics seem dubious, although they may be valuable for their stimulation and educational effects on both the profession and the public, and they may lead to more systematic programmes being developed later.

Case finding at primary care level

This means questioning a patient who visits their primary care provider for another reason about recent skin changes, or offering a partial or full skin examination. This can be promoted both by encouraging the general public to ask for it and encouraging GPs to offer it. Any general education or self-screening campaign will also tend to encourage this behaviour. Improved case finding, allied to improved referral decisions, and prompt and accurate management at the referral level, is probably the most important management tool to reduce melanoma mortality. Many countries have documented considerable improvements in survival over time, together with improvements in depth distribution and diagnosis, and it seems likely that this is a result of a combination of increased public awareness of the early signs, better management by primary care doctors, and better and faster hospital referrals and treatment. However, documentary evidence from controlled studies is almost non-existent, and there are few specific studies of the effects of efforts to improve case finding at primary care level.

There is evidence in high-risk countries that the level of expertise in GPs is high. In a survey of a large representative sample of GPs in New Zealand, over 95% described the correct management for three presented scenarios involving early melanoma, and the responses were not greatly different from those of a small sample of specialist dermatologists [41]. Skill levels were higher in younger than in older GPs, and were increased in those who had dealt personally with at least one melanoma patient. In Australia, the effect of a one-day training course for GPs on their diagnostic abilities was tested by examination of patients at clinics set up with a higher than normal proportion of subjects with suspicious lesions [42]. The training had no significant effect on the sensitivity, specificity or predictive value of the screening. In general, the sensitivity was high but specificity low: many subjects with non-malignant lesions were referred for further assessment.

The scope for further improvements in case finding and primary care may be limited in high-risk areas unless screening activities are added. However, it seems likely that there is considerable potential for improvement in moderate- and low-risk countries where the level of public awareness, the expertise in primary care management, and the speed and appropriateness of referral practices may all have room for improvement. In the UK, delays both in the presentation of suspicious lesions to GPs and in the referral process have been documented, and setting up specific pigmented lesion clinics may have some success [10,43,44].

Self-screening

This goes considerably further than public education, although obviously there is an overlap. While any campaign which attempts to educate about the early signs of melanoma must encourage people to be aware or look at their skin, some initiatives specifically encourage a specific self-screening protocol. This can range from a simple checklist [45] to the comprehensive regular screening promoted by the American Cancer Society [46].

Self-screening has been assessed in a case–control study in Connecticut [47]. This study compared subjects with 'lethal' (fatal or advanced) melanoma with population controls, assessing the history of self-examination, defined as 'a careful, deliberate and purposeful examination of the skin', by questionnaire. The results showed a substantial but non-significant reduction in the risk of 'lethal' melanoma among melanoma patients (risk ratio 0.58, 95% CI = 0.31–1.11), which is consistent with a beneficial effect. However, the study also showed a reduction in total melanoma incidence associated with screening (risk ratio 0.66, 95% CI = 0.44–0.99), which is counterintuitive. The main way in which incidence could be reduced is by the recognition and removal of precursor lesions, which seems an unlikely effect and there is no direct evidence of this from the study [48]. By assuming both effects are valid, the authors estimated that self-examination may reduce mortality from melanoma by 63% (risk ratio 0.37, 95% CI = 0.16–0.84). However, the reduction in incidence suggests bias or confounding with the study, raising questions about the validity of the other results. While this is a carefully performed study, assessing screening by case–control methods is inherently difficult, and further assessment of screening by analytical studies or preferably by randomized trials is required.

Recent Australian data show a high level of screening. In New South Wales, 48% of subjects reported self-screening and 17% reported having had a GP skin check in the previous year [49]. However, screening involving a systematic whole body assessment is much less common. In a Queensland survey [50,51], 60% of subjects reported that they practised self-screening, but the authors felt that many or most of the examinations would be inadequate. In a telephone survey of a national sample in the USA [52], almost half the respondents reported that they conducted skin self-examination and, of those that did, the majority reported that they examined their skin at least weekly or even daily. It is questionable whether weekly or daily screening is a healthy behaviour, but the thoroughness of the self-examination was not described. In the USA, performance of self-screening (ever) was positively associated with self-perceived risk and with having discussed skin cancer with health professionals [53].

Thus there is some evidence for benefit from self-screening and further assessment is warranted. Evaluating the practice of self-screening is difficult because it is under individual control; the vigorous promotion of self-screening on an individual or population basis could be evaluated in a trial.

Invitation-based screening by the primary health care provider

The term 'screening' can be confusing [54]. The essential difference between screening and case finding is that case finding is opportunistic, adding an extra question or examination, but only for those people visiting the GP for other reasons. In contrast, screening, as it is used in other disease contexts, implies a deliberate visit to the GP (or other screener) for that purpose. There will need to be a specific programme to encourage people to come for screening. Thus, a GP practising case finding would offer skin examination to all patients who visit his or her premises, while a GP practising skin screening would use the age–sex register to invite all patients in the practice (perhaps over a certain age) for screening at regular intervals. Skin screening is therefore a new programme in addition to normal care, with financial and organizational implications. A specific invitation-based screening service by the primary care provider has considerable potential and deserves fuller assessment. No trials of such a programme have been published.

New screening services outside normal care provision

A new screening service outside the normal care provision mechanism could consist of a screening clinic, allied to a programme to ensure that all residents in the area were made aware of the new facility and encouraged to attend. This could involve media publicity or a personal invitation, analogous to the methods used in breast or cervical screening. Such a system apparently has yet to be tried in any large general population in regard to melanoma. Screening has been used in England in a privately funded (BUPA) general health screening centre [55]. A complete skin check was carried out by a doctor, usually a GP, and the position and characteristics of any pigmented lesion regarded as suspicious or changing were marked on a skin chart, and assessed by the seven-point checklist system. All lesions were then photographed using Polaroid cameras, and the picture assessed independently by two consultant dermatologists. Of 39 922 subjects screened, 948 (2.4%) had at least one skin lesion assessed and photographed. Of the 1052 lesions in these subjects, 231 were assessed as requiring follow-up and amongst these there were 11 melanomas, but follow-up was incomplete. The authors conclude that photography greatly reduced the need for specialist referral, but their estimate of sensitivity was only 37%.

Selective screening of high-risk groups

All the above have dealt with general population approaches, which may be restricted by age but not in other ways. Other approaches are designed to target high-risk subgroups. The impact on the whole disease depends on both the impact on the selected subgroup, and also how that subgroup is selected and what proportion of all melanomas in the population occur within the group. Most of the above methods, particularly the free access clinics, have an element of high-risk selection, although this is unsystematic and subjective. Systematic attempts to identify high-risk groups on a population basis are more complex, as they require a preselection process for risk which is itself a form of screening.

The highest risk groups are subjects with a previous melanoma, the dysplastic naevus syndrome, or specific genetic markers; these are dealt with elsewhere in this book. Careful regular surveillance, based on clinical observation supplemented by photography, has been shown to result in improved depth distribution of subsequent melanomas [56–58]. There are no randomized trials of alternative types of follow-up surveillance in high-risk groups. The value of screening for less well-defined risk groups, such as subjects with some dysplastic naevi or a high total naevus count, is less clear [59–61].

Limitations of screening

A major limitation of melanoma screening is that it is simply using unaided observation. Most current efforts are based on the clinical signs and symptoms of melanoma, which are non-specific and have a low predictive value. In New South Wales, a population survey showed that 12% of adults had had within the previous 12 months a lesion fitting the ABCD criteria for a suspicious lesion [49]. A study of 21-year-olds in New Zealand showed a 20% frequency of the same phenomenon, with approximately half of these subjects having sought a primary care opinion [62]. In a general practice in England, self counting of naevi was compared with a naevus count carried out by trained GPs [63]. The authors report that self-counts could be useful in self-identification of risk, and note that in this group 13% had reported some change in a mole in the previous 3 months and 5% had reported a major change.

Instruments such as the dermatoscope, and techniques of computer image analysis [64–68] are likely to be valuable, mainly in regard to the diagnosis of referred patients and in the regular follow-up of high-risk subjects with specific lesions. The application of these methods for population screening requires much further development and evaluation in a population context. Simpler technology may be valuable; a randomized trial in Queensland showed that providing GPs with a simple algorithm and a cheap camera to assist their follow-up of patients with suspicious skin lesions gave a reduction in excision rates of benign lesions, with no change in the excision rates of melanoma [69].

Number needed to screen per death prevented

A very approximate estimate can be produced from simple calculations. Consider a high-risk general population, Australia, and the age range 50–69, in both sexes, as a feasible target for screening. Their annual mortality rate from melanoma (1996) is 10 per 100 000. Suppose, optimistically, a 30% reduction in mortality from a screening test every 2 years for which the positivity rate (the proportion of screenees requiring further investigation) is 5% on the first screen, reducing to 2% on the second screen. Assume that the cost per screen is $A24, and the cost for the investigation of each positive subject is $A140 [70]. On this basis, to prevent one death would require screening 1700 persons (number needed to screen; NNS) and performing some 18 000 screens. The cost would be around $A500 000 and the number of false-positives to be investigated would be somewhat over 400. If we assume a life saved equates to 20 years of lives saved, the cost per year of life saved would be about $A25 000 (approximately £10 000), which is comparable to the costs of breast or colorectal cancer screening. As the mortality rate is higher in men, the NNS is around 1200 for men and 2600 for women in this age group. However, a full assessment is much more complex, as it needs to assess the marginal costs and benefits of screening compared with current practice, which includes a high level of less systematic assessment, many GP visits, referrals and biopsies, and needs to use appropriate discounting.

A cost effectiveness analysis has been published [70] for the Australian situation which assumes mortality reductions of 15–34% with either 5- or 2-yearly screening, starting at age 50. This produces costs per year of life saved, with appropriate analytical assumptions including discounting, of from $A6800 (men: 5-yearly, 60% sensitivity, 27% mortality reduction) to $A31 000 (women: 2-yearly, 30% sensitivity, 24% mortality reduction). These costs are comparable to those of breast cancer screening. The critical assumption is that screening does produce a substantial reduction in mortality. Further, generally similar, estimates have also been given [42].

One of the main contributions to the cost is the fact that the death rate from melanoma, even in high-risk countries, is relatively small compared, for example, to the death rate from breast cancer or colorectal cancer. If the above simple calculation is based on UK annual mortality rates for subjects aged 50–69 (approximately 3.5 per 100 000), the number needed to be screened to prevent one death is about 4800, with 48 000 screens. Positivity rates should be lower; using 2% for a first screen and 1% thereafter gives about 500 positives to be assessed per death prevented, and a cost per year of life saved of around $A60 000 (£24 000). Obviously, the results of these calculations will be more favourable if the mortality rate is increased, as would be possible if a high-risk group is defined, but it is then important to add in the costs, and the accuracy or otherwise, of whatever method is used to define the high-risk group.

The evidence base for melanoma screening

Screening for cancer on a population basis requires strong evidence. Screening for breast cancer and colorectal cancer is supported by evidence from large-scale population-based randomized trials; screening for uterine cervical cancer does not have randomized trial evidence, but has a large number of strong cohort and case–control studies to support it. In other cancer screening situations, for example ovarian cancer, the predominant view is that screening should not be undertaken until the results of current randomized trials become available. In contrast, the evidence base for screening for melanoma is extremely weak (Table 9.2). There are no available results from randomized trials or cohort studies, and the only analytical study result being the single case–control study. The main argument for the effectiveness of screening is based on the assumption that earlier diagnosis will produce mortality and morbidity benefits, which in turn is based on the large differences in postdiagnosis survival with depth of invasion, for patients diagnosed in normal clinical practice. These assumptions may be correct, but the lack of empirical evidence of benefit needs to be acknowledged.

Conclusions

In high-risk and high awareness countries, such as Australia and New Zealand, the further potential for media education on the early signs of

Table 9.2 Levels of evidence (from the Physician Data Query of the US National Cancer Institute) applied to cancer screening

Level of evidence	Cancer screening application
1 Evidence obtained from at least one RCT	Breast, colorectal (several RCTs)
2 Evidence obtained from controlled trials that use allocation methods other than randomization (e.g. by birth date or hospital chart number)	Cervix (many studies)
3 Evidence obtained from cohort or case–control analytic studies, preferably from more than one centre or research group	Melanoma (one case–control study)
4 Evidence obtained from multiple time series with or without intervention (quasi-experimental designs)	
5 Opinions of respected authorities based on clinical experience, descriptive studies, or reports of expert committee	

Abbreviation: RCT, randomized controlled trial.

melanoma is probably limited and open access clinics are of dubious value. Case finding in primary care, while it may be quite good at present, has considerable potential for further development, and innovative programmes could be useful. The promotion of self-screening may be of value; assessing costs and outcomes is a priority. Invitation-based screening in primary care should be developed on a pilot basis and assessed. Invitation-based screening as a new service is probably not very valuable in countries with a well-developed primary care service, if assessed in terms of skin screening alone. The potential for an integrated invitation-based screening service for a number of chronic diseases is greater.

In lower risk countries with lower levels of public and professional awareness, such as the UK, improved public and professional education has been shown to be valuable, and programmes including spot checks and specific professional training may be useful. While the frequency of the disease is lower, the relatively low levels of awareness increases the potential benefits of education and screening programmes.

Further development should pay great attention to evaluation, using the most rigorous methods which are feasible. The best method of assessment is a randomized trial, and a large randomized trial of a community-based programme using education, self-screening and doctor screening is being developed in Queensland (J. Aitken, personal communication). Other randomized trials would be valuable. Carefully performed evaluations using cohort, case–control, or time series designs will be valuable if control groups are used, and attention is paid to bias and confounding.

References

1 Rigel DS, Friedman RJ, Kopf AW. The incidence of malignant melanoma in the United States: issues as we approach the 21st century. *J Am Acad Dermatol* 1996; **34**: 839–47.

2 Giles GG, Armstrong BK, Burton RC, Staples MP, Thursfield VJ. Has mortality from melanoma stopped rising in Australia? Analysis of trends between 1931 and 1994. *Br Med J* 1996; **312**: 1121–5.

3 Roush GC, McKay L, Holford TR. A reversal of the long-term increase in deaths attributable to malignant melanoma. *Cancer* 1992; **69**: 1714–20.

4 Roder DM, Luke CG, McCaul KA, Esterman AJ. Trends in prognostic factors of melanoma in South Australia, 1981–92: implications for health promotion. *Med J Aust* 1995; **162**: 25–9.

5 Balch CM, Soong SJ, Shaw HM, Urist MM, McCarthy WH. An analysis of prognostic factors in 8500 patients with cutaneous melanoma. In: Balch CM, Houghton AN, Milton GW, Sober AJ, Soong SJ, eds. *Cutaneous Melanoma*. Philadelphia: J.B.Lippincott, 1992: 165–87.

6 Häffner AC, Garbe C, Burg G, Büttner P, Orfanos CE, Rassner G. The prognosis of primary and metastasising melanoma: an evaluation of the TNM classification in 2495 patients. *Br J Cancer* 1992; **66**: 856–61.

7 Burton RC, Coates MS, Hersey P, *et al*. An analysis of a melanoma epidemic. *Int J Cancer* 1993; **55**: 765–70.

8 Burton RC, .Armstrong BK. Recent incidence trends imply a non-metastasizing form of invasive melanoma. *Melanoma Res* 1994; **4**: 107–13.

9 Burton RC. Analysis of public education and the implications with regard to nonprogressive thin melanomas. *Curr Opin Oncol* 1995; **7**: 170–4.
10 Whitehead SM, Wroughton MA, Elwood JM, Davison J, Stewart M. Effects of a health education campaign for the earlier diagnosis of melanoma. *Br J Cancer* 1989; **60**: 421–5.
11 Doherty VR, MacKie RM. Experience of a public education programme on early detection of cutaneous malignant melanoma. *Br Med J* 1988; **297**: 388–91.
12 MacKie RM, Hole D. Audit of public education campaign to encourage earlier detection of malignant melanoma. *Br Med J* 1992; **304**: 1012–15.
13 MacKie RM. Strategies to reduce mortality from cutaneous malignant melanoma. *Arch Dermatol Res* 1994; **287**: 13–15.
14 MacKie RM. Melanoma prevention and early detection. *Br Med Bull* 1995; **51**: 570–83.
15 Herd RM, Cooper EJ, Hunter JA, *et al.* Cutaneous malignant melanoma: publicity, screening clinics and survival—the Edinburgh experience 1982–90. *Br J Dermatol* 1995; **132**: 563–70.
16 Melia J. Early detection of cutaneous malignant melanoma in Britain. *Int J Epidemiol* 1995; **24**: S39–S44.
17 Bonerandi JJ, Grob JJ, Cnudde N, Enel P, Gouvernet J. Campaign of early detection of melanoma in the Provence–Alpes–Cote-d'Azur area 1989: lessons of an experience. *Ann Dermatol Venereol* 1992; **119**: 105–9.
18 Bulliard J-L, Raymond L, Levi F, *et al.* Prevention of cutaneous melanoma: an epidemiological evaluation of the Swiss campaign. *Rev Epidemiol Sante Publique* 1992; **40**: 431–8.
19 Graham-Brown RAC, Osborne JE, London SP, *et al.* The initial effects on workload and outcome of a public education campaign on early diagnosis and treatment of malignant melanoma in Leicestershire. *Br J Dermatol* 1990; **122**: 53–9.
20 Del Mar CB, Green AC, Battistutta D. Do public media campaigns designed to increase skin cancer awareness result in increased skin excision rates? *Aust N Z J Public Health* 1997; **21**: 751–3.
21 Marks R. Two decades of the public health approach to skin cancer control in Australia: why, how and where are we now? *Australas J Dermatol* 1999; **40**: 1–5.
22 McCarthy WH. Secondary prevention of skin cancer in Australia. In: MacKie RM, ed. *Primary and Secondary Prevention of Malignant Melanoma*. Basel: Karger, 1996: 31–42.
23 Howell JB, Cockerell CJ. Melanoma self-examination day: Melanoma Monday, May 1, 1995. *J Am Acad Dermatol* 1996; **34**: 837–8.
24 Koh HK, Caruso A, Gage I, *et al.* Evaluation of melanoma/skin cancer screening in Massachusetts. *Cancer* 1990; **65**: 375–9.
25 Koh HK, Geller AC, Miller DR, Caruso A, Gage I, Lew RA. Who is being screened for melanoma/skin cancer? Characteristics of persons screened in Massachusetts. *J Am Acad Dermatol* 1991; **24**: 271–7.
26 Koh HK. Geller AC. Melanoma control in the United States: current status. [Review] *Recent Results Cancer Res* 1995; **139**: 215–24.
27 Koh HK, Norton LA, Geller AC, *et al.* Evaluation of the American Academy of Dermatology's national skin cancer early detection and screening program. *J Am Acad Dermatol* 1996; **34**: 971–8.
28 Rampen FHJ, van Huystee BEWL, Kiemeney LALM. Melanoma/skin cancer screening clinics: experiences in the Netherlands. *J Am Acad Dermatol* 1991; **25**: 776–7.
29 Rampen FH, Casparie-van Velsen JI, van Huystee BE, Kiemeney LA, Schouten LJ. False-negative findings in skin cancer and melanoma screening. *J Am Acad Dermatol* 1995; **33**: 59–63.
30 de Rooij MJ, Rampen FH, Schouten LJ, Neumann HA. Skin cancer screening focusing on melanoma yields more selective attendance. *Arch Dermatol* 1995; **131**: 422–5.
31 de Rooij MJ, Rampen FH, Schouten LJ, Neumann HA. Volunteer melanoma screenings: follow-up, compliance, and outcome. *Dermatol Surg* 1997; **23**: 197–201.
32 Katris P, Crock JG, Gray BN. Research note: the Lions Cancer Institute and the Western Australian Society of Plastic Surgeons skin cancer screening

programme. *Aust N Z J Surg* 1996; **66**: 101–4.

33 Taylor DW, Haynes RB, Sackett DL, Gibson ES. Long-term follow-up of absenteeism among working men following the detection and treatment of their hypertension. *Clin Invest Med* 1981; **4**: 173–7.

34 Kricker A, English DR, Randell PL, *et al.* Skin cancer in Geraldton, Western Australia: a survey of incidence and prevalence. *Med J Aust* 1990; **152**: 399–407.

35 Rigel DS, Friedman RJ, Kopf AW, *et al.* Importance of complete cutaneous examination for the detection of malignant melanoma. *J Am Acad Dermatol* 1986; **14**: 857–60.

36 de Rooij MJ, Rampen FH, Schouten LJ, Neumann HA. Total skin examination during screening for malignant melanoma does not increase the detection rate. *Br J Dermatol* 1996; **135**: 42–5.

37 Leffell DJ, Chen Y-T, Berwick M, Bolognia JL. Interobserver agreement in a community skin cancer screening setting. *J Am Acad Dermatol* 1993; **28**: 1003–5.

38 Bolognia JL, Berwick M, Fine JA. Complete follow-up and evaluation of a skin cancer screening in Connecticut. *J Am Acad Dermatol* 1990; **23**: 1098–106.

39 Katris P, Donovan RJ, Gray BN. Nurses screening for skin cancer: an observation study. *Aust N Z J Public Health* 1998; **22**: 381–3.

40 Törnberg S, Månsson-Brahme E, Lindén D, *et al.* Screening for cutaneous malignant melanoma: a feasibility study. *J Med Screen* 1996; **3**: 211–15.

41 McGee R, Elwood M, Sneyd MJ, Williams S, Tilyard M. The recognition and management of melanoma and other skin lesions by general practitioners in New Zealand. *N Z Med J* 1994; **107**: 287–90.

42 Burton RC, Howe C, Adamson L, *et al.* General practitioner screening for melanoma: sensitivity, specificity, and effect of training. *J Med Screen* 1998; **5**: 156–61.

43 Doherty VR, MacKie RM. Reasons for poor prognosis in British patients with cutaneous malignant melanoma. *Br Med J* 1986; **292**: 987–9.

44 Kirkpatrick JJ, Taggart I, Rigby HS, Townsend PL. A pigmented lesion clinic: analysis of the first year's 1055 patients. *Br J Plast Surg* 1995; **48**: 247–51.

45 Fitzpatrick TB, Rhodes AR, Sober AJ, Mihm CM Jr. Primary malignant melanoma of the skin: the call for action to identify persons at risk; to discover precursor lesions; to detect early melanomas. In: Elwood JM, ed. *Naevi and Melanoma: Incidence, Interrelationships and Implications*; *Pigment Cell no. 9*. Basel: Karger, 1988: 110–17.

46 Friedman RJ, Rigel DS, Silverman MK, Kopf AW, Vossaert KA. Malignant melanoma in the 1990s: the continued importance of early detection and the role of physician examination and self-examination of the skin. *CA Cancer J Clin* 1991; **41**: 201–26.

47 Berwick M, Begg CB, Fine JA, Roush GC, Barnhill RL. Screening for cutaneous melanoma by skin self-examination. *J Natl Cancer Inst* 1996; **88**: 17–23.

48 Elwood JM. Skin self-examination and melanoma. *J Natl Cancer Inst* 1996; **88**: 3–5.

49 Girgis A, Campbell EM, Redman S, Sanson-Fisher RW. Screening for melanoma: a community survey of prevalence and predictors. *Med J Aust* 1991; **154**: 338–43.

50 Del Mar CB, Stanton WR, Gillespie AM, Lowe JB, Balanda KP. What use do people make of physicians in checking their skin for cancer? *Cancer Detect Prev* 1996; **20**: 325–31.

51 Baade PD, Balanda KP, Lowe JB. Changes in skin protection behaviors, attitudes, and sunburn: in a population with the highest incidence of skin cancer in the world. *Cancer Detect Prev* 1996; **20**: 566–75.

52 Miller DR, Geller AC, Wyatt SW, *et al.* Melanoma awareness and self-examination practices: results of a United States survey. *J Am Acad Dermatol* 1996; **34**: 962–70.

53 Robinson JK, Rigel DS, Amonette RA. What promotes skin self-examination? *J Am Acad Dermatol* 1998; **39**: 752–7.

54 Koh HK, Lew RA, Prout MN. Screening for melanoma/skin cancer: theoretic and practical considerations. *J Am Acad Dermatol* 1989; **20**: 159–72.

55 Edmondson PC, Curley RK, Marsden RA, Robinson D, Allaway SL, Willson CD. Screening for malignant melanoma using

instant photography. *J Med Screen* 1999; **6**: 42–6.

56 Rhodes AR. Intervention strategy to prevent lethal cutaneous melanoma: use of dermatologic photography to aid surveillance of high-risk persons. *J Am Acad Dermatol* 1998; **39**: 262–7.

57 Masri GD, Clark WH Jr, Guerry DIV, Halpern A, Thompson CJ, Elder DE. Screening and surveillance of patients at high risk for malignant melanoma result in detection of earlier disease. *J Am Acad Dermatol* 1990; **22**: 1042–8.

58 MacKie RM, McHenry P, Hole D. Accelerated detection with prospective surveillance for cutaneous malignant melanoma in high risk groups. *Lancet* 1993; **341**: 1618–20.

59 Tucker MA, Halpern A, Holly EA, *et al.* Clinically recognized dysplastic nevi. *J Am Med Assoc* 1997; **277**: 1439–44.

60 Jackson A, Wilkinson C, Ranger M, Pill R, August P. Can primary prevention or selective screening for melanoma be more precisely targeted through general practice? A prospective study to validate a self-administered risk score. *Br Med J* 1998; **316**: 34–8.

61 Grob JJ, Gouvernet J, Aymar D, *et al.* Count of benign melanocytic nevi as a major indicator of risk for nonfamilial nodular and superficial spreading melanoma. *Cancer* 1990; **66**: 387–95.

62 Douglass HM, McGee R, Williams S. Are young adults checking their skin for melanoma? *Aust N Z J Public Health* 1998; **22**: 562–7.

63 Little P, Keefe M, White J. Self screening for risk of melanoma: validity of self mole counting by patients in a single general practice. *Br Med J* 1995; **310**: 912–16.

64 Green A, Martin N, McKenzie G, *et al.* Computer image analysis of pigmented skin lesions. *Melanoma Res* 1991; **1**: 231–6.

65 Binder M, Kittler H, Seeber A, Steiner A, Pehamberger H, Wolff K. Epiluminescence microscopy-based classification of pigmented skin lesions using computerised image analysis and an artificial neural network. *Melanoma Res* 1998; **8**: 261–6.

66 Hall PN, Claridge E, Smith JD. Computer screening for early detection of melanoma: is there a future? *Br J Dermatol* 1995; **132**: 325–38.

67 Kopf AW, Salopek TG, Slade J, Marghoob AA, Bart RS. Techniques of cutaneous examination for the detection of skin cancer. *Cancer* 1995; **75**: 684–90.

68 Seidnari S, Pellacani G, Pepe P. Digital videomicroscopy improves diagnostic accuracy for melanoma. *J Am Acad Dermatol* 1998; **39**: 175–81.

69 Del Mar CB, Green AC. Aid to diagnosis of melanoma in primary medical care. *Br Med J* 1995; **310**: 492–5.

70 Girgis A, Clarke P, Burton RC, Sanson-Fisher RW. Screening for melanoma by primary health care physicians: a cost effectiveness analysis. *J Med Screen* 1996; **3**: 47–53.

Part 3: Management

10: Excision of primary cutaneous melanoma

Michael J. Timmons

Introduction

Complete surgical excision with histological examination of the tumour is the best and most effective treatment of a primary cutaneous melanoma. Management of the regional lymph nodes and the role of adjuvant therapies are discussed later in this book. The most challenging question to address here is whether or not further adjuvant surgery after a narrow margin excision biopsy will reduce the risk of local recurrences, more distant metastases or death.

Melanoma *in situ*

The diagnosis of melanoma *in situ* may be made after an excision biopsy of a suspicious skin lesion. As Kirkham discusses in Chapter 7, the histological diagnosis of melanoma *in situ* can be difficult for pathologists [1]. Depending on who performed the biopsy and the margins of excision, the clinician may decide after histological confirmation of complete excision that no further treatment is required. If there are any doubts, then further excision of the biopsy site is recommended. Only a small excision margin of normal skin is needed. Based on a review of 121 cases of melanoma *in situ*, Bartoli *et al.* [2] concluded that for lesions up to 2 cm in diameter 3 mm margins are adequate. Multidisciplinary panels in the USA and Australia recommend a 5 mm margin [3,4].

Lentigo maligna is one form of melanoma *in situ* [5]. Lentigo malignas occur more commonly in older patients, mainly on the face, and may be large when first seen by a doctor. They usually grow slowly but may rapidly progress to invasive lentigo maligna melanoma. The lifetime risk of developing an invasive melanoma is not known; one study calculated that the lifetime risk with a lesion appearing at age 45 years is 4.7% [6]. This makes for a therapeutic challenge and explains the wide variety of treatments from surgery to treatments such as cryotherapy, radiotherapy, laser ablation and the topical application of azelaic acid, which have all been used for lentigo maligna [5].

The alternatives to surgery have three major disadvantages: failure to treat deep periadnexal atypical melanocytes; inability to detect atypical melanocytes beyond the clinical margin; and lack of a surgical specimen to detect invasive melanoma.

Many authors believe that surgical excision is the treatment of choice for lentigo malignas. Lentigo malignas sometimes have vague edges and can recur after apparently complete surgical excision and the difficulty here is to decide what excision margins to use. The margin of 5 mm recommended for other melanomas *in situ* is also recommended for lentigo malignas by the multidisciplinary panels in the USA and Australia. One of the histological criteria for lentigo maligna is the presence of atypical melanocytes along the basal layer of the epidermis, arranged in solitary units and small nests [5]. Atypical melanocytes can extend beyond the clinical margins of lentigo malignas and this may be a cause of local recurrences. Because of this, Mohs' micrographic surgery to ensure complete excision of all atypical melanocytes has been advocated.

There can be difficulties in interpreting the frozen sections used in Mohs' microsurgery and permanent paraffin sections are needed in some cases. Another difficulty for Mohs' microsurgery is that it involves excision of atypical melanocytes outside the main clinical lesion. The significance of these is not known and in addition there are no universally agreed criteria about which atypical melanocytes should be excised; for example, is it all of them or just those in clumps? This debate has echoes of the attempts made from the 19th century to base the extent of wide excision of invasive malignant melanomas on pathology [7]. For example, increased melanocyte density 5 cm from the edge of seven of 12 primary malignant melanomas studied by Wong [8] was used by others to justify 5 cm margins; increased melanocyte numbers and mild atypia around malignant melanomas are now attributed to chronic sun exposure [9]. What is certain is that Mohs' microsurgery can paradoxically result in much larger defects than excision with a 5 mm margin; in one series of 45 patients, the mean lesion size was 1.7×1.7 cm and the mean defect size to achieve clear margins was 4.2×4.5 cm [5].

Nevertheless, Mohs' microsurgery does achieve high complete excision and low recurrence rates. A study of 16 patients treated by Mohs' microsurgery and followed up for at least 5 years reported only one recurrence (8 years after excision of a 4 cm diameter lentigo maligna with a 1 cm margin); the author concluded that the study confirmed the recommendation of excision of lentigo malignas with 5 mm–1 cm margins but 5 mm was most applicable to lesions less than 2 cm in diameter [10].

Given that the lifetime risk of any individual lentigo maligna developing an invasive melanoma is not known, excision of a lentigo maligna with the recommended 5 mm margin is reasonable, although in some sites (e.g. close to the eye), a narrower margin may have to be accepted. Mohs' microsurgery is not necessary for all lentigo malignas but should be considered for assessment of the defect edges after excision of large lentigo malignas and for recurrent lentigo malignas.

Malignant melanoma

The maximum thickness of the tumour determines the prognosis for a patient with AJCC/UICC pTNM stage I or II malignant melanoma, gives an indication of the need for adjuvant treatment and is useful in deciding how long to follow up the patient after treatment. This is why an excision biopsy of the whole tumour is important. Incisional biopsies do not appear to adversely affect the prognosis in terms of local recurrence and mortality, provided they are followed by complete tumour excision [11], and are occasionally useful (e.g. for a possible subungual melanoma or a large tumour for which an excision biopsy would leave a defect needing a skin graft). After complete excision of a melanoma with a narrow skin margin (e.g. 2 mm), will wide excision of the excision biopsy site improve the prognosis for thin or thick melanomas?

While it is certain that the thicker the melanoma the greater the risk of metastases and death [12], opinions vary about what are 'thin', 'thick' and 'intermediate thickness' melanomas and what are 'narrow' and 'wide' excision margins.

From the 19th century to the 1970s wide local excision, if possible with 5 cm margins of normal skin, was routinely performed to improve the chances of survival [13]. However, there is no clear evidence from retrospective studies that increasing excision margins improves survival; indeed what is striking about the results of past radical surgery with wide excision is not how good the survival rates were but how bad they were, presumably because thick melanomas were being treated [7].

Two prospective randomized trials have confirmed that wide excision margins do not improve overall and disease-free survival for melanomas up to 4 mm thick. In the World Health Organization (WHO) Melanoma Group's study of 612 primary cutaneous melanomas 0.1–2 mm thick the narrow margin excision biopsy sites were excised with either a 1 cm or a 3 cm margin of skin (together with an additional 1–2 cm margin of subcutaneous fat down to the muscle fascia in both groups) [14]. The reported overall and disease-free survival rates were the same for the narrow (1 cm) and wide (3 cm) margin groups (8-year overall survival: 89.6% and 90.3% respectively; 8-year disease-free survival: 81.6% and 84.4%, respectively). In a multi-institutional trial from the USA, Canada and Denmark (Intergroup

Melanoma Trial), patients with melanomas 1–4 mm thick had their melanoma excision site excised with either a 2 cm (narrow) or a 4 cm (wide) excision margin [15]. The trial design was complex because patients were also randomized to have or not have elective regional lymph node dissections. In the 462 patients evaluated, the median 5-year overall and disease-free survival rates were not significantly different: 79.5% overall survival for the narrow margin patients and 83.7% for the wide margin patients.

These narrow excision margins do not adversely affect survival but do reduce the need for skin grafts or flaps in the excision sites. In the Intergroup trial of melanomas of the trunk and the limbs proximal to the elbow or knee, 46% of patients with 4 cm margins but only 11% of patients with 2 cm margins required a split thickness skin graft.

Local recurrences

Local recurrence of a tumour is unpleasant and frightening. Even though wide excision margins do not improve survival, it would be reasonable to use them if they could at least reduce local recurrences.

The first problem is to decide what is a local recurrence. In many studies, local recurrence is not defined. Some distinguish between a local recurrence with an epidermal *in situ* component and a local metastasis without such an *in situ* component [16]. For some, local recurrences are recurrences within or contiguous with the excision scar or graft [17]. For some, local 'metastases' can be in the scar or skin graft, at the edge of the scar/graft and in transit [18], while for others local 'metastases' or 'recurrences' are within 5 cm from the perimeter of the primary scar or skin graft [19,20]. In the WHO trial, local recurrences were defined as cutaneous or subcutaneous nodules that appeared along the scar or in an area of 1 cm or less in radius from the surgical scar. In the Intergroup trial, a local recurrence was defined as a pathologically documented melanoma that recurred within 2 cm of the surgical scar after a definitive excision of the primary melanoma. Whatever their definition, if any, of local recurrence, retrospective studies of various excision margins show that local recurrence of melanomas less than 1 mm thick is rare and that local recurrence of the thickest melanomas occurs in about 12% of patients.

At a mean follow-up of 8 years, there were four local recurrences as the first site of relapse in the WHO trial. All four were in patients with melanomas more than 1 mm thick and all four patients had 1 cm margin excisions. The local recurrence rate was low and, in contrast, 21 patients with 1 cm margins and 24 patients with 3 cm margins had regional lymph node metastases as the first site of relapse.

In the Intergroup trial, at a median follow-up of 6 years, it was reported that there was no increase in local recurrence rates with increasing tumour thickness. There were two local recurrences in the 2 cm margin group and four in the 4 cm margin group. From this and because local recurrences only occurred after 1 cm margin excisions for 1.1–2 mm thick melanomas in the WHO trial, it was argued that while 1 cm margins are sufficient for melanomas < 1 mm thick, they may be inadequate for melanomas > 1 mm thick and 2 cm margins should be used whenever possible for 1–2 mm thick melanomas [15].

However, review of the Intergroup trial results at a median follow-up of 91 months [21], comparable to the WHO trial at 96 months, showed that there were then more local recurrences after excision of thicker tumours, as there were in the WHO trial. Accepting that the definition of a local recurrence was different in the two trials, it is interesting that the 2% recurrence rate for the 1–2 mm thick melanomas excised with 2 cm margins in the Intergroup trial was similar to the 3.5% recurrence rate for the 113 patients in the WHO trial who had 1.1–2 mm thick melanomas excised with 1 cm margins. In the 146 patients who had 1–2 mm thick melanomas excised with 2 cm margins in the Intergroup trial there were three local recurrences but there were no local recurrences in the 141 patients who had 1–2 mm thick melanomas excised with 4 cm margins.

From these figures, mathematical logic would dictate that if 1 cm margins are not safe for 1–2 mm thick melanomas then 2 cm margins are equally not safe and 4 cm margins should be used. The biology of melanoma suggests otherwise. In the Intergroup trial, six of the eight local recurrences of melanomas after excision of 2.01–4 mm thick melanomas were in the 4 cm margin group, with all three recurrences of 3.01–4 mm thick melanomas being in the 4 cm margin group; wide excision does not reduce local recurrence in these patients. It is safe to use 2 cm margins for melanomas 2.01–4 mm thick and it is equally safe to use 1 cm margins for melanomas 1–2 mm thick.

A retrospective study of 214 patients with melanomas more than 4 mm thick compared the outcomes after excision with margins of 2 cm or less (n = 134) and margins more than 2 cm (n = 80) [22]. Although the study was retrospective, the known prognostic factors for melanoma were distributed equally between the two excision margin groups. Local recurrence was defined as disease recurrence within 3 cm of the wide local excision surgical scar. At a median follow-up of 27 months, overall survival and local recurrence rates were not significantly different in the two groups; 11.1% local recurrence after excision margins of 2 cm or less and 12.2% local recurrence after excision margins of > 2 cm. This suggests that 2 cm may be the maximum excision margin required for all melanomas more than 2 mm thick.

Unfortunately, even melanomas < 0.76 mm thick can be fatal [23] and wide excision of melanomas does not improve survival. Wide excision with 4 or 5 cm margins is no guarantee against local recurrence [15,18]. There is no clear evidence that wide excision reduces the risk of local recurrence. The average thickness of melanomas in the WHO trial was about 1 mm and the average thickness of the tumours in the Intergroup trial was 1.96 mm. It is hoped that the Melanoma Study Group/British Association of Plastic Surgeons prospective randomized trial of 1 cm and 3 cm excision margins for melanomas 2 mm or more in thickness will show whether or not wide excision reduces local recurrences of such melanomas or whether 1 cm margins are safe for all primary cutaneous melanomas.

Patients with local recurrence after complete excision of an invasive melanoma usually have a poor prognosis [20]. Local recurrence after complete excision is probably an indicator not a cause of the poor prognosis. Until the 1990s, this was also considered to be true for breast cancer; trials of post-operative radiotherapy for breast cancer showed significant reductions in locoregional recurrences but no significant improvement in overall survival [24]. However, two prospective randomized trials reported in 1997 showed that the addition of radiotherapy to adjuvant chemotherapy after total mastectomy and axillary dissection for high-risk breast cancer not only reduces locoregional recurrences but also improves survival [25,26]. This is not an argument for adjuvant radical surgery for melanoma (unlike radiotherapy in breast cancer it has no proven benefit for either locoregional recurrences or survival) but it is a challenge to oncologists to find effective non-surgical adjuvant treatments for high-risk melanomas.

Subungual and other acral melanomas

On the face, the ears and the distal limbs the debate about narrow and wide excision margins is different because 3 cm skin margins are often not anatomically feasible in these regions.

The skin of the hands and feet, including the palms, soles and nail-beds, can develop the same types of melanoma as the skin in other areas. Acral melanomas are those which occur in the glabrous skin of the hands and feet [27]. In addition to superficial spreading and nodular melanomas, the glabrous skin can also develop acral lentiginous melanoma *in situ* [illegible] and acral lentiginous melanoma [27]. Most acral lentiginous melanomas occur on the soles of the feet. Survival of patients with acral melanomas depends on the same factors as other types of melanoma; acral melanomas tend to have a poor prognosis but this is because they present at an advanced stage. Acral lentiginous melanomas do not have a worse prognosis than other histological types of acral melanoma of the same thickness [27].

Excision of acral melanomas should be based on the same criteria as excision of melanomas in other sites. The defect after even a 1 cm margin excision of a melanoma from the sole of the foot usually requires a skin graft or a local flap or free flap to close it. If a skin graft is used on the foot or elsewhere on the leg, the skin graft can be taken from the same leg so the patient has one leg free from surgery to stand on [28]. Surgical tradition dictated that skin grafts should be taken from the other leg to reduce the risk of metastatic melanoma in the skin graft donor site. However, such metastases are rare and are just as likely to develop in the contralateral limb [28,29]; they are a sign of a poor prognosis.

Subungual melanomas are rare, about 1–3% of all melanomas [30–33]. They occur mainly on the thumb and the great toe. They have a variety of histological features, the most common being acral lentiginous melanoma [30,33]. Subungual melanomas may be amelanotic; in a series of 38 patients in Sydney with subungual melanomas of the hand, 14 cases had amelanotic melanomas [33]. This can lead to a delay in diagnosis and in the Sydney patients lack of pigmentation was the most significant prognostic indicator. Delay in presentation with a thick tumour also makes the prognosis worse for subungual melanomas; the mean tumour thicknesses in three series with a total of 162 patients were 3.05 [33] and 4.7 mm [30,31]. The most common site for recurrence of subungual melanoma is in the regional lymph nodes, as with other cutaneous melanomas [31–33].

The only effective treatment for subungual melanomas is surgery. There is not enough evidence to allow detailed analysis of the surgical options. Amputation through or proximal to the metacarpophalangeal joints of the fingers and thumbs was recommended in early studies of subungual melanoma [33]. Overall survival has not been affected by less radical amputations [31–33]. Recent reports recommend amputation through the neck of the proximal phalanx of the thumb, through the middle phalanx or the proximal interphalangeal joint of the fingers and at or proximal to the metatarsophalangeal joint of the toes [31–35]. With this policy there are a few local recurrences, which emphasizes that it is important not to compromise the excision because of concern about the extent of the amputation. However, local recurrences can also occur with more extensive amputations (e.g. through the metacarpophalangeal joint of the thumb [32] or a metatarsal of the foot [31]). Excision of the primary tumour must at least include the nail-bed and the underlying cortex of the distal phalanx together with a margin of normal tissue. It is possible that more distal excisions may be adequate for selected tumours but there are no long-term studies of such limited surgery.

At many sites, such as the face and distal limbs, defects after excision of malignant melanomas with relatively narrow (1 cm) margins may require reconstructive surgery (e.g. skin grafts or flaps). Even partial amputation of a digit, especially the thumb, can cause major problems with function as well as appearance. Patients with subungual melanomas and other malignant melanomas of the hand should therefore be referred to a surgeon experienced in reconstructive surgery of the hand.

Conclusions

Surgery is curative for most thin primary cutaneous melanomas and for many thicker melanomas.

There is some evidence that excision margins less than 1 cm are safe for melanomas < 0.76 mm thick [36,37]. Although there have been no published long-term follow-up studies of such narrow margins, there is a case for excision of minimally invasive small melanomas with a total margin of 3–5 mm of normal skin, treating them similarly to melanoma *in situ*. However, the WHO trial of 1 cm and 3 cm margins included 112 patients with melanomas 0.1–0.5 mm thick and published guidelines recommend 1 cm margins for these very thin melanomas. For all melanomas > 0.76 mm thick, the minimum excision margin is 1 cm, unless there are anatomical reasons to prevent this. The maximum excision margin for melanomas 1 mm or less in thickness is 1 cm. The Australian guidelines recommend 1 cm as the maximum margin for pT1 and pT2 melanomas up to 1.5 mm thick and others consider that this is also the maximum for melanomas up to 2 mm thick. For melanomas more than 2 mm and up to 4 mm thick, the maximum margin is 2 cm. For melanomas more than 4 mm thick, the maximum recommended margin at present is 3 cm.

Prospective studies are still needed to find out if wide excision has any value in the treatment of primary cutaneous melanomas. The main challenge in the management of the primary tumour is to discover a method of identifying those melanomas which are not cured by surgery and to develop an effective adjuvant treatment for them.

References

1 Skov L, Clemmensen O, Baadsgaard O. Thin cutaneous malignant melanoma and the MIN terminology. *Lancet* 1997; **350**: 1264–5.

2 Bartoli C, Bono A, Clemente C, Del Prato I, Zurrida S, Cascinelli N. Clinical diagnosis and therapy of cutaneous melanoma *in situ*. *Cancer* 1996; **77**: 888–92.

3 National Institutes of Health Consensus Development Panel on Early Melanoma. Diagnosis and treatment of early melanoma. *J Am Med Assoc* 1992; **268**: 1314–19.

4 Australian Cancer Network. *Guidelines for the Management of Cutaneous Melanoma*. Epping: The Stone Press, 1997.

5 Cohen LM. Lentigo maligna and lentigo maligna melanoma. *J Am Acad Dermatol* 1995; **33**: 923–36.

6 Weinstock MA, Sober AJ. The risk of progression of lentigo maligna to lentigo maligna melanoma. *Br J Dermatol* 1987; **116**: 303–10.

7 Timmons MJ. Malignant melanoma excision margins: plastic surgery audit in Britain and Ireland, 1991, and a review. *Br J Plast Surg* 1993; **46**: 525–31.

8 Wong CK. A study of melanocytes in the normal skin surrounding malignant melanomata. *Dermatologica* 1970; **141**: 215–25.

9 Fallowfield ME, Cook MG. Epidermal melanocytes adjacent to melanoma and the field change effect. *Histopathology* 1990; **17**: 397–400.

10 Robinson JK. Margin control for lentigo maligna. *J Am Acad Dermatol* 1994; **31**: 79–85.

11 Lees VC, Briggs JC. Effect of initial biopsy procedure on prognosis in Stage I invasive cutaneous malignant melanoma: review of 1086 patients. *Br J Surg* 1991; **78**: 1108–10.

12 MacKie R, Hunter JAA, Aitchison TC, *et al*. Cutaneous malignant melanoma, Scotland, 1979–89. *Lancet* 1992; **339**: 971–5.

13 Timmons MJ. Malignant melanoma excision margins: making a choice. *Lancet* 1992; **340**: 1393–5.

14 Veronesi U, Cascinelli N. Narrow excision (1-cm margin): a safe procedure for thin cutaneous melanoma. *Arch Surg* 1991; **126**: 438–41.

15 Balch CM, Urist MM, Karakousis CP, *et al*. Efficacy of 2-cm surgical margins for intermediate-thickness melanomas (1 to 4 mm): results of a multi-institutional randomized surgical trial. *Ann Surg* 1993; **218**: 262–9.

16 Kelly JW, Sagebiel RW, Calderon W, Murillo L, Dakin RL, Blois MS. The frequency of local recurrence and microsatellites as a guide to reexcision margins for cutaneous malignant melanoma. *Ann Surg* 1984; **20**: 759–63.

17 Milton GW, Shaw HM, McCarthy WH. Resection margins for melanoma. *Aust NZ J Surg* 1985; **55**: 225–6.

18 Griffiths RW, Briggs JC. Incidence of locally metastatic ('recurrent') cutaneous malignant melanoma following conventional wide margin excisional surgery for invasive clinical stage I tumours: importance of maximal primary tumour thickness. *Br J Surg* 1986; **73**: 349–53.

19 Roses DF, Harris MN, Rigel D, Carrey Z, Friedman R, Kopf AW. Local and in-transit metastases following definitive excision for primary cutaneous malignant melanoma. *Ann Surg* 1983; **198**: 65–9.

20 Ames FC, Balch CM, Reintgen D. Local recurrences and their management. In: Balch CM, Houghton AM, Milton GW, Sober AJ, Soong S-j, eds. *Cutaneous Melanoma*, 2nd edn. Philadelphia: Lippincott, 1992: 287–94.

21 Karakousis CP, Balch CM, Urist MM, Ross MI, Smith TJ, Bartolucci AA. Local recurrence in malignant melanoma: long-term results of the multiinstitutional randomized surgical trial. *Ann Surg Oncol* 1996; **3**: 446–52.

22 Heaton KM, Sussman JJ, Gershenwald JE, *et al*. Surgical margins and prognostic factors in patients with thick (>4 mm) primary melanoma. *Ann Surg Oncol* 1998; **5**: 322–8.

23 Briggs JC, Ibrahim NBN, Hastings AG, Griffiths RW. Experience of thin cutaneous melanomas (<0.76 mm and <0.85 mm thick) in a large plastic surgery unit: a 5 to 17 year follow-up. *Br J Plast Surg* 1984; **37**: 501–6.

24 Fisher B, Anderson S, Fisher ER, *et al*. Significance of ipsilateral breast tumour recurrence after lumpectomy. *Lancet* 1991; **338**: 327–31.

25 Overgaard M, Hansen PS, Overgaard J, *et al*. Postoperative radiotherapy in high-risk premenopausal women with breast cancer who receive adjuvant chemotherapy. *N Engl J Med* 1997; **337**: 949–55.

26 Ragaz J, Jackson SM, Le N, *et al*. Adjuvant radiotherapy and chemotherapy in node-positive premenopausal women with breast cancer. *N Engl J Med* 1997; **337**: 956–62.

27 Slingluff CL, Vollmer R, Seigler HF. Acral melanoma: a review of 185 patients with identification of prognostic variables. *J Surg Oncol* 1990; **45**: 91–8.

28 Flook D, Horgan K, Taylor BA, Hughes LE. Surgery for malignant melanoma: from which limb should the graft be taken? *Br J Surg* 1986; **73**: 793–5.

29 McLean NR, Boorman JG. Secondary malignant melanoma arising in a contralateral thigh donor site. *Br J Plast Surg* 1984; **37**: 386–7.

30 Rigby HS, Briggs JC. Subungual melanoma: a clinico-pathological study of 24 cases. *Br J Plast Surg* 1992; **45**: 275–8.

31 Park KGM, Blessing K, Kernohan NM. Surgical aspects of subungual malignant melanomas. *Ann Surg* 1992; **216**: 692–5.

32 Heaton KN, El-Naggar A, Ensign LG,

Ross MI, Balch CM. Surgical management and prognostic factors in patients with subungual melanoma. *Ann Surg* 1994; **219**: 197–204.

33 Quinn MJ, Thompson JE, Crotty K, McCarthy WH, Coates AS. Subungual melanoma of the hand. *J Hand Surg* 1996; **21A**: 506–11.

34 Ross MI, Balch CM. Surgical treatment of primary melanoma. In: Balch CM, Houghton AN, Sober AJ, Soong S-j, eds. *Cutaneous Melanoma*, 3rd edn. St.Louis: Quality Medical Publishing, 1998: 141–53.

35 Hayes IM, Thompson JF, Quinn MJ. Malignant melanoma of the toenail apparatus. *J Am Coll Surg* 1995; **180**: 583–8.

36 Breslow A, Macht SD. Optimal size of resection margin for thin cutaneous melanoma. *Surg Gynecol Obstet* 1977; **145**: 691–2.

37 Evans J, McCann BG. A new protocol for the treatment of stage I cutaneous malignant melanoma: interim results of the first 806 patients treated. *Br J Plast Surg* 1990; **43**: 426–30.

11: Imaging and investigation of melanoma patients

Razvan A. Popescu, Poulam M. Patel and John Spencer

Introduction

The incidence of cutaneous malignant melanoma continues to rise rapidly, increasing demands on evaluation and treatment at diagnosis. As a larger proportion of patients is being identified earlier in their disease [1], with better outcomes, the prevalence of individuals with a past history of melanoma is also increasing. In an increasingly financially restricted medical environment, optimal strategies for staging, treatment and follow-up are needed.

This chapter addresses issues of diagnostic imaging in malignant melanoma. Other investigations, such as blood tests, are not discussed, except in relation to imaging. Routine blood tests, although frequently ordered both for staging and surveillance of this disease [2], have been shown to contribute little in their own right to detection of melanoma metastases in patients with thin and intermediate thickness melanoma [3–5]. Recommendations on their usefulness, particularly of lactate dehydrogenase (LDH), a relatively inexpensive test, diverge [3–8].

Cutaneous malignant melanoma is almost always diagnosed by physical examination followed by pathological analysis of the primary tumour, and diagnostic imaging rarely contributes to diagnosis. The radiological contribution to the management of this disease lies in the initial staging of the disease, assessment of response to therapy and in monitoring freedom from relapse (surveillance). The entire spectrum of imaging techniques has been used. This chapter addresses some particular aspects of imaging techniques in melanoma and then discusses the current evidence for use of these techniques according to stage of disease and pertinent risk factors. We aim to provide a rational and practical approach to familiar clinical situations, recognizing that contradictory research evidence and clinical experience will always result in some controversy and variation in practice.

Imaging in melanoma

Over recent years a range of new imaging modalities has become available, complementing conventional radiological procedures. Technological improvements in apparatus and novel scanning techniques have increased the level of definition of established techniques, such as ultrasound, computed tomography (CT) and magnetic resonance imaging (MRI). Imaging modalities such as scintigraphy, single proton emission computed tomography (SPECT) and, more recently, positron emission tomography (PET) which rely on differences in metabolism and function, complement the anatomical imaging techniques.

Chest radiography is a widely available and inexpensive test. It is reasonable for all patients who require staging to have a baseline chest radiograph. If lung metastases are shown this may serve to assess response (Fig. 11.1).

Abdominal ultrasound is also widely available and may be used to assess the liver, spleen and upper abdominal lymph nodes. Some retroperitoneal sites and the pelvic sidewall are difficult to assess. Ultrasound is an operator-dependent technique.

The ability to examine large tissue volumes rapidly and reproducibly makes CT the preferred option for staging patients with metastatic disease and in clinical trials. It also facilitates external review of imaging. However, it imposes a significant radiation burden on patients.

MRI produces unrivalled soft tissue contrast and allows multiplanar imaging. It may be particularly helpful for characterizing melanoma

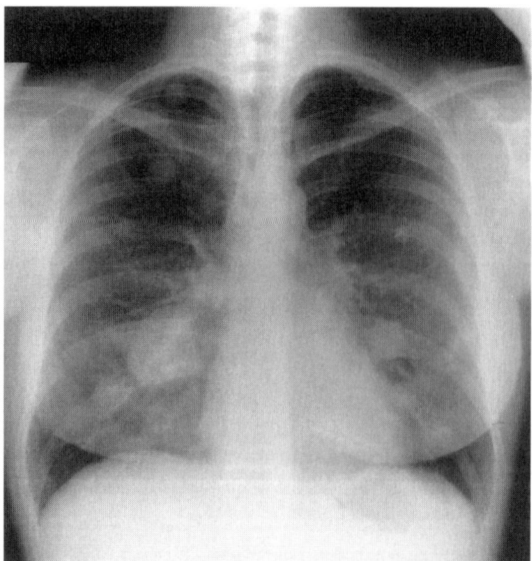

Fig. 11.1 Chest radiograph showing multiple pulmonary metastases, many exceeding 5 mm in size. In such a patient chest radiography could be used for follow-up.

metastases as the paramagnetic effect of melanin results in high T1 and low–intermediate T2 signal. It is not widely available and is best reserved as a problem solving tool or for site specific indications defined by multidisciplinary discussion (e.g. for head and neck melanomas).

Nuclear medicine has had little clinical impact on management of melanoma. Exclusion of skeletal metastases is not part of routine staging but is best performed by scintigraphy. Recent reports of PET scanning in melanoma patients are promising but at present access to PET scanning is even more limited than for MRI.

Factors influencing choice of imaging modalities

Decisions regarding investigation of melanoma require knowledge of its natural history and prognostic factors and an understanding of the prevalence of lymph node or visceral metastases in the various populations at risk. Furthermore, choice of imaging modalities will depend on their technical limitations, their local availability, the expertise in their use and, importantly, the safety and convenience for and tolerance by the patient. Choice will be a reflection of the type and extent of information that is sought, as well as its clinical context and impact.

In deciding the type and extent of information required, there is an essential difference between detection and characterization of radiological abnormalities. With modern cross-sectional imaging, detection of very small lesions is possible but their characterization is difficult. Multiplicity of lesions often indicates metastatic disease but in the lungs granulomas from prior infection may produce identical findings. Indeterminate small lesions bedevil radiologists. In the liver, small cysts and haemangiomas may be indistinguishable from metastases. If such lesions were present on comparable imaging studies prior to the diagnosis of melanoma or are stable over more than 6 months, this usually indicates benignity. Another test or biopsy may be useful to further characterize indeterminate lesions, and these options should be discussed in multidisciplinary reviews. Frequently one is left with watchful waiting to see how lesions progress.

The number and extent of investigations required depends on the clinical context. With clinically obvious stage IV disease, a chest radiograph may be sufficient to identify disease that can act as a marker of response to palliative treatment. When the treatment considered is radical excision of distant metastases, the patient requires exhaustive exclusion of other disease using the most accurate tests available.

It is important to understand some of the terms used in test analysis, including prevalence, sensitivity, specificity, positive and negative predictive value, likelihood ratios and accuracy. The prevalence (prior probability) of a characteristic is the proportion of patients with that characteristic in the total patient population studied. The test sensitivity is the likelihood that a patient with the disease would have a positive test, while the specificity is the probability that patients without the disease would have negative test results. The positive predictive value reflects the proportion of true-positive test results in all positive test results, while the negative predictive value reflects the proportion of true-negative test results in all negative test results. Both sensitivity and specificity of imaging tests depend on often arbitrarily chosen thresholds, above which disease is considered present and below which it is considered absent. This threshold represents a compromise.

Consider an impalpable regional lymph node identified by CT in a patient with melanoma. A threshold of 10 mm for maximum short axis dimension is widely used. Some nodes smaller than the threshold size will harbour microscopic metastasis; others larger than it will be reactive benign nodes. Thresholds used may vary with treatment intent. If the unit policy were only to remove nodes definitely considered metastatic, a higher threshold would be appropriate. This would improve specificity (reduce the number of reactive nodes removed). If the unit policy were for aggressive removal of all potentially metastatic nodes, use of a lower threshold would improve sensitivity—but reduce specificity. This relationship between sensitivity and specificity can be evaluated by developing a receiver-operated characteristic (ROC) curve, which displays the changing ratios of sensitivity and specificity as the threshold changes. Sensitivity and specificity not only depend on thresholds used to define abnormality—and the technical limitations of the imaging modality—but also on the population in which they are defined. Finally, post test probabilities are greatly influenced by prevalence (prior probability) of a characteristic, and thus the usefulness of detecting metastatic disease even for the most sensitive test available will *a priori* be very limited in patient populations where this finding is rare, for instance in stage I patients. For a further discussion of test analysis we refer the reader to the pertinent texts [9,10].

Prior probabilities are defined by known prognostic factors, which given their clinical relevance are incorporated in staging systems. The most important prognostic factors in melanoma are pathological parameters of the primary tumour: depth of invasion and presence or absence of ulceration. The Breslow thickness is thought to be more reproducible than the level of invasion according to Clark, and a more powerful prognostic indicator. The analyses of Vollmer [11], Balch [12], Morton *et al.* [13], Buttner *et al.* [14] and, more recently, Buzaid *et al.* [15] have confirmed that there is a continuous correlation between tumour thickness and survival. Grouping patients according to Breslow thickness of 1, 2 and 4 mm was suggested to correlate better with outcome [14], and these values were proposed as prognostically more relevant cut-off points for the new 2001 AJCC staging system [15]. Ulceration was shown to have a significantly adverse effect, especially in very thin or thick lesions [11,12].

For patients with regional lymph node involvement, the most powerful prognostic factor reported is the number of involved lymph nodes rather than their size [16]. Until recently, for most patients assessment of lymph node involvement was clinical, but some centres now perform sentinel lymph node dissection in patients with thick primary tumours, because the prevalence of lymph node involvement is greatest in these patients. In series reporting outcome of clinically N0 patients with primaries of 4 mm or thicker, pathologically N0 patients have, not surprisingly, been shown to have a better outcome than pathologically N1 patients and the entire cohort [15]. In-transit and satellite metastases have similar prognostic significance to nodal metastases [15]. The number of metastatic sites and their location (e.g. visceral involvement), remission duration and LDH as a measure of disease burden are important factors in patients with metastatic melanoma [17].

All these prognostic factors have been used with various cut-offs to generate probabilities for survival and disease recurrence rates. They can also be used to guide decisions about the need for and extent of staging and surveillance imaging.

Staging and surveillance of melanoma patients

Pathological information from the primary tumour (Breslow thickness and presence or absence of ulceration) and clinical information of lymph node status are the main parameters on which further staging investigations are based.

The ideal staging process requires the use of the best imaging modalities available using the fewest steps. Staging works best when there are agreed protocols that work for the majority of patients but are flexible enough to accommodate unusual presentations of disease. Both clinician and radiologist must recognize the limitations and weaknesses of their investigation protocols. Currently, wide variations occur in the use of imaging studies in the treatment of malignant melanoma for staging and follow-up [2].

Stage I and II melanoma

Staging

Most patients with melanoma present with stage I or II disease according to the American Joint Committee on Cancer (AJCC) 1992 classification based on the characteristics of the primary tumour on pathological analysis and clinical examination of locoregional skin and lymph nodes. Five-year median survival rates for stage I and II disease are 85 and 65%, respectively [16]. Thus in many patients, micrometastases are already present at the time of resection.

A careful history and complete medical examination, as well as full blood count, electrolytes and creatinine, liver function tests and LDH are often determined at the first clinic visit. Various investigative procedures have been used in staging these patients, including chest radiographs, radionuclide scanning, upper gastrointestinal series and barium enemas, as well as, more recently, abdominal sonography, CT of chest, abdomen, pelvis or brain and MRI. It is vital that the radiologist is fully appraised of the surgery performed prior to staging. Various groups have retrospectively assessed the value of these imaging tests in asymptomatic patients.

In an early study [18], the records of 393 patients seen at the Princess Margaret Hospital in Toronto between 1978 and 1982 were reviewed. Of these, 347 had tumours thinner than 4 mm. A total of 969 imaging investigations were performed at presentation and during follow-up in asymptomatic patients with normal physical examinations. Of these, 67 were false-positive and only two bipedal lymphangiograms were true-positive. Over a median follow-up of 3 years, 64 recurrences were detected, of which 58 by clinical examination and six by chest radiographs. Imaging investigations included 337 chest radiographs (8 false-positives), 169 whole lung tomograms, 187 liver–spleen scans, 109 bone scans (7 false-positives), 50 chest CTs (9 false-positive) and 51 CTs of the brain. The investigators reviewed previous data on usefulness of chest radiographs, lung tomography, radionuclide scanning, upper gastrointestinal series and barium enemas, intravenous pyelograms, and considered this together with their own results and concluded that these investigations are not helpful in initial staging of patients with malignant melanoma. They suggested that initial staging should be restricted to history and physical examination, together with chest radiograph.

Terhune *et al.* [19] retrospectively analysed 876 of 1032 (85%) asymptomatic patients with localized melanoma who had an initial staging chest radiograph performed. Of these, 130 (15%) of patients had suspicious findings, but follow-up radiological findings suggested that only 1 of 876 (0.1%) had a true-positive chest radiograph demonstrating lung metastasis. Here is a key example where prevalence (prior probability) of true disease was very low and thus 'positive' findings were more likely to be false than true. Of note is that the vast majority of patients (836) had melanomas thinner than 4 mm. Addition of lateral chest radiographs to the standard posteroanterior chest radiograph is not of value in staging or surveillance of melanoma [20].

Buzaid *et al.* [21] retrospectively evaluated the role of CT of chest and abdomen in 151 patients seen in the Yale Melanoma Unit between 1984 and 1991, of which 63 were AJCC clinical stage I, 61 were stage II (14 patients

T4N0) and 23 were stage III. Investigations were ordered as part of adjuvant study protocols, at patients' insistence or at the discretion of the attending physician, but all patients were asymptomatic, had normal physical examinations and routine blood tests including LDH. Twenty-nine patients (19%) had scans considered suspicious for metastases, most abnormalities being single liver lesions or lung nodules. In eight patients, invasive diagnostic procedures were performed, the others were followed up with repeat CT scans or liver ultrasound. Two patients had true-positive findings, and in three others a second primary tumour was diagnosed (two lymphomas, one stage I renal cell carcinoma). The other 21 abnormalities on scan were false-positive. Of the 124 patients with stage I and II disease, one had cervical lymph node involvement that was undetected clinically, and none had distant organ metastases by CT, although four patients eventually had disease recurrence in regional lymph nodes and 26 developed distant metastases. Of 23 patients with stage III disease, four regional and nine of 10 distant metastases which subsequently developed were not detected by CT scans. Retrospective review of all scans in patients who relapsed failed to show any false-negative scans. The authors concluded that CT scans were not useful in detecting a significant number of occult metastases in asymptomatic patients at initial staging, and that abnormalities were more likely to represent other pathology or benign changes.

In these studies of patients with stage I and II disease the number with deeply invasive non-metastatic melanomas (>4 mm, stage IIB) is small, reflecting their rarity. Some clinicians regard these patients at high risk of developing distant metastases although data on the usefulness of imaging remains limited. When management of such patients is similar to those with stage III disease it is reasonable that investigation reflects this.

Surveillance

Surveillance recommendations for patients with thin or intermediate thickness melanomas without clinical lymph node involvement have varied [3–8,22–25] and their discussion is beyond the scope of this chapter, except for some general comments about usefulness of investigations. Blood tests have not been found to be the sole indicators of relapse [3,4] and may be unnecessary for thin melanomas. Most recurrences were detected by constitutional symptoms or locoregional recurrence that was noted on physical examination [4,5]. When repeatedly instructed about symptoms and signs of recurrence, patients themselves detected melanoma recurrences in the vast majority of cases [26]. In two series, imaging revealed only one-tenth of recurrences. Out of 528 patients with stage I melanoma undergoing regular follow-up [4], 115 recurred. Six recurrences were only picked up by chest radiograph and six by abdominal ultrasound, but in only one patient was curative resection recommended. The authors calculated that the cost to detect one metastasis was 9, 20 or 36 times higher when chest radiograph, abdominal ultrasound or both were used, as compared to regular clinical examination. Weiss *et al.* [3] investigated how recurrence was diagnosed in 145 patients treated in a clinical study. In 99 patients (68%) symptoms signalled the recurrence of disease, and physical examination of asymptomatic patients led to the detection of recurrence in 37 patients (26%). Only nine patients (6%) with recurrent disease had abnormal chest radiographs.

A retrospective analysis of 1004 patients with stage I or II malignant melanoma treated at Roswell Park Cancer Institute between 1971 and 1995 analysed impact of method of recurrence detection on survival [5]. Of note in this series only 7% of patients had AJCC pT4 tumours. Constitutional symptoms heralded 17% of 154 recurrences, physical examination 72% (over half patients detected) and chest radiograph 11% (17 patients). Overall survival curves were superimposable for patients who detected their recurrence themselves and those whose recurrence was detected by the physician. Survival was identical in patients whose pulmonary recurrence was picked up by chest radiograph or by symptoms. However, nine of the 17 patients with recurrences detected by chest radiograph alone underwent curative surgical excision with median survival of 24 months from diagnosis of recurrence, compared to 15 months in patients who received chemotherapy for unresectable disease. We estimate that, for the 1004 patients followed up according to protocol for a median of 6.1 years, with 174 recurring at a median of 2.5 years and 830 patients not recurring during reported follow-up, over 10 000 chest radiograph investigations would have been performed to detect the 17 recurrences. Although the patient dose from a single chest radiograph is minimal, the cumulative dosage over the study period for say 10 radiographs is not. Unfortunately, no information was provided about false-positive chest radiograph results and the follow-up investigations to clarify those further.

The risk of recurrence and death from melanoma can be calculated for patients according to the thickness of their primary lesion, and has been reported as a function of time since diagnosis [23–29]. For all melanomas, the risks of first recurrence and death are highest in the first years following excision and fall gradually over the next 10 years. However, a small risk of death from melanoma relapse persists at 10 years for even the thinnest melanomas. Most recurrences are diagnosed by physical examination and the patients can be taught to perform this proficiently themselves [26]. To date there are no prospective studies to assess the use of imaging in follow-up, and so the use of imaging in surveillance will ultimately depend on clinicians' interpretation of the published retrospective data and available financial resources. The published evidence argues strongly against follow-up imaging of any sort in patients with stage I and II disease.

Stage III melanoma

Staging

Sentinel node dissection (SND) is increasingly used to determine pathological nodal status in patients with intermediate or thick primaries. The rationale of SND is the demonstration of orderly progression of melanoma nodal metastases, coupled with the ability to identify the first draining node using intraoperative lymphatic mapping guided by vital blue dye or radiolymphoscintigraphy. SND is now variously accepted as standard practice in Europe and the USA, but most studies of the value of imaging in stage III patients have included patients that were conventionally staged, rather than by SND.

Patients with clinical lymph node involvement by melanoma often have thicker primaries and their risk of harbouring further metastases is substantially higher than for stage I and II patients. Buzaid *et al.* [30] were the first to analyse the value of staging CT scans in patients with lymph node involvement at diagnosis or first recurrence. They reviewed the records of 89 asymptomatic patients with stage III disease and with normal LDH and chest radiograph who underwent staging CTs. A further 10 patients were described who were excluded from analysis based on either symptoms suggestive of distant disease, raised LDH or positive chest radiograph. Overall, even in group of 'high risk' patients, the positive predictive value of CT was less than 25%. True-positive findings were seen in six patients, false-positive in 20 and true-negative in 63 patients.

Kuvshinoff *et al.* [31] published the Memorial Sloan Kettering experience with 347 asymptomatic patients, of which 136 had CT scans of chest, abdomen and pelvis. A total of 788 scan results were analysed retrospectively, with 33 (4.3%) confirmed instances of metastatic melanoma and 66 (8.4%) false-positives. Body CT scans further identified five second primaries, four at early stages. When only the patients who had combined scans of chest, abdomen and pelvis were analysed separately, the overall yield was of 11 true-positive scans (8.1%) for melanoma and three for second primaries. When patients with abnormal LDH or chest radiograph were excluded, the diagnostic yield for melanoma was 4.4% (or for melanoma and second primaries 5.9%). Management of nine of 14 patients with positive findings was altered by the CT findings, and in three patients a complete resection of identified tumour was possible. Pertinently, the authors also analysed the diagnostic yield of scans as affected by the location of the primary tumour. Pelvic scans were of no use for primaries above the diaphragm, and the yield of chest scans was lowest for patients with lower extremity primaries and inguinal lymphadenopathy.

A further study analysed the value of CT in detecting neck node metastases in patients with thin and intermediate thickness head or neck melanoma [32]. Twenty-six patients, of whom 18 had clinically involved lymph nodes, had CT evaluation before undergoing neck dissections. Although the diagnostic accuracy was greater than palpation, in seven patients small nodal metastases were missed on the scan when pathology data were reviewed.

Recently, the use of 2-fluoro-2-deoxyglucose (FDG)-PET scanning was reported for detection of melanoma metastases [33,34]. Although access to PET is at present limited, it is a promising tool in staging of melanoma which appears to have a higher sensitivity and specificity than CT. Between 1994 and 1996, 100 patients with melanomas thicker than 1.5 mm underwent an extensive staging programme [33], consisting of chest radiograph, abdominal ultrasound and high-resolution sonography of regional nodes, CT of chest and abdomen and MRI of the brain, together with whole body PET scans. Overall, sensitivity, specificity and accuracy of PET (91.8, 94.4 and 92.1%, respectively) were significantly higher than for conventional imaging, the other modalities combined (57.5, 45 and 55.7%, respectively). PET was superior in imaging of lymph nodes, abdomen and mediastinum, while CT was superior for definition of lung nodules. The authors concluded that a single PET scan would replace all other conventional imaging techniques for staging malignant melanoma. One reason for the superiority of PET is that metabolic changes often precede morphological changes, and foci of melanoma smaller than the threshold above which disease is considered present on CT already are visualized by PET imaging. Superior sensitivity (94.2%) and specificity (83.3%) for PET scans compared to CT (55.3 and 84.4%, respectively) is also claimed by another group [34], who indicated 5 mm as the threshold of detection melanoma size.

FDG-PET staging of regional lymph nodes prior to SND was investigated. In contrast to an earlier report [35], Wagner *et al.* [36] claimed that PET was an insensitive indicator of occult nodal disease in 70 patients when compared to histological results of SND and clinical course. Sensitivity was merely 16.7%, with median tumour volume of 4.3 mm^3. However, specificity was very good (95.8%), which may be of relevance in those centres where SND is not routinely performed, as this makes FDG-PET still the most accurate non-invasive method of lymph node assessment.

Surveillance

Patients with AJCC stage III melanoma have a chance of relapse of approximately two-thirds, with two-thirds of those occurring at distant sites [37]. Furthermore, the majority of relapses occur early. Surveillance practice varies widely [2] and involves use of chest radiograph, CT of chest, abdomen, pelvis and brain or MRI. There may be benefits in early detection of recurrence, and preliminary reports on earlier identification of relapse in high-risk patients followed up by PET scans than conventional imaging are encouraging. It is to be hoped that prospective randomized studies evaluating clinical and survival impact of PET surveillance compared to conventional follow-up will be forthcoming.

Stage IV melanoma

Staging and response assessment

As curative approaches to patients with extensive melanoma spread are lacking, for some patients receiving conventional treatment assessment by chest radiograph or abdominal ultrasound may be sufficient. Differential responses are rare, and extrapolation of response in the imaged metastases to the others is reasonable. For monitoring of response, reproducibility is of key importance, and thus repeat imaging should be the same as initial evaluation. More extensive imaging may be required for patients treated in the context of clinical studies.

The ability to examine large tissue volumes rapidly and reproducibly makes CT the preferred option. MRI may be useful as a problem solving tool or for specific indications (e.g. cord compression, leptomeningeal metastasis). The role of PET is unclear in patients with evident metastases.

For some treatment regimens, toxicity may result from treatment of unsuspected brain metastases. These patients will usually be investigated with contrast enhanced CT of the body and examination of the brain at the end of the body examination suffices to assess metastatic disease.

Problem solving by multidisciplinary meeting

For most patients the information provided from imaging will confirm the clinical impression of disease activity and extent. For a few there are discrepancies or other problems requiring clinicopathoradiological discussion. Such discussion works best within a multidisciplinary team which meets regularly to review problem cases. An understanding of the sites and appearance of melanoma metastases is key to their recognition (e.g. advanced melanoma may spread to uncommon sites, such as spleen and muscle) (Figs 11.2 and 11.3). Familiarity with these patterns avoids investigation for alternative causes.

What are the options for dealing with uncertainty? Often the fuller discussion within the multidisciplinary meeting of the clinical problem suffices. As discussed, imaging involves first detection of abnormalities and then their

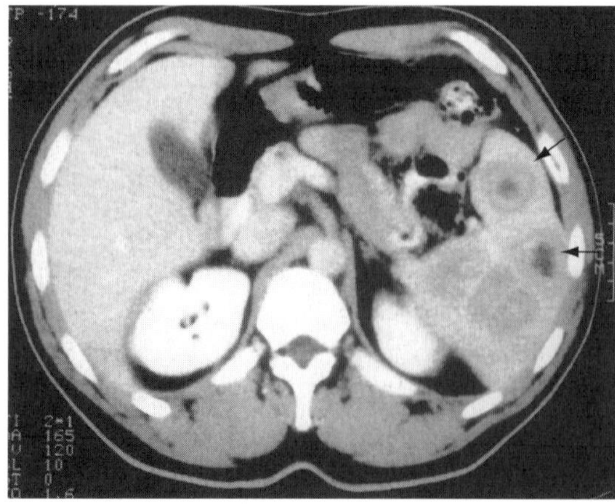

Fig. 11.2 Contrast enhanced upper abdominal CT showing splenic metastases (arrows).

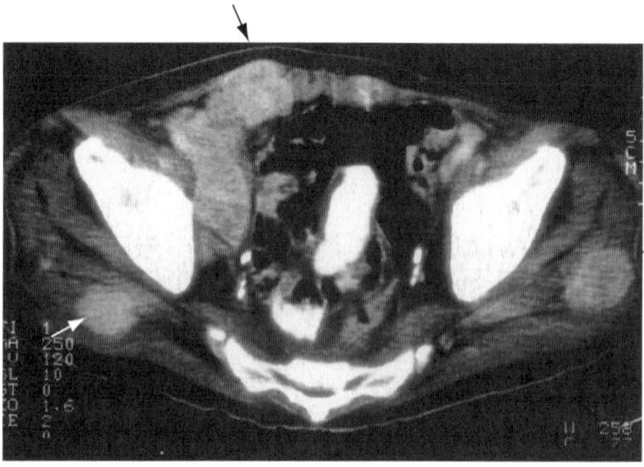

Fig. 11.3 Contrast enhanced pelvic CT showing left inguinal nodal metastases (arrows) and unsuspected bilateral buttock metastases.

characterization. However, the characterization has a clinical context and management impact. Thus, if a lesion is detected which might be metastatic in a patient already committed to systemic chemotherapy, its characterization would not alter management. However, its characterization is important to determine context; would such treatment be in an adjuvant or metastatic setting?

Definitive characterization requires histological analysis following surgical excision or image guided biopsy. Only a positive biopsy result is reliable, as sampling error as well as technical failure may result in false-negative findings. In certain circumstances, addition of another imaging test may be diagnostic. In staging it is usual to use the best and most rapid methods for detection and characterization of metastatic disease but there is a compromise to be reached between using many specialized tests or a single multipurpose examination (e.g. CT). MRI is a valuable supplementary test for melanoma metastases as they may have characteristic high signal on T1-weighted images (Fig. 11.4).

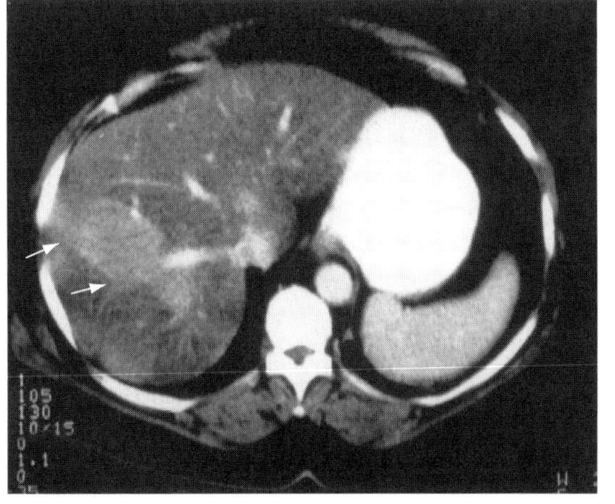
(a)

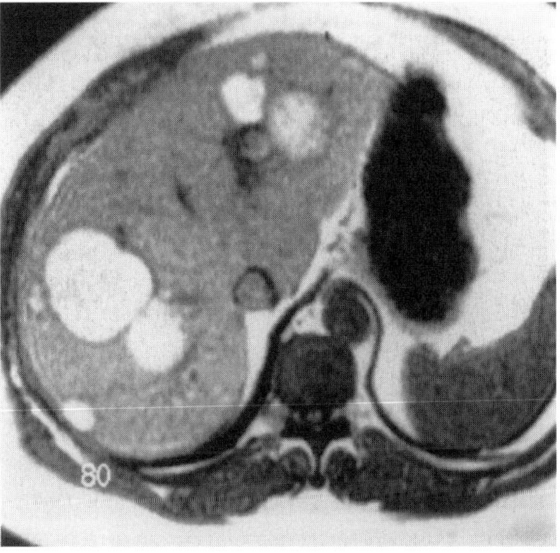

(b)

Fig. 11.4 (a) Contrast enhanced upper abdominal CT showing hyperdense liver metastases (arrows); and (b) contemporaneous T1-weighted MRI of the liver at a similar level showing high signal change within these and additional lesions not seen with CT. Diagnosis: melanoma metastases in a patient with a previous breast cancer and melanoma.

If the nature of abnormalities cannot be ascertained by any of these methods—or if biopsy is considered too invasive—the other option is a wait and watch policy. This is particularly suitable when a patient is asymptomatic or when active management would not be prejudiced by a delay in characterization—during which interval the lesion may grow or others may appear. Small pulmonary nodules can cause problems of characterization for CT (Fig. 11.5) as well as chest radiography. Other common indeterminate lesions are subcentimetre liver nodules which could represent benign entities (cyst, haemangioma) and adrenal nodules.

Recommendations for use of imaging in melanoma patients

For patients not treated or followed up in the context of clinical trials, imaging

(a)

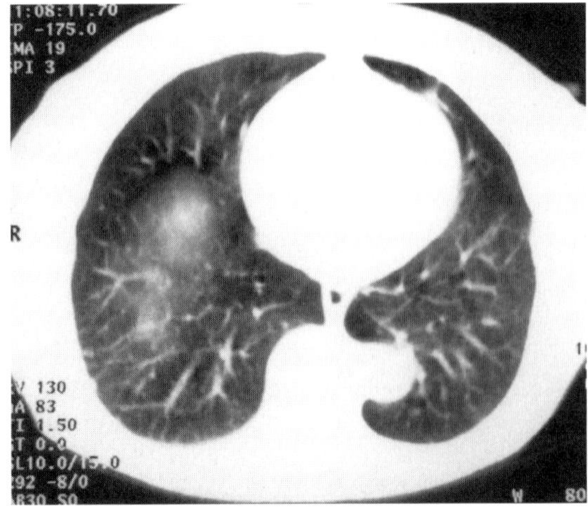

(b)

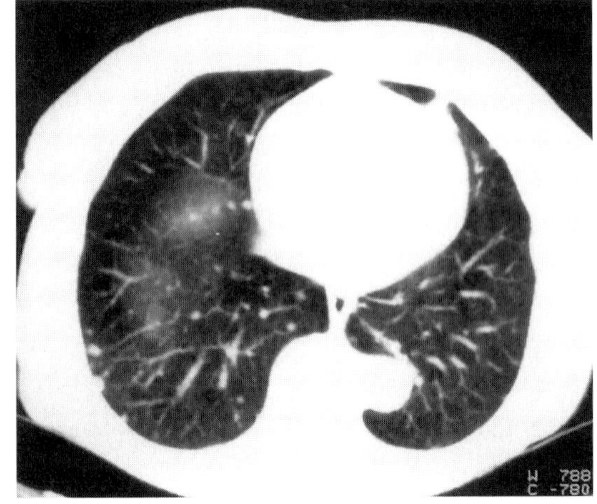

Fig. 11.5 Lung CT showing: (a) indeterminate subpleural nodules; and (b) after 2 months of observation showing an increase in the size and number of nodules suggesting metastatic disease.

protocols should be based on the prevalence of metastases in the corresponding risk group, based on pathological criteria for the primary lesion and in-transit, satellite and locoregional lymph node metastases (Table 11.1). There are few prospective trials that allow estimates of sensitivity and specificity of imaging modalities in the various risk groups, and these are urgently needed.

In the past, increasing availability and perceived higher sensitivity of newer imaging techniques led to their use in many patients with melanoma in the absence of any evidence that they improve staging and outcome in early stage melanoma. There is little evidence to support use of any radiological investigations in patients with thin melanoma. For stage I and IIA melanomas (primary tumours <4 mm thickness), chest radiograph and CT scans have a poor ratio of true-positive : false-positive findings. Stage I patients do not benefit from any form of imaging for staging, while use of chest radiograph and

Table 11.1 Practical recommendations for initial staging investigations

Stage	Location of primary tumour	Recommendation
I, IIA	Any	Chest radiograph as baseline If abnormal repeat in 2–3 months. No other imaging unless clearly abnormal film with high index of suspicion
IIB, III	Head and neck	CT chest* CT neck if no lymph node dissection planned
IIB, III	Thorax, upper extremities	CT chest*, liver No indication for CT pelvis
IIB, III	Lower torso, lower extremities	CT chest*, abdomen and pelvis
IV	Any	CT chest*, abdomen and pelvis *or* Chest radiograph and abdominal ultrasound

* Also chest radiograph if metastases > 1 cm present, as this may substitute for follow-up.
Abbreviation: CT, computed tomography.

CT scans for stage II is controversial and both diagnostic accuracy and yield are poor. We thus recommend that these patients have a baseline chest radiograph only, against which future suspected relapse can be assessed. Occasionally, clear-cut pulmonary metastases will be revealed. More likely, indeterminate nodules will be found and will require a repeat radiograph in 2–3 months.

Patients with melanomas thicker than 4 mm (stage IIB) have a higher risk of subclinical metastases. There are thus grounds to investigate them similarly to clinical stage III but at present principally in the context of clinical trials. More data are required on the use of imaging in staging and surveillance of stage IIB disease.

For asymptomatic stage III patients with normal baseline blood tests, chest radiograph and CT tailored to the primary site seem warranted, given that these investigations will pick up clinically occult disease in 10–20% of patients. This is the group of patients who may be offered adjuvant interferon therapy, a toxic and expensive treatment, justifying the need to exclude metastatic disease. PET scans, where available, may be a better tool than CT for staging and surveillance in these high-risk patients.

Choice of imaging modality in patients with distant metastases will be informed by the goals of treatment, either radical or palliative.

References

1 Balch CM, Reintgen DS, Kirkwood JM, *et al.* In: de Vita VT, Hellman S, Rosenberg SA, eds. *Cancer Principles and Practice of Oncology,* 5th edn. Philadelphia: Lippincott-Raven, 1997; 1947–94.

2 Provost N, Marghoob AA, Kopf AW, DeDavid M, Wasti Q, Bart RS. Laboratory tests and imaging studies in patients with cutaneous malignant melanomas: a survey of experienced physicians. *J Am Acad Dermatol* 1997; **36**: 711–20.

3 Weiss M, Loprinzi CL, Creagan ET, Dalton RJ, Novotny P, O'Fallon JR. Utility of follow-up tests for detecting recurrent disease in patients with malignant melanomas. *J Am Med Assoc* 1995; **274**: 1703–5.

4 Basseres N, Grob JJ, Richard MA, *et al.* Cost-effectiveness of surveillance of stage I melanoma: a retrospective appraisal based on a 10-year experience in a dermatology department in France. *Dermatology* 1995; **191**: 199–203.

5 Mooney MM, Kulas M, McKinley B, Michalek AM, Kraybill WG. Impact on survival by method of recurrence detection in stage I and II cutaneous melanoma. *Ann Surg Oncol* 1998; **5**: 54–63.

6 Rumke P, van Everdingen JE. Consensus on the management of melanoma of the skin in the Netherlands, Dutch Melanoma Working Party. *Eur J Cancer* 1992; **28** (2–3): 600–4.

7 Orfanos CE, Jung EG, Rassner G, Wolff HH, Garbe C. Position and recommendations of the Malignant Melanoma Committee of the German Society of Dermatology on diagnosis, treatment and after-care of malignant melanoma of the skin. Status 1993–94. *Hautarzt* 1994; **45**: 285–91.

8 Ross MI. Staging evaluation and surveillance for melanoma patients in a fiscally restrictive medical environment: a commentary [Review with 43 references]. *Surg Clin North Am* 1996; **76**: 1423–32.

9 Sackett DJ, Haynes RB, Guyatt GH, *et al.* *Clinical Epidemiology: A Basic Science for Clinical Medicine*, 2nd edn. London: Little, Brown, 1991.

10 Kuhns LR, Thornbury JR, Fryback DG. *Decision Making in Imaging*. Chicago: Yearbook Medical, 1989.

11 Vollmer RT. Malignant melanoma: a multivariate analysis of prognostic factors. *Pathol Annu* 1989; **24**: 383–407.

12 Balch CM. Cutaneous melanoma: prognosis and treatment results worldwide. *Semin Surg Oncol* 1992; **8**: 400–14.

13 Morton DL, Davtyan D, Wanek LA. Multivariate analysis of the relationship between survival and the microstage of primary melanoma by Clark level and Breslow thickness. *Cancer* 1993; **71**: 3737–43.

14 Buttner P, Garbe C, Bertz J, *et al.* Primary cutaneous melanoma: optimized cutoff points of tumor thickness and importance of Clark's level for prognostic classification. *Cancer* 1995; **75**: 2499–506.

15 Balch CM, Buzaid AC, Soong S *et al.* Final version of the American Joint Committee on cancer staging system for cutaneous melanoma. *J Clin Oncol* 2001; **19**: 3635–48.

16 Balch CM, Soong S, Shaw HM, Balch CM, Houghton AN, Milton GW, eds. An analysis of prognostic factors in 8500 patients with cutaneous melanoma. In: *Cutaneous Melanoma*, 2nd edn. Philadelphia: Lippincott Co, 1992: 439–67.

17 Barth A, Wanek LA, Morton DL. Prognostic factors in 1521 melanoma patients with distant metastases. *J Am Coll Surg* 1995; **181**: 193.

18 Kersey PA, Iscoe NA, Gapski JA, *et al.* The value of staging and serial follow-up investigations in patients with completely resected, primary, cutaneous malignant melanoma. *Br J Surg* 1985; **72**: 614–7.

19 Terhune MH, Swanson N, Johnson TM. Use of chest radiography in the initial evaluation of patients with localized melanoma [see comments]. *Arch Dermatol* 1998; **134**: 569–72.

20 Collins CD, Padley SP, Greenwell F, Phelan M. The efficacy of a single posteroanterior radiograph in the assessment of metastatic pulmonary melanoma. *Br J Radiol* 1993; **66**: 117–19.

21 Buzaid AC, Sandler AB, Mani S, *et al.* Role of computed tomography in the

staging of primary melanoma. *J Clin Oncol* 1993; **11**: 638–43.
22 Moloney DM, Gordon DJ, Briggs JC, Rigby HS. Recurrence of thin melanoma: how effective is follow-up? *Br J Plast Surg* 1996; **49**: 409–13.
23 Mooney MM, Mettlin C, Michalek AM, Petrelli NJ, Kraybill WG. Life-long screening of patients with intermediate-thickness cutaneous melanoma for asymptomatic pulmonary recurrences: a cost-effectiveness analysis. *Cancer* 1997; **80**: 1052–64.
24 Johnson RC, Fenn NJ, Horgan K, Mansel RE. Follow-up of patients with a thin melanoma. *Br J Surg* 1999; **86**: 619–21.
25 Kanzler MH. Initial evaluation of melanoma: don't stop getting that chest X- ray . . . Yet [letter]. *Arch Dermatol* 1999; **135**: 1121–2.
26 Jillella A, Mani S, Nair B, *et al.* The role for close follow-up of melanoma patients with AJCC stages I-III: a preliminary analysis [Abstract]. *Proc Am Soc Clin Oncol* 1995; **14**: 413.
27 Soong SJ, Shaw HM, Balch CM, McCarthy WH, Urist MM, Lee JY. Predicting survival and recurrence in localized melanoma: a multivariate approach. *World J Surg* 1992; **16**: 191–5.
28 Slingluff CL, Dodge RK, Stanley WE, Seigler HF. The annual risk of melanoma progression. *Cancer* 1992; **70**: 1917.
29 Sylaidis P, Gordon D, Rigby H, Kenealy J. Follow-up requirements for thick cutaneous melanoma. *Br J Plast Surg* 1997; **50**: 349–53.
30 Buzaid AC, Tinoco L, Ross MI, Legha SS, Benjamin RS. Role of computed tomography in the staging of patients with local–regional metastases of melanoma. *J Clin Oncol* 1995; **13**: 2104–8.
31 Kuvshinoff BW, Kurtz C, Coit DG. Computed tomography in evaluation of patients with stage III melanoma. *Ann Surg Oncol* 1997; **4**: 252–8.
32 van den Brekel MW, Pameijer FA, Koops W, Hilgers FJ, Kroon BB, Balm AJ. Computed tomography for the detection of neck node metastases in melanoma patients. *Eur J Surg Oncol* 1998; **24**: 51–4.
33 Rinne D, Baum RP, Hor G, Kaufmann R. Primary staging and follow-up of high risk melanoma patients with whole-body 18F-fluorodeoxyglucose positron emission tomography: results of a prospective study of 100 patients [see comments]. *Cancer* 1998; **82**: 1664–71.
34 Holder WD Jr, White RL Jr, Zuger JH, Easton EJ Jr, Greene FL. Effectiveness of positron emission tomography for the detection of melanoma metastases. *Ann Surg* 1998; **227**: 764–9; discussion 769–71.
35 Macfarlane DJ, Sondak V, Johnson T, Wahl RL. Prospective evaluation of 2-[18F]-2-deoxy-D-glucose positron emission tomography in staging of regional lymph nodes in patients with cutaneous malignant melanoma. *J Clin Oncol* 1998; **16**: 1770–6.
36 Wagner JD, Schauwecker D, Davidson D, *et al.* Prospective study of fluorodeoxyglucose-positron emission tomography imaging of lymph node basins in melanoma patients undergoing sentinel node biopsy. *J Clin Oncol* 1999; **17**: 1508–15.
37 Calabro A, Singletary SE, Balch CM. Patterns of relapse in 1001 consecutive patients with melanoma nodal metastases. *Arch Surg* 1989; **124**: 1051–5

12: The management of regional lymph node relapse in melanoma

David Ross and Merrick I. Ross

Introduction

It has been recognized for over a century that management of the regional lymph nodes may have an important role in the assessment and treatment of primary melanoma [1]. Surgical excision of palpable nodal disease (therapeutic lymph node dissection, TLND) can cure a small but significant group of patients and will usually obtain local control. However, more patients are presenting with stage I and II disease and, in this instance, the role of node dissection becomes both contentious and obscure.

Approximately 90% of patients presenting with primary melanoma are clinically node-negative at the time of presentation, but 20% of these patients will harbour micrometastases in their regional nodes [2,3]. Furthermore, regional nodes are the most common sites for relapse occuring in 70% of patients with recurrent disease [4]. A number of retrospective studies have suggested that elective lymph node dissection (ELND) may improve survival, particularly for intermediate thickness melanomas, although this has not been supported from the findings of prospective randomized trials as yet.

Consequently, controversy surrounds exactly how clinically node-negative patients with potential micrometastases should be managed and several important questions remain. How can patients most at risk of early spread be detected and treated? What surgical technique should be employed and what is the optimal timing of surgery? In addition, does ELND influence outcome and, if so, is this benefit confined to a subgroup of patients?

This chapter aims to outline the evidence for present surgical strategy and review areas of future development.

Management of metastatic disease in regional nodes

Over the last decade, our definitions and concepts of nodal relapse have changed. Traditionally, nodal metastases were recognized as palpable clinically obvious masses, usually found at follow-up or by the patient. Presence of palpable nodes, usually confirmed on fine needle aspiration biopsy, is an indication for clearance of the nodes within that basin (TLND). Relapse in the regional node basin is associated with a worse prognosis, and outcome is influenced by the number of lymph nodes involved and evidence of extracapsular spread [5,6] (Fig. 12.1). Node dissections are usually confined to the groin, axilla and cervical region, although occasionally the epitrochlear and popliteal basins may also warrant clearance [7,8]. TLND is thus directed at removing recurrent disease, with the added aim of achieving local control and possible cure. Surgical techniques are well described elsewhere, and are usually safe, but associated with significant morbidity. This includes prolonged lymphatic drainage, particularly following groin dissection, wound infection, delayed healing and lymphoedema. Despite these problems, node clearance and formal restaging represents the optimum management in the face of established metastases, and the benefits of treatment outweigh those risks noted above.

At present, considerable controversy remains as how best to manage the regional node basin in the majority of patients with primary melanoma, with potential occult metastases. This question remains the most contentious issue in contemporary surgical management of melanoma. The risk of micrometastases led many centres worldwide to remove clinically negative regional lymph nodes at the time of primary surgery (ELND). The beneficial role of ELND is based on several assumptions.

1 Micrometastases may occur in regional nodes without spread elsewhere.

2 Removal of micrometastases is better than waiting for larger volume, palpable disease to develop.

3 Removal of early metastases prevents further distant spread and also recurrent disease in the dissected basin.

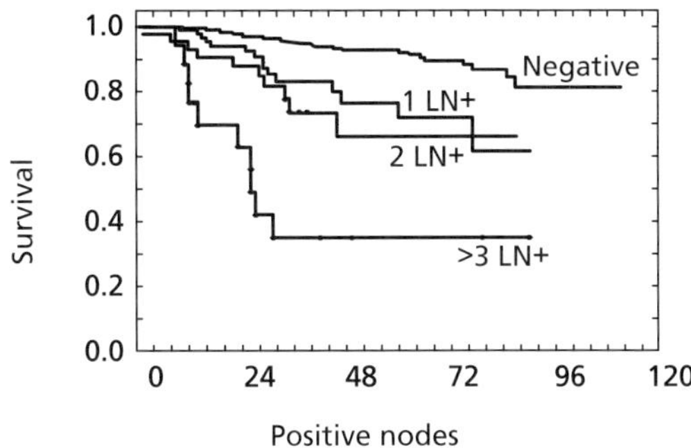

Fig. 12.1 Graph to show survival vs. number of involved nodes.

The detection of early spread was given even greater impetus by the early optimism surrounding adjuvant interferon [9].

Role of elective lymph node dissection

An improved understanding of the natural history of melanoma and the predictive value of tumour-related factors, such as primary thickness and ulceration, identified subsets of patients at increased risk of harbouring occult regional lymph node metastases. Primary tumour thickness was subcategorized into < 1, 1–4 and > 4 mm and classified as low, intermediate and high risk, respectively [10,11]. Specifically, the intermediate thickness group of patients have been proposed potentially to benefit by the complete removal of microscopic nodal disease in order to prevent future distant failure [10,11]. Thin melanomas are considered to be of low metastatic potential, whereas thick tumours are likely to have spread by additional haematogenous routes. Intermediate thickness tumours are considered to have an elevated risk of nodal metastases and are the group thought to most benefit from ELND; it is this contention that lies at the centre of the controversy.

The benefit of ELND has been debated for decades. Surgeons, reporting data from a variety of retrospective studies, were equally divided between those who supported early removal of regional lymph nodes and those who believed that lymphadenectomy should be confined to patients with clinical regional disease (Table 12.1). TLND reduces the number of unnecessary lymphadenectomies and may not prejudice the chance for cure. Both Duke University and the Sydney Melanoma Unit reversed their treatment protocols, from ELND to TLND, based on further retrospective analyses performed after longer follow-up [12,13]. The results of these retrospective series, however, do support the previous contentions, based on prognostic variables that the intermediate thickness group of patients could potentially benefit from ELND. As a result, the appropriate patient populations to study in a prospective and randomized fashion were identified.

Elective lymph node dissection and prospective randomized trials

The long-term results of the first prospective randomized trial investigating ELND vs. TLND, conducted by the World Health Organization (WHO) Melanoma Program, did not demonstrate any benefit from ELND [14,15]. This trial investigated almost 600 patients in a well-designed randomized study, but was concluded prior to the establishment of the critical prognostic primary tumour factors (tumour thickness) and therefore specific subgroups were not stratified. The cohort mainly comprised females with distal extre-

Table 12.1 Elective lymph node dissection (ELND) trials

Trial [Reference]	Design	Result
Retrospective Studies		
Memorial Sloan-Kettering, 1975 [16]	Retrospective	Benefit for intermediate thickness group
University of Alabama, 1982 [17]	Retrospective	Benefit for intermediate thickness group
Duke University, 1983 [18]	Retrospective	Benefit for intermediate thickness group
Sydney Melanoma Unit, 1985 [19,20]	Retrospective	Benefit for intermediate thickness group
University of Pennsylvania [21]	Retrospective	No benefit for intermediate thickness group
Rompel et al, 1995 [22]	Retrospective (matched pair)	Survival benefit for intermediate thickness group
Sydney Melanoma Unit, 1995 [13]	Retrospective	No benefit
Drepper et al, 1993 [23]	Retrospective (multi-centre)	Survival benefit for intermediate thickness group
Prospective Studies		
WHO, 1977 [14,15]	Prospective/randomised (N = 553)	No benefit
Mayo Clinic [24]	Prospective/randomised (N = 171)	No benefit
Intergroup Melanoma, 1996 (1–4 mm, all sites) [25]	Prospective/randomised (N = 740)	Benefit for 1–2 mm subset and patients <60 years of age

mity lesions of mixed depth and thickness (predominantly thin). Identical survival rates were observed for patients receiving ELND compared with those treated with wide local excision (WLE) alone. However, it is conceivable that any benefit afforded to higher risk subsets could have been masked by the overwhelming majority of low-risk patients. A separate subset analysis performed retrospectively identified a small group of patients with intermediate thickness tumours as the beneficiaries of improved survival after ELND. A subsequent, smaller prospective randomized trial conducted by the Mayo Clinic also failed to reveal any survival benefit using ELND [24].

The design of two recent trials were intended to overcome the limitations inherent in previous randomized trials as well as attempting to verify retrospective data demonstrating that patients with higher risk primaries could potentially benefit from ELND. The WHO Trunk Trial [26] only accrued patients with melanomas thicker than 1.5 mm, to receive ELND vs. WLE alone. Patients were stratified according to gender and tumour thickness (1.5–4 vs. >4 mm). Long-term follow-up, published in 1998, confirmed the results of earlier randomized trials in failing to observe a statistically significant difference in survival between ELND- and TLND-treated patients. However, this study also compared outcome in those patients undergoing ELND who were clinically node-negative, but subsequently found to have nodal micrometastases, compared to patients managed with TLND. In this instance, survival was significantly greater in the ELND group, with a 5-year survival of 48.2 vs. 26.6% ($P=0.04$).

The more recently concluded prospective randomized trial conducted by the Intergroup Melanoma Committee included patients only with melanomas between 1 and 4 mm in thickness from any anatomic subsite. In this trial, patients with trunk melanomas underwent preoperative lymphoscintigraphy to identify nodal basins at risk. In addition, patients were prospectively stratified according to tumour thickness (1–2, 2–3 and 3–4 mm), the presence or absence of ulceration and by anatomic subsite (extremity vs. trunk vs. head and neck) [25,27]. This study made a number of interesting observations, concluding that ELND benefited male patients less than 60 years of age, with tumours between 1 and 2 mm thick. Throughout the period that many of these studies were conducted it was recognized that indiscriminate application of ELND led to many patients being overtreated, incurring additional costs and morbidity. Therefore, the challenge arose as to how to identify those patients with early subclinical node relapse and select those patients that might benefit from early node dissection (Fig. 12.2a,b).

Sentinel node biopsy and selective lymphadenectomy

In an effort to resolve the controversy between ELND and TLND, Morton and Cochrane drew upon animal models [28] and the earlier work of Cabanas [29] to postulate the concept of lymphatic mapping and sentinel node biopsy for melanoma. This technique relies on the concept that finite regions of skin drain specifically to an initial sentinel node within the regional nodal basin via an organized array of specific afferent lymphatic channels. In theory, each lymph node within a nodal basin potentially represents a sentinel node draining different regions of the skin. The identification and biopsy of the sentinel node may thus determine disease status within a specific lymph node basin and would allow identification of those patients who harbour occult disease. In this way, patients could be selected to undergo complete lymphadenectomy and spare the remaining patients the costs and morbidity of an unnecessary procedure.

Scientific rationale for the sentinel node concept

Lymphatic mapping, as it applies to melanoma, relies on the hypothesis that dermal lymphatic drainage from specific cutaneous areas to the regional lymph node basin occurs in an orderly and definable process. Furthermore, it

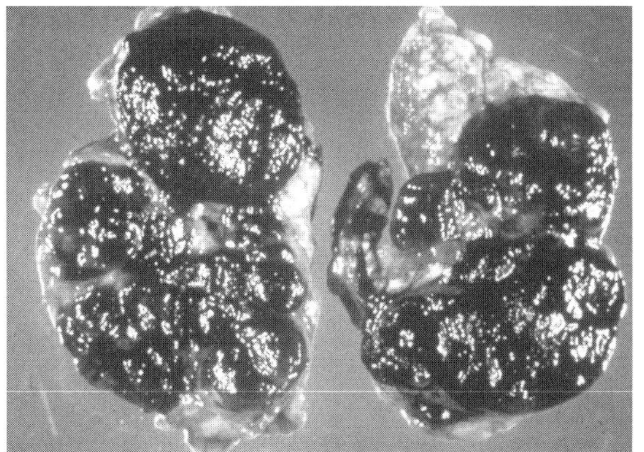
(a)

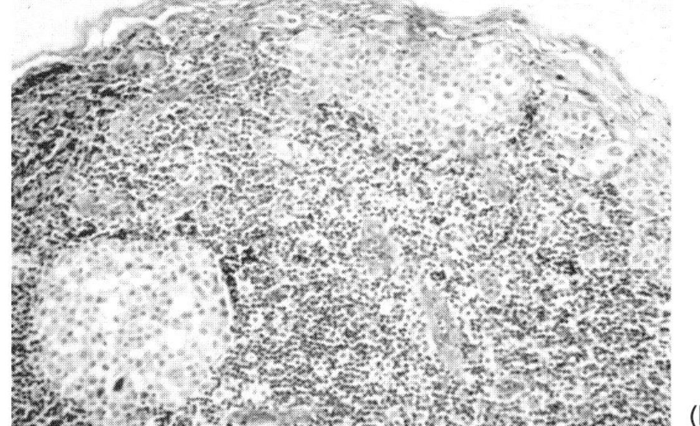
(b)

Fig. 12.2 (a) Lymph node containing relatively high volume disease. This node was detected by clinical examination at routine follow-up. (b) Micrometastases within the subcapsular sinus detected following sentinel node biopsy. Intuitively, it would seem better to treat nodal disease at this stage, rather than that shown in (a).

is postulated that these lymphatic drainage patterns should mimic the metastatic spread of melanoma cells within the lymphatic compartment, such that the first lymph node(s) receiving lymphatic drainage are the most likely nodes to contain metastatic disease. In theory, each lymph node within a formal basin may represent a sentinel node, but for different and finite regions of the skin. Consequently, melanomas that arise within a site that has drainage to more than one lymph node basin (e.g. the trunk or head and neck), will potentially have sentinel nodes in each basin.

To confirm this hypothesis, sentinel node identification had to be established as reliable and repeatable. Animal studies evaluated a variety of dyes that could be injected intradermally and transported through the lymphatic system to the regional lymph node basin, thereby providing a visualization of the sentinel node upon surgical exploration of the lymph node basin. Morton *et al.* demonstrated that two dyes were most effective: isosulfan blue (Lymphazurin) and patent blue V. Initial clinical studies were performed in melanoma patients to determine sentinel node identification rates and the accuracy of the sentinel node in establishing the presence or absence of regional nodal metastases.

The first report, published in 1992, evaluated 237 consecutive patients following intradermal injection of Lymphazurin around the intact primary melanoma or excision biopsy site [28]. The authors demonstrated an 82% sentinel node identification rate and an average of 1.3 sentinel nodes per basin and similar findings were confirmed from elsewhere. The accuracy of the sentinel node was assessed by performing completion lymphadenectomy at the time of sentinel node biopsy. In this way, the false-negative rate could be determined (defined as detection of microscopic disease in a non-sentinel node accompanying a negative sentinel node). Accordingly, the false-negative rate was then calculated as the number of false-negative events divided by the total number of patients with microscopic nodal disease. Collectively, these initial studies evaluated 402 patients with successful sentinel lymph node localization, 86 of who were found to have regional node metastases. Of these 86 patients, 81 patients had one or more positive sentinel lymph nodes and five additional patients had disease in a non-sentinel lymph node identified by completion clearance; producing a false-negative rate of 5%. These data strongly supported the sentinel lymph node concept.

Morton's initial study also established that frozen section analysis was unreliable for detection of melanoma micrometastases, and that a considerable learning curve was essential in order to become technically proficient. Two subsequent series, a collaborative study between the MD Anderson Cancer Center (MDACC) and the Moffit Cancer Center, and the other from the Sydney Melanoma Unit, confirmed the results of Morton's initial trial, describing sentinel node identification rates >85% [30,31]. Patients eligible for lymphatic mapping in this series were similarly stage I and II patients with melanomas >0.76 or 1 mm in thickness. Overall, micrometastases were identified in approximately 20% of patients.

This early experience has led to the adoption of sentinel lymph node biopsy (SNLB) worldwide [32,33]. Patients with a histologically positive sentinel node are offered therapeutic lymphadenectomy, while those with a negative sentinel node are observed. This large clinical experience yielded significant improvements in sentinel node localization techniques [33], generated additional findings that supported the sentinel lymph node concept, and provided valuable insights into the biological significance of the sentinel node.

Since then it has been recognized that SNLB is most accurate when performed with an excision margin < 1 cm. With margins > 1 cm the accuracy of the technique is decreased, as the lymphatic drainage of the remaining skin may be different to the skin adjacent to the original primary melanoma. Accordingly, lymphoscintigraphy may label nodes draining sites other than that of the tumour. Several small series suggest lymphatic mapping may still be accurate in these patients and can be offered selectively, provided the patient recognizes that true false-negative rates have not yet been established.

Present indications for SNLB include:

- tumour thickness ≥ 1 mm;
- Clark's level IV or above, regardless of tumour thickness;
- histological evidence of primary tumour ulceration; and
- histological evidence of extensive regression.

Other clinical scenarios can arise where SNLB is used.

1 In patients who develop a local recurrence subsequent to a relatively narrow excision as primary treatment of a primary melanoma.

2 Where exact tumour thickness is difficult to establish, either because of biopsy technique, problems during histological preparation or regression.

3 When the pathological diagnosis of an atypical melanocytic lesion is ambiguous but the differential diagnosis includes primary melanomas > 1 mm in thickness.

4 In patients who have already received a formal wide excision with or without a skin graft and then wish to have accurate assessment of their draining lymph node basins.

The initial promising results with this technique elicited considerable interest and further attempts were made to increase the accuracy of sentinel node identification and limit the learning curve. Advances have occurred as a result of cooperation between surgeons, nuclear physicians and pathologists and have been in three main areas:

1 preoperative evaluation of the site and number of nodes using lymphoscintigraphy;

2 the introduction of a hand-held γ probe to aid peroperative localization of sentinel nodes; and

3 the application of intensive histological molecular technologies to detect minimal volume micrometastases.

Preoperative lymphoscintigraphy has become an established prerequisite for SNLB [34] to determine nodal basins at risk in patients with primaries located in ambiguous drainage sites, such as on the trunk and the head and neck. The use of anatomical proximity or historical lymphatic drainage, as established by Sappey [35], to target basins at risk is often inaccurate [34]. Lymphoscintograms are obtained using an intradermal injection of technetium-labelled sulphide, antimony colloid or human serum albumin followed by nodal scanning with a γ-counter. Rather than obtaining only static views of the nodal basin at specific time points after injection of the radiolabel, dynamic real-time studies of lymphatic flow can be performed at early time points subsequent to injection. The sentinel node is always defined as the initial node concentrating the radiolabel. Using this technology, nuclear medicine physicians identify nodal basins at risk, the number and location of the sentinel nodes (Fig. 12.3). These site(s) are then marked on the overlying skin. These high-resolution scans provide preoperative road maps for the sur-

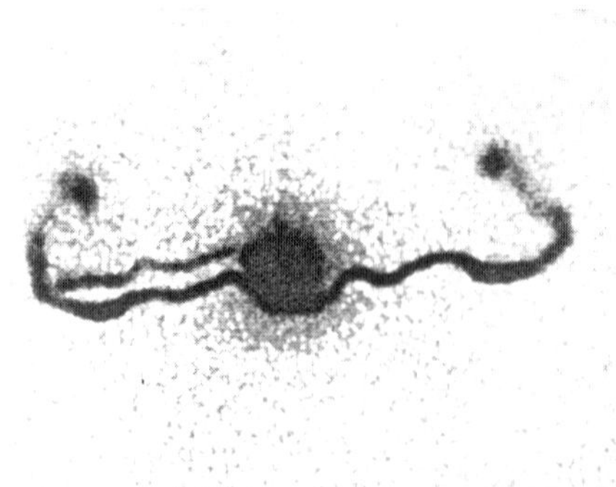

Fig. 12.3 Preoperative lymphoscintigraphy of a melanoma in the lower mid-back. This image demonstrates drainage to sentinel nodes in both inguinal basins.

Table 12.2 Sentinel node identification rates and methods of detection

Reference	No. of patients	Identification sentinel node (%)	Method (D/GP)	Metastases detected (% patients)	False-negative rate (%)
Morton *et al.* [28]	223	82	D	21	1
Morton *et al.* [36]	72	90	D	15	0
Lingam *et al.* [37]	15	100	D	27	0
Thompson *et al.* [31]	118	87	D	23	0
Albertini *et al.* [38]	106	96	GP & D	15	0
Mudun *et al.* [39]	25	100	GP	24	Not given
Kapteijn *et al.* [40]	110	99.5	GP & D	23	2.7

Abbreviations: D, dye; GP, γ probe.

geon and aid in the intraoperative identification of the blue-stained sentinel node(s).

Development of an intraoperative hand-held γ probe, capable of detecting the accumulation of intradermally injected radiolabelled colloid within sentinel nodes, provided the next important technical advance. This allows the surgeon to transcutaneously localize the sentinel node prior to incision and acts as an essential adjunct to the visual cues required to localize the blue-stained sentinel node at the time of surgery. As a result, the learning curve for successful SNLB is both shorter and less steep. Several studies have now shown sentinel node detection rates in excess of 99% (Table 12.2). The greatest benefit, and improvement, has been in facilitating successful harvest in traditionally difficult areas, such as the head and neck or axilla.

Perhaps the most significant developments in SNLB to date have been in pathological detection of micrometastases. Studies at the MDACC and elsewhere have established that simple bivalving of the lymph node is insufficient to determine disease status accurately. Gershenwald *et al.* [41] reported a study of 10 patients who had relapsed in the regional nodal basin following a negative mapping. The original paraffin blocks of the previously 'negative' sentinel nodes were subjected to haematoxylin and eosin (H&E) examination of 25 μm step sections and immunohistochemical staining HMB45 and S-100. Microscopic disease, initially undetected by conventional histological techniques, was identified in eight of the 10 patients. Therefore only two of these nodal failures can be truly classified as false-negative events, resulting in an actual overall false-negative rate of <1%. Accordingly, it is now recommended that nodes be carefully sectioned and then subjected to immunohistochemistry if negative.

In addition, there is a small but robust and growing body of evidence to suggest that nodes should then be screened with polymerase chain reaction (PCR) for tyrosinase messenger RNA (mRNA) and other melanoma-specific markers [34,42]. The most obvious advantage of PCR analysis is that the entire lymph node can be potentially evaluated. The clinical relevance of PCR findings are still under investigation, but preliminary data suggest that PCR-positive–H&E-negative lymph node patients have survival rates intermediate between those patients who are PCR- and H&E-positive and those who are both PCR- and H&E-negative [43] (Fig. 12.4). These observations emphasize

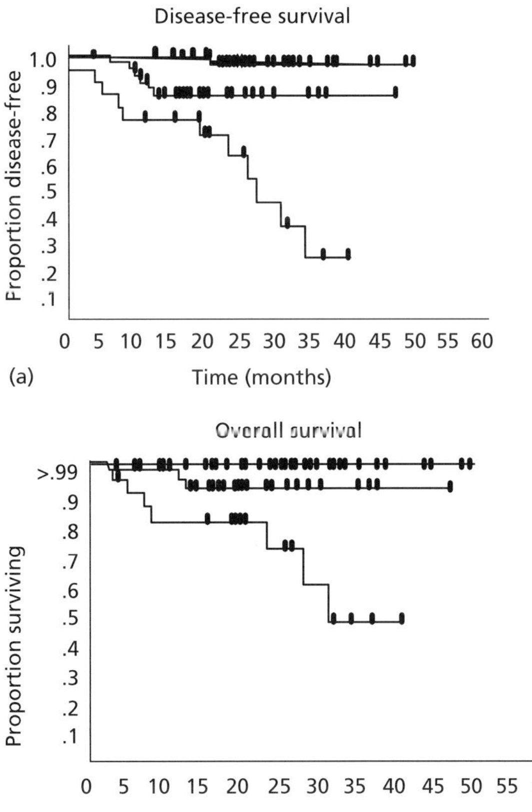

Fig. 12.4 Survival vs. polymerase chain reaction (PCR) status for tyrosinase messenger mRNA (mRNA). The upper curve demonstrates survival in patients with sentinel nodes negative with both haematoxylin and eosin (H&E) and PCR. The middle curve shows survival in patients with PCR-positive–H&E-negative nodes. The lower survival curve is in patients with both H&E- and PCR-positive nodes [43].

the necessity for multidisciplinary involvement in SLNB and adequate funding, particularly for pathology expertise and time.

Current surgical technique for sentinel node biopsy

Immediately prior to primary or wide local excision, 2–4 mL of patent blue dye, or Lymphazurin, is injected intradermally around the tumour or the biopsy site. A small incision is then made at the lymphoscintigraphy-indicated site and dye-stained afferent lymphatics sought. Nodes are usually identified with the dye alone, particularly in the groin (Fig. 12.5). However, if this is not possible, then the hand-held γ probe can be used to detect emission and identify the node. In this way, sentinel node detection rates are very reliable and have increased to almost 100%. Crucially, once the node is harvested, γ emission is confirmed with the probe and the count recorded. The probe is then reintroduced into the basin to ensure no other sentinel nodes are present (average 1.8 sentinel nodes per basin).

The delineation of lymphatic drainage has revealed a number of aberrant routes at variance with that proposed by Sappey [35]. Lymphoscintigraphy has shown that about 25% of upper back melanomas drain to a node within the triangular space [44]. Rarely, back tumours may drain to paravertebral of retroperitoneal nodes [45]; Uren *et al.* [44] noted drainage through the body wall in 14 of 542 patients (2.6%) presenting with posterior trunk melanomas. Triangular space nodes should be biopsied and, if found positive, then the ipsilateral axilla is cleared. However, harvesting of retroperitoneal nodes is particularly invasive and it is generally felt that these nodes should be regularly imaged to observe early signs of change. As experience with lymphoscintigraphy grows, it is evident that individual variations in drainage patterns are not uncommon and should be anticipated.

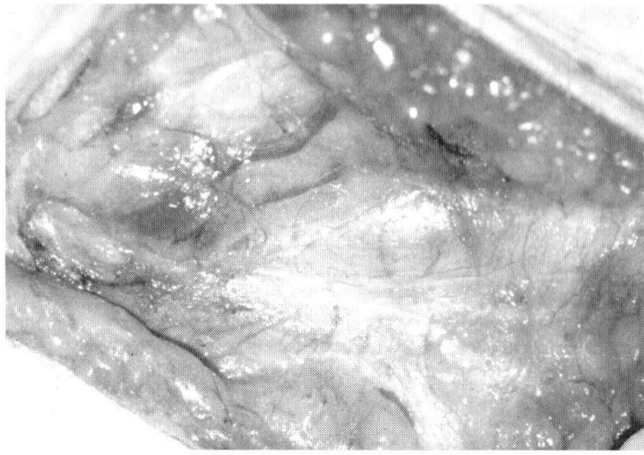

Fig. 12.5 Once the dye-stained afferent lymphatic has been identified, it can be followed to the sentinel node.

Biological significance of the sentinel node

As experience has accrued with this technique, it has become evident that SNLB may contribute significant additional information, other than selecting patients for lymph node dissection. Studies have demonstrated the incidence of sentinel node metastases correlates with increasing tumour thickness. This correlation is strong and similar to that noted between incidence of microscopic nodal disease in ELND specimens and tumour thickness. Other known primary tumour factors, such as anatomic location, ulceration and Clark's level, also predict sentinel node involvement. In a multivariate analysis, the two variables that independently predicted sentinel node involvement were tumour thickness and ulceration. Accordingly, the most powerful primary tumour prognostic factors are also the best predictors of sentinel node metastases and offer further evidence that sentinel node involvement is a biologically important and non-random event. Subsequent studies have confirmed that sentinel node status is the most important clinical determinant of prognosis identified to date [46] (Fig. 12.6).

Sentinel node status also allows accurate staging of disease in the patient and this has been recognized in the most recent modifications to the American Joint Committee on Cancer (AJCC) and TNM classifications, where micrometastastases are separated into their own categories. This is clinically relevant in the design and implementation of clinical trials; in the past it is likely that a proportion of stage I and II patients harboured micrometastases and were incorrectly downstaged. SNLB will play a crucial part in future adjuvant clinical trials to ensure that treatment groups are correctly matched.

Further support for the sentinel node concept is provided from long-term follow-up of patients following negative sentinel node biopsy. In a cohort of

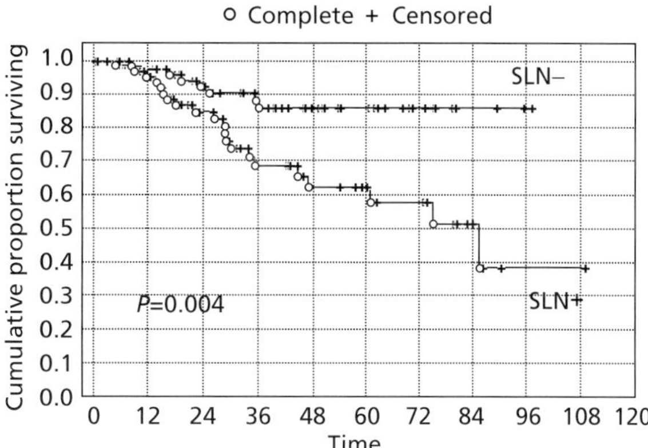

Fig. 12.6 Sentinel node status and survival.

almost 250 patients followed for over 3 years, only 3% of the patients have died of recurrent disease, 10% of the patients have had some type of recurrence, and 4% developed failure within the previously mapped regional nodal basin as the sole site or a component of the first site of failure. Such regional nodal basin failures represent another type of false-negative event. Three mechanisms have been proposed to explain nodal failure (recurrence in a negatively mapped basin) after a negative sentinel node biopsy.

1 *Technical failure*: lymphatic mapping did not identify the primary draining node and a non-sentinel node was removed. Residual micrometastases within the true sentinel node act as a source of recurrent disease within that basin.

2 *Pathological failure*: one of the sentinel nodes was removed and contained microscopic disease undetected by conventional histological techniques. An additional sentinel node or a non-sentinel node with disease remained as the source of subsequent clinical failure.

3 *Biological or natural history-type failure*: at the time of the initial surgery, the correct sentinel node was removed and no metastatic disease was present; however, nodal failure occurred because of subclinical intralymphatic in-transit disease present since diagnosis.

As a result of the experience noted above, SNLB has become established as an investigative technique in most cancer centres within the USA and Australia. At this stage, mature data are not available to confirm a therapeutic role for selective lymphadenectomy, although SNLB has already made significant contributions to the surgical rationale and approach to melanoma surgery. It provides a reliable method for detecting early nodal spread, accurate staging and prognostic information. This has led to its application in the assessment of several other tumour types, including cancer of the breast and bowel.

Clinical trials

SLNB/SNLB provides an opportunity to investigate and clarify several key issues in melanoma and its management. These include:

1 the natural history and staging of clinical stage I and II patients;

2 the effect of early therapeutic node dissection on local–regional control and/or survival;

3 the long-term regional nodal basin failure rate following a negative sentinel node biopsy; and

4 the role for systemic adjuvant therapy in patients with subclinical nodal disease.

The Multicentre Selective Lymphadenectomy Trial, sponsored by the National Cancer Institute, is an ongoing prospective randomized study with a target accrual of 1200 patients. Eligible patients are randomized to LM/SNLB vs. WLE alone. Patients with positive sentinel nodes undergo therapeutic lymphadenectomy while sentinel node-negative patients are observed. Patients who are initially managed with WLE alone will undergo a therapeutic dissection if clinical regional nodal failure develops. The following questions will be specifically addressed.

1 Is there a survival benefit for patients who undergo early lymphadenectomy?
2 What is the false-negative rate as determined by failure in nodal basin after a negative sentinel lymph node biopsy?

Another multi-institutional study, the 'Sunbelt Melanoma Trial', attempts to address issues related to the clinical significance of microscopic nodal disease as determined by different histological methods:

1 conventional histology;
2 serial sectioning and immunohistology; and
3 PCR analysis using four molecular markers (MAGE III, MART I, GP 100 and tyrosinase).

This study aims not only to elucidate the natural history of these subsets of patients, but also to examine the potential benefit of high-dose interferon administered to patients with low nodal burden metastatic disease.

Future clinical trials will stratify patients into homogenous prognostic groups based on sentinel node evaluation. In this way, one can better select the highest risk patients for aggressive adjuvant therapy, determine if less toxic adjuvant regimens may be effective in lower risk groups, and spare the most favourable groups (H&E-negative, step section-negative, PCR-negative) the morbidity and cost of any adjuvant therapy.

Site of relapse and surgical technique

Dissection of the axilla usually involves a level 2 clearance, although this may be extended to all three levels in the face of palpable bulky disease. Similarly, in the neck no objective evidence exists to indicate that a radial clearance provides superior local control to a functional dissection.

There is still uncertainty as to how best to treat inguinal disease and protocols vary around the world. Patients with micrometastases are usually offered a superficial inguinal dissection. This removes all those nodes lying in the femoral triangle and immediately above the inguinal ligament. However, variation occurs in the face of obvious nodal disease, the practice at MDACC is to perform an ilioinguinal (deep) dissection. At St Thomas' Hospital, patients with obvious nodal disease undergo a computed tomography (CT) scan of the inguinal region and ilioinguinal dissection is only offered if deep nodes are seen to be involved.

Others have used the presence of disease in Cloquet's node as an indication for deep dissection. This node lies within the femoral ring and was thought to be a common passage for cells to metastasize from the superficial to the deep inguinal system. Several anatomical studies have shown that Cloquet's node is not the only route between femoral and iliac nodes. Furthermore, involvement of this node is not a reliable indicator of deep disease [47].

No prospective trials have been performed to compare these techniques in the face of palpable disease and this is likely to be addressed in forthcoming studies. In the absence of such data, no firm recommendations can be made. However, several points are worth considering. It has not been our experience to find pelvic relapse common after superficial clearance, although it may be argued that residual disease is left to source elsewhere. Secondly, deep dissection does involve a more radical procedure, extending to clear nodes along the iliac and obturator systems. In centres where this is commonly practised, complication rates between the two methods, however, are similar, although the extended procedure involves greater dissection.

Reconstructive surgery and the management of nodal relapse

In the UK, plastic surgeons play an important part in the management of both primary and metastatic melanoma. They are often required to perform the wider excision and reconstruction. In the face of advanced fungating nodal disease, more advanced reconstructive techniques are required, where the aim of treatment is to improve local control and quality of life. Furthermore, these masses may lie close to, or involve neurovascular bundles and produce considerable pain or bleeding. In these situations, overlying skin is usually involved and requires removal together with the mass. In order to provide cover it is essential that they use local or regional flaps. Accordingly, the groin can be resurfaced with the tensor fascia lata flap. The axilla can be covered with several flaps, including the pectoralis major myocutaneous flap (Fig. 12.7) or the latissimus dorsi.

Conclusions

Management of the regional node basin in patients with primary melanoma remains a contentious issue. Evidence suggests that patients with intermediate tumours may benefit from ELND, and SNLB has allowed identification of micrometastases and selection of those patients most likely to benefit from regional clearance. The main established trial initiated to answer this question should provide mature data within 5 years. In the mean time, SNLB has proven of benefit in other aspects of patient assessment, and should not be regarded as an 'experimental' technique. The status of the sentinel node has been shown to be of prognostic significance and early findings have suggested the

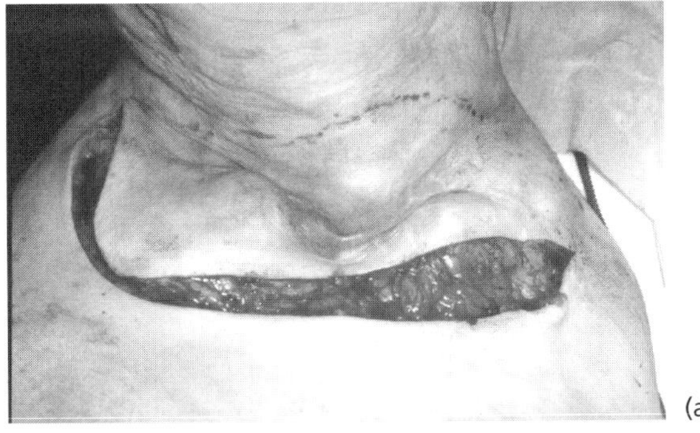
(a)

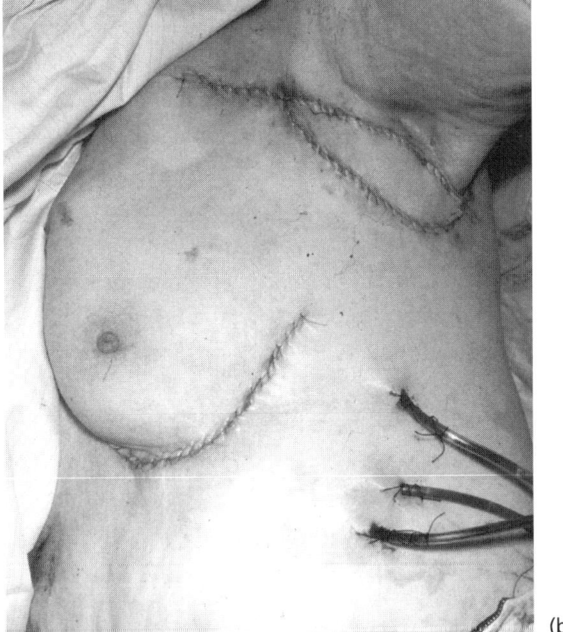
(b)

Fig. 12.7 This patient, a 77-year-old female, presented with distant disease and painful fungating nodal metastases in the left axilla. Following excision and debulking of the axilla (a), the defect was resurfaced with an ipsilateral pectoralis major myocutaneous flap (b). The patient made an uneventful recovery and died of distant disease. Note the donor site on the inferomedial aspect of the breast.

potential for molecular diagnostic techniques in identifying the earliest evidence of metastatic spread. A further important application of SNLB lies in accurate staging of patients for clinical trials. This latter role will be crucial in future trials of adjuvant therapies for stage I–III melanoma.

References

1 Snow H. Melanotic cancerous disease. *Lancet* 1892; **2**: 872.

2 Balch CM, Soong SJ, Shaw HM *et al.* Changing trends in the clinical and pathologic features of melanoma. In: Balch CM, Houghton AN, Milton GW, Sober AJ, Soong, SJ, eds. *Cutaneous Melanoma*, 2nd edn. Philadelphia: JB Lippincott, 1992: 40–5.

3 Karakousis CP, Emrich LJ, Rao U. Groin dissection in malignant melanoma. *Am J Surg* 1985; **152**: 491–5.

4 O'Rourke MG, Louis A. Metastasis in malignant melanoma. *Aust N Z J Surg* 1982; **52**: 154–8.
5 Kissin MW, Simpson DA, Easton DA *et al.* Prognostic factors related to survival and groin recurrence following therapeutic lymph node dissection for lower limb malignant melanoma. *Br J Surg* 1987; **74**: 1023–6.
6 Cascinelli N, Vaglini M, Nava M *et al.* Prognosis of skin melanoma with regional node metastases (stage 2). *J Surg Oncol* 1984; **25**: 240–7.
7 Tanabe KK. Lymphatic mapping and epitrochlear lymph node dissection for melanoma. *Surgery* 1997; **121**: 102–4.
8 Karakousis P. The technique of popliteal lymph node dissection. *Surg Gynae Obs* 1980; **151**: 421–3.
9 Kirkwood J, Strawderman M, Ernstoff M *et al.* Interferon-alfa-2b adjuvant therapy of high-risk resected cutaneous melanoma: the Eastern Cooperative Oncology Group Trial EST 1684. *J Clin Oncol* 1996; **14**: 7–17.
10 Balch CM, Murad TM, Soong SJ *et al.* Tumor thickness as a guide to surgical management of clinical stage I melanoma patients. *Cancer* 1979; **43**: 883–8.
11 Balch CM *et al.* A prospective randomised trial of 742 melanoma patients comparing the efficacy of elective node dissection (immediate) versus observation. Abstract presented at the American Surgical association Meeting, Phoenix, AZ, April 17–20, 1988.
12 Slingluff CL Jr, Stidham KR, Ricci WM *et al.* Surgical management of regional lymph nodes in patients with melanoma: experience with 4682 patients [see comments]. *Ann Surg* 1994; **219**: 120–30.
13 Coates AS, Ingvar CI, Petersen-Schaefer K *et al.* Elective lymph node dissection in patients with primary melanoma of the trunk and limbs treated at the Sydney Melanoma Unit from 1960 to 1991. *J Am Coll Surg* 1995; **180**: 402–9.
14 Veronesi U, Adamus J, Bandiera DC *et al.* Inefficacy of immediate node dissection in stage I melanoma of the limbs. *N Engl J Med* 1977; **297**: 627–30.
15 Veronesi U, Adamus J, Bandiera DC *et al.* Delayed regional lymph node dissection in stage I melanoma of the skin of the lower extremities. *Cancer* 1982; **49**: 2420–30.
16 Wanebo HJ, Woodruff J, Fortner JG. Malignant melanoma of the extremities: a clinicopathologic study using levels of invasion (microstage). *Cancer* 1975; **35**: 666–76.
17 Balch CM, Cascinelli N, Milton GW *et al.* Elective node dissection: pros and cons. In: Balch CM, Milton GW, eds. *Cutaneous Melanoma: Clinical Management and Treatment Results Worldwide*. Philadelphia: Lippincott, 1985: 131–58.
18 Reintgen DS, Cox EB, McCarty KS Jr. *et al.* Efficacy of elective lymph node dissection in patients with intermediate thickness primary melanoma. *Ann Surg* 1983; **198**: 379–84.
19 McCarthy WH, Shaw HM, Milton GW. Efficacy of elective lymph node dissection in in 2347 patients with clinical stage I malignant melanoma. *Surg Gynecol Obstet* 1985; **161**: 575–80.
20 Milton GW, Shaw HM, McCarthy WH *et al.* Prophylactic lymph node dissection in clinical stage I cutaneous malignant melanoma: results of surgical treatment in 1319 patients. *Br J Surg* 1982; **69**: 108–11.
21 Elder DE, Guerry DIV, VanHorn M *et al.* The role of lymph node dissection for clinical stage I malignant melanoma of intermediate thickness (1.51–3.99 mm). *Cancer* 1985; **56**: 413–8.
22 Rompel R, Garbe C, Buttner P *et al.* Elective lymph node dissection in primary malignant melanoma: a matched-pair analysis. *Melanoma Res* 1995; **5**: 189–94.
23 Drepper H, Kohler CO, Bastian B *et al.* Benefit of elective lymph node dissection in subgroups of melanoma patients: results of a multicenter study of 3616 patients. *Cancer* 1993; **72**: 741–9.
24 Sim FH, Taylor WF, Pritchard DJ, Soule EH. Lymphadenectomy in the management of stage I malignant melanoma: a prospective randomised study. *Mayo Clin Proc* 1986; **61**: 697–705.
25 Balch C, Soong S, Bartolucci A *et al.* Efficacy of an elective regional lymph node dissection of 1–4 mm thick melanomas for patients 60 years of age and younger. *Ann Surg* 1996; **224**: 255–63.
26 Cascinelli N, Morabito A, Santinami M, MacKie RM, Belli F. Immediate or delayed dissection of regional nodes in patients

with melanoma of the trunk: a randomised trial. *Lancet* 1998; **351**: 793–6.

27 Balch CM, Soong S, Ross MI *et al.* Long-term results of a multi-institutional randomized trial comparing prognostic factors and surgical results for intermediate thickness melanomas (1.0–4.0 mm). Intergroup Melanoma Surgical Trial. *Ann Surg Oncol* 2000; 7 (2): 87–97.

28 Morton DL, Wen DR, Wong JH *et al.* Technical details of intraoperative lymphatic mapping for early stage melanoma. *Arch Surg* 1992; **127**: 392–9.

29 Cabanas RM. An approach for the treatment of penile carcinoma. *Cancer* 1977; **39**: 456–66.

30 Reintgen D, Cruse C, Wells K *et al.* The orderly progression of melanoma nodal metastases. *Ann Surg* 1994; **220**: 759–67.

31 Thompson J, McCarthy W, Bosch C *et al.* Sentinel lymph node status as an indicator of the presence of metastatic melanoma in regional lymph nodes. *Melanoma Res* 1995; **5**: 255–60.

32 Ross M, Reintgen D, Balch C. Selective lymphadenectomy: emerging role for lymphatic mapping and sentinel node biopsy in the management of early stage melanoma. *Semin Surg Oncol* 1993; **9**: 219–23.

33 Ross MI. Surgical management of stage I and II melanoma patients: approach to the regional lymph node basin. *Semin Surg Oncol* 1996; **12**: 394–401.

34 Norman J, Cruse CW, Espinosa C *et al.* Redefinition of cutaneous lymphatic drainage with the use of lymphoscintigraphy for malignant melanoma. *Am J Surg* 1991; **162**: 432–7.

35 Sappey MP. *Injection, preparation, et conservation des vaisseaux lymphatique.* These pour le doctorat en medecine, no. 241. Dissertation, Paris: Rignoux, Imprimeur de la Faculte de Medecine, 1843.

36 Morton DL, Wen DR, Foshag LJ, Essner R, Cochran A. Intraoperative lymphatic mapping and selective cervical lymphadenectomy for early-stage melanomas of the head and neck. *J Clin Oncol* 1993; **11**: 1751–6.

37 Lingam MK, Mackie RM, Mackay AJ. Intraoperative lymphatic mapping using patent blue V dye to identify nodal micrometastases in malignant melanoma. *Reg Cancer Treat* 1994; **7**: 144–6.

38 Albertini JJ, Cruse CW, Rapaport D *et al.* Intraoperative radiolymphoscintigraphy improves sentinel lymph node identification for patients with melanoma. *Ann Surg* 1996; **130**: 654–8.

39 Mudun A, Murray DR, Herda SC *et al.* Early stage melanoma: lymphoscintigraphy, reproducibility of sentinel node detection, and effectiveness of the intraoperative γ probe. *Radiology* 1996; **199**: 171–5.

40 Kapteijn BAE, Nieweg OE, Liem IH *et al.* Localising the sentinel node in cutaneous melanoma: γ probe detection versus blue dye. *Ann Surg Oncol* 1997; **2**: 335–40.

41 Gershenwald J, Colome M, Lee JE *et al.* Pattern of recurrence following a negative sentinel lymph node biopsy in 243 patients with stage I or II melanoma. *J Clin Oncol* 1998; **16** (6): 2253–60.

42 Wang X, Heller R, VanVoorhis N *et al.* Detection of submicroscopic lymph node metastases with polymerase chain reaction in patients with malignant melanoma. *Ann Surg* 1994; **220** (6): 768–74.

43 Shivers SC, Wang X, Li W *et al.* Molecular staging of malignant melanoma: correlation with clinical outcome. *J Am Med Assoc* 1998; **280** (16): 1410–5.

44 Uren R, Howman-Giles R, Thompson J *et al.* Lymphoscintigraphy to identify sentinel lymph nodes in patients with melanoma. *Melanoma Res* 1994; **4**: 395–9.

45 Thompson JF, Uren RF, Shaw HM *et al.* Location of sentinel lymph nodes in patients with cutaneous melanoma: new insights into lymphatic anatomy. *J Am Coll Surg* 1999; **189** (2): 195–204.

46 Gershenwald J, Thompson W, Mansfield PF *et al.* Multi-institutional melanoma lymphatic mapping experience: the prognostic value of sentinel lymph node status in 612 stage I or II melanoma patients. *J Clin Oncol* 1999; **17** (3): 976–83.

47 Strobbe LJA, Wauters CAP, Nieuwenhoven EJ *et al.* Is there an anatomical rationale for a combined lymph node dissection of the groin in stage III melanoma? *Br J Surg* 2000.

13: Congenital melanocytic naevi

Julia A. Newton Bishop and Rudolf Happle

Introduction

Congenital melanocytic naevi (CMN) are important because of their cosmetic implications and because of the potential for malignant transformation. The majority of such naevi are small (Fig. 13.1). Rarely, large ones, even giant naevi are seen, covering a significant proportion of the body surface (Figs 13.2 and 13.3). The congenital naevus spilus or speckled naevus (Fig. 13.4) is considered to be a separate type. Studies commonly differentiate naevi on the basis of size but differ in the definitions used. Most now use the American National Institutes of Health (NIH) consensus definition in which small naevi are defined as under 1.5 cm in diameter, large as having a diameter between 1.5 and 20 cm and naevi with a diameter of 20 cm or more as 'giant' [1].

Natural history

A congenital melanocytic naevus is, by definition, a pigmented lesion of the skin which contains increased numbers of melanocytes and which is present at birth. They are most common on the trunk. Studies have suggested that such naevi are present in around 1% of live births [2–4]. Confusingly, naevi which are clinically and histologically similar to congenital ones may develop after birth, presumably because of delayed pigmentation or cell division of previously inapparent naevus cells. Such naevi, which may be large, are known as 'tardive CMN' [5]. Giant congenital naevi occur in only 1 in 20 500 births [6]. CMN are to be distinguished from other pigmented lesions seen on neonatal skin, such as *café au lait* spots.

Congenital naevi may be flat or raised at birth, but typically change as the child grows. Generally speaking, they are most pigmented at birth or soon after it, becoming less pigmented with age. Often, marked loss of pigmentation may occur quickly, in the first few weeks. In other patients, the loss of pigmentation occurs slowly as the naevus matures in the same way that acquired naevi mature, as they become dermal with age.

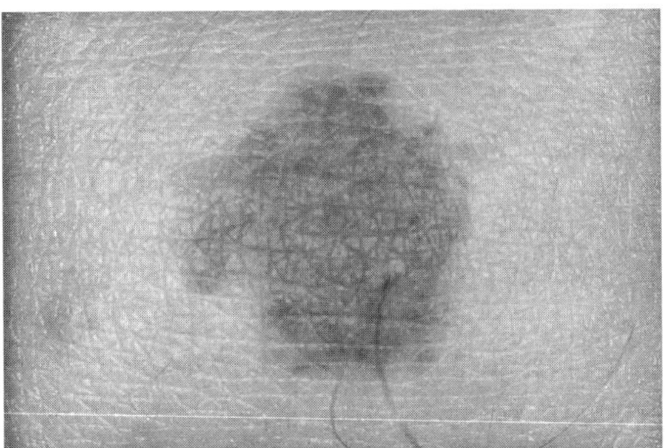

Fig. 13.1 A small congenital naevus which has become paler with time.

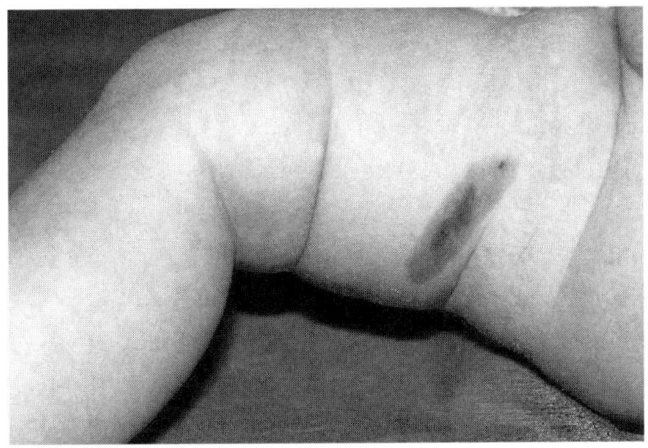

Fig. 13.2 This is by definition a large congenital naevus, being > 1.5 cm in but < 20 cm in diameter.

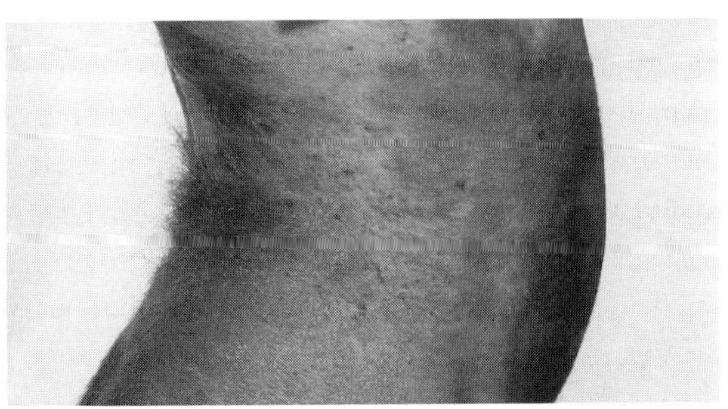

Fig. 13.3 A giant congenital naevus involving predominantly the torso of a child. The large amount of terminal hair is obvious. The depth of pigmentation visible in this naevus has diminished progressively with time. Some areas of central scarring are seen in the dorsal area after surgery carried out early in life.

It would appear that most congenital naevi grow in surface area in proportion to the growing child, although some seem to stay the same in size and therefore may appear in relative terms to become smaller with time. If an individual naevus appears to grow in size relative to the child then this should probably cause concern. The emergence of tardive CMN is, in our experience, more common in children with giant naevi in whom small distant naevi, simi-

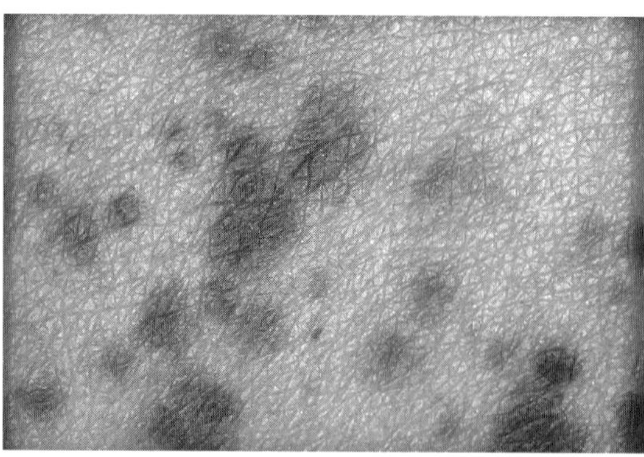

Fig. 13.4 This photograph shows part of a speckled naevus.

lar in appearance to true congenital naevi, seem to develop at distant sites, such as on the face, as the child ages. These may be referred to as 'satellite naevi'.

Congenital naevi often have clinically obvious hair at birth but the growth of terminal hair often becomes particularly obvious with time. As the child ages, the surface of the naevus commonly becomes uneven: either mammillated or nodular, particularly giant naevi. These normal changes understandably often cause concern in families previously advised to keep the naevus under review in case of malignant change. Generally speaking, as for acquired naevi, the slow almost imperceptible development of nodules is reassuring, whereas rapid growth over weeks is worrying. Rarely, plexiform neurofibroma-like new growths develop [7].

In summary, most congenital naevi become paler in colour with time and, although the skin surface may become more warty and more hairy with time, the majority of congenital naevi become a less serious cosmetic problem than they are at birth. In a proportion, the naevus remains deeply pigmented and may actually grow proportionally in surface area, and these are the most worrying cosmetically and in terms of risk of melanoma.

Aetiology

Congenital naevi may be more common in black or Asian children [8]. There may be an excess in females [7].

Families with more than one case of large congenital pigmented naevi have rarely been described, suggesting a possible genetic origin. The presence of a large naevus was said to have existed in four second-degree relatives of 80 patients with giant naevi (>20 cm in diameter) reported by Ruiz-Maldonado *et al.* [7]. While it would seem appropriate to acknowledge this to patients seeking genetic counselling advice, the significance of this remains to be established.

As a genetic basis of giant CMN, the concept of a lethal mutation surviving by mosacism has been proposed [9]. Cells carrying the mutation would survive only in a mosiac state, in close proximity with normal cells. This would explain why giant CMN exclusively occur sporadically, and why identical twins may be discordant for this trait [10]. If this hypothesis holds true, the exceptional occurrence of a large naevus in relatives of a patient with a giant naevus would best be explained by paradominant inheritance [11]. Heterozygous individuals would be, in general, clinically unaffected, which is why the mutation would be transmitted, unrecognized, through many generations. The trait would only become manifest when a postzygotic event of allelic loss gave rise to a homozygous or hemizygous cell clone forming a mosiac patch.

However, it should be emphasized that this concept cannot be applied to a small or medium sized CMN which most likely have a polygenic basis as similarly proposed for acquired naevi, both of a dysplastic or non-dysplastic type [12].

In normal development of melanocytes *in utero*, pigment cell precursors known as melanoblasts, derived from the neural crest, appear to populate the dermis [13]. In several case reports in the literature, naevus cell aggregates have been reported in the placenta of mothers giving birth to babies with giant pigmented naevi [14]. Similarly, cellular proliferations of melanocytes may be seen in the central nervous system in babies, usually presenting with hydrocephalus: a proportion of whom also have giant congenital naevi [15]. It has been suggested that these melanocytic proliferations in skin, central nervous system and placenta may result from aberrant migration of neural crest cells to primitive mesoderm early in embryogensis [14]. The presumption is that in such an aberrant site, differentiation of cells would be abnormal. Congenital naevi may therefore represent a developmental anomaly in which excessive melanocyte proliferation occurs as a result of aberrant migration of cells from the neural crest during embryogenesis.

Histological characteristics

Congenital naevi tend to be larger and thicker than acquired naevi and more commonly exhibit naevus cells in or around skin appendages and vasculature [16]. Such may be the depth of large naevi that cells may be seen extending well into fat and skeletal muscle. Some authors have described the infiltration of single naevus cells between collagen bundles and a naevus-cell-poor subepidermal zone. Everett [17] reviewed all of these characteristics in 39 congenital naevi and concluded that the differences between congenital and acquired naevi were confirmed for large but not for small naevi. This would parallel our observations of the clinical appearance of the vast majority of small naevi which appear to behave like acquired naevi in many ways.

The giant naevi may well have the more or less 'characteristic' histological appearances listed above, but they may also have complex and variegated mixtures of tissues histologically consistent with their origin as hamartomas of the ectoderm. There may be cells exhibiting neural differentiation. The melanocytic structures may have the appearance of Spitz tumours or blue naevi. The benign nodules which develop within giant naevi and malignant tumours may all exhibit pleomorphic patterns which causes diagnostic difficulty for pathologists. Bizarre tumours with a malignant-looking histology may behave in a benign fashion so that the morphological distinction between benign and malignant may be blurred [18]. The term nodular proliferative neurocristic hamartoma may be used to describe massive rapidly enlarging ulcerative masses present at birth in which the histological appearances are of diverse tissues of neural or mesoenchymal appearance, but which still behave in a benign fashion.

In normal individuals melanomas nearly always arise from junctional cells. True origin from dermal cells is excessively rare if it happens at all. In giant congenital naevi, however, origin from dermal cells has been reported [19,20].

The interpretation of the histological appearance of giant naevi demands close correlation with the clinical behaviour of the naevus. If the histology of a nodule suggests malignancy but it has been clinically stable, then the prognosis may be less somber, although wider excision should be carried out. The reporting of histological appearances of these naevi is the province of an expert.

Complications, or sequelae

Psychological problems are common in patients with large naevi because of the cosmetic deficit suffered. Attempts to improve cosmesis will be discussed subsequently.

When large naevi occur on a limb there is, not uncommonly, demonstrably reduced growth in that limb. Less significantly, there may be an absence of subcutaneous fat underlying truncal naevi.

Proliferation of melanocytes within the central nervous system may lead to hydrocephalus, developmental delay or even central nervous system melanoma [15] but these are uncommon. In a series of 80 Mexican patients with giant naevi, only one case of hydrocephalus was reported [7]. In patients with giant naevi, central nervous system involvement should nevertheless be sought for prognostic purposes clinically and with ultrasound scan when the naevus lies in the midline. The possibility of using a magnetic resonance image (MRI) scan and lumbar puncture should be considered.

There is undoubtedly an increased risk of melanoma arising in congenital naevi; however, the controversy rages as to the definite risk. More data are available for the giant naevi. The lifetime risk in these patients has been estimated at between 4 and 14%: most frequently at around 5% [7,21]. It would appear that the risk of malignancy in this group of patients is highest in the first 10 years of life [7,22,23], but malignancy can occur at any time subsequently [24]. In one series both melanomas reported occurred in the patients' early 20s [21]. One of the difficulties in assessing the suggestion that malignancies occur predominantly in early life is in differentiating melanoma from the simulants of melanoma, which may occur in childhood, as discussed above. Rarely, malignant tumours of neural origin or mesenchymanl origin, such as rhabdomyosarcomas and liposarcomas, develop in giant naevi [7,18].

For the clinician managing these patients, the great difficulty is that the melanoma may be difficult to diagnose clinically and indeed may present as nodal disease or even widespread metastases.

The risk to patients with smaller naevi is unclear. Certainly, melanomas do arise in congenital naevi as they do in acquired naevi. The public health issues concern the level of risk for naevi which are present in 1% of the population. There are no means of estimating the lifetime risk from these naevi but the risk is likely to be very small. In these patients, whole-scale removal prophylactically would be costly both in terms of health service costs and cosmesis to the patient. In the UK the perception is that the data do not support the prophylactic excision of such naevi [25].

It is the authors' view that the risk of melanoma in all individuals is proportional to the melanocyte mass. In patients with atypical naevi, this may present clinically as multiple and atypical naevi. In patients with congenital naevi, the risk is likely to be further determined by the proportion of melanocytes which remain proliferative. We think it likely therefore that risk is proportional to the volume of junctional melanocytes. If surgery is to be considered for prophylactic excision in order to reduce the risk of melanoma, rather than for cosmesis, which naevi should be removed?

- Small naevi which remain pigmented and are in sites which are difficult to monitor, such as the scalp.
- Medium or large-sized naevi in which excision with primary closure may be accomplished with good cosmetic results.
- Partial excision may be considered in giant naevi which remain pigmented in such a way as to improve the cosmetic appearance of the naevus.

Surgical treatment

The purpose of treatment of these naevi is to reduce the risk of malignancy and to improve cosmesis. In terms of reduction of risk, any reduction in the volume of proliferative melanocytes is likely to be of benefit. For patients with large or giant naevi then there may be some benefit from most surgical treatments of all naevi. However, any procedure must be balanced against the cosmetic result of the operation. Many naevi fade progressively with time, and teenage and adult patients then commonly feel that the most cosmetically troublesome areas are the scars from early reconstructive attempts. For this reason our view of when surgery should be attempted, in an attempt to prevent melanoma, is presented above.

The need to improve the cosmetic appearance of large naevi is usually the preoccupation of both patient and doctor and the literature is full of differing surgical approaches to the problem. If considering surgery, however, we must always remember that patients often do well with no intervention at all from a cosmetic point of view.

If surgery is planned for large or giant naevi then the aims must be to reduce melanoma risk *and* improve the cosmesis. There are numerous approaches in the literature and indeed one of the problems is that the rarity of giant naevi is such that few clinicians have a large experience of their management.

An attempt has been made to summarize the approaches usually taken to the surgery of giant naevi by reconstructive surgeons. The techniques used depend on the site. Tissue expansion is viewed as superior cosmetically than serial excision or grafting [26] but although it is the preferred option on the head and neck, it is unsuitable for the extremities and buttocks. On the trunk in an infant it may be possible to perform abdominoplasty: the naevus is widely excised down to fatty abdominal muscle and the wound closed by primary intention by greatly undermining the adjacent normal skin and stretching the expansile infantile skin [27]. Some authors have reported the use of cryopreserved or cultured epithelium to cover cutaneous defects [28] but others found this to be disappointing cosmetically [26]. Many authors advocate early intervention, as soon as infants can safely tolerate general anaesthesia, to take advantage of the relative excess of skin early in infancy and the excellent elasticity and healing of infantile skin [27].

A large series of 78 patients with giant naevi treated surgically at the Childrens' Hospital in Chicago was reported by Bauer & Vicari [29]. Their approach to surgery is summarized in Table 13.1.

A number of centres have developed a different approach to surgical treatment: the very early removal of naevus cells from the epidermis and the epidermodermal junction using a technique either of curettage or dermabrasion [30,31]. It has been found that by removing the tissue in this way in the newborn period, or certainly within the first year of life, reasonable cosmetic results may be obtained without grafting or the use of tissue expanders (Fig. 13.5a–c). The rationale was the probably mistaken view that melanocytes are more superficial at birth and then descend. The fact that newborns do better with these techniques than adults may in fact reflect the nature of their skin:

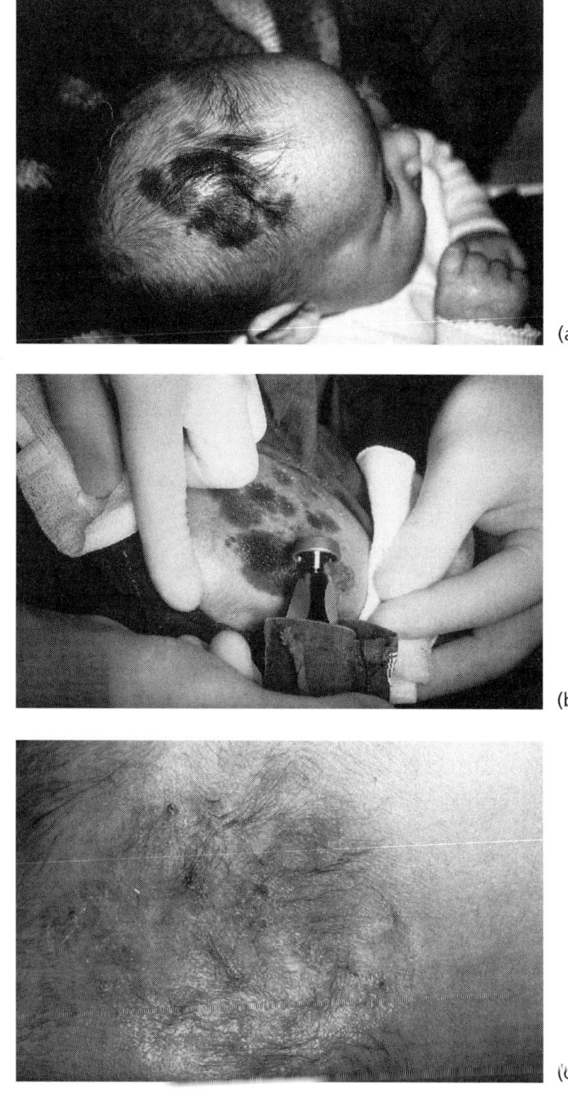

Fig. 13.5 (a) Congenital melanocytic naevus in a 2-month-old girl. (b) Dermabrasion under general anaesthesia. (c) Result 5 months later. No recurrence and and no disturbance of hair growth was noted during a follow-up period of 12 months. (Courtesy of Dr Arne König, Marburg, Germany.)

the suggestion of a natural plane of cleavage in the upper dermis in infancy which may be exploited using the curette [32]. These techniques appear to produce a loss of pigmentation without the scars of reconstructive surgery. However, clearly deep dermal naevus cells will be left in place with this technique so the impact on reduction of risk of malignancy is not clear and there have been concerns expressed that the dermal scarring which results from the procedure could obscure developing melanoma in deeper tissues [32].

The Q-switched ruby laser has been used experimentally to depigment congenital naevi although the congenital naevus cells appear to persist histo-

Table 13.1 Surgical approaches for the treatment of giant melanocytic naevi as proposed by Bauer & Vicari [29]

Site	Preferred technique	Notes
Scalp	Tissue expansion	Often begun at 3 months of age
Face	Tissue expansion	
Back and buttocks	Early large segment excision and immediate sheet grafting	
Anterior trunk	Abdominoplasty, tissue and skin grafting combined	
Extremities	Excision and skin grafting	Usually circumferential lesions excised in two phases, extensor and flexor surfaces

logically [33]. There are therefore concerns about this treatment, both because of the recurrence of pigmentation and because of the unknown effects this treatment has on the risks of malignancy.

Conclusions

In summary, the use of surgery to remove congenital naevi may be carried out to reduce the risk of malignancy but the effects on the cosmetic appearance of the naevus must be considered. In choosing the surgical approach, the site of the naevus is critical and Table 13.1 shows the preferred techniques for different sites. The choice available to the family and the clinician at birth is either to wait and see what happens in the first 6–12 months, given that many naevi become significantly paler in this time, with the possibility of reconstructive surgery later, or to try early curettage or dermabrasion, with an uncertain effect on risk.

References

1 Concensus Conference. Precursors to malignant melanoma. *J Am Med Assoc* 1984; **251** (14): 1864–6.

2 Walton R, Jacobs A, *et al.* Pigmented lesions in newborn infants. *Br J Dermatol* 1976; **95**: 389–96.

3 Alper J, Holmes L, *et al.* Birthmarks with serious significance. *J Pediatr* 1979; **95**: 696–700.

4 Kroon S, Clemmensen OJ, *et al.* Incidence of congenital melanocytic nevi in newborn babies in Denmark. *J Am Acad Dermatol* 1987; **17**: 422–6.

5 Rhodes AR. Congenital nevomelanocytic nevi: histologic patterns in the first year of life and evolution during childhood. *Arch Dermatol* 1986; **122**: 1257–62.

6 Castilla E, Dutra M, *et al.* Epidemiology of congenital pigmented nevi: incidence rates and relative frequencies. *Br J Dermatol* 1981; **104**: 307–15.

7 Ruiz-Maldonado R, Tamayo L, *et al.* Giant pigmented nevi: clinical, histopathologic, and therapeutic considerations. *J Pediatr* 1992; **120**: 906–11.

8 Castilla E, Da Graca Dutra M, *et al.* Epidemiology of congenital pigmented naevi: risk factors. *Br J Dermatol* 1981; **104**: 421–7.

9 Happle R. Lethal genes surviving by mosiacism: a possible explanation for sporadic birth defects involving the skin. *J Am Acad Dermatol* 1987; **16**: 899–906.

10 Amir J, Metzker A, *et al.* Giant pigmented nevus occurring in one identical twin. *Arch Dermatol* 1982; **118**: 188–9.

11 Happle R. Loss of heterozygosity in human skin. *J Am Acad Dermatol* 1999; **41**: 143–61.

12 Happle R. Dysplastic nevus syndrome: the emergence and decline of an erroneous concept. *J Eur Acad Dermatol* 1993; **2**: 275–80.

13 Bennett DC. Genetics, development and malignancy of melanocytes. *Int Rev Cytol* 1993; **146**: 191–260.

14 Antaya R, Keller R, *et al.* Placental nevus cells associated with giant congenital pigmented nevi. *Pediatr Dermatol* 1995; **12**: 260–2.

15 Reyes-Mugica M, Chou P, *et al.* Nevomelanocytic proliferations in the central nervous system in children. *Cancer* 1993; **72**: 2277–85.

16 Rhodes AR, Silverman RA, *et al.* A histologic comparison of congenital and acquired nevomelanocytic nevi. *Arch Dermatol* 1985; **121**: 1266–73.

17 Everett M. Histopathology of congenital pigmented nevi. *Am J Dermatopathol* 1989; **11**: 11–12.

18 Hendrickson M, Ross J. Neoplasms arising in congenital giant nevi. *Am J Surg Pathol* 1981; **5**: 109–35.

19 Rhodes A, Wood W, *et al.* Nonepidermal origin of malignant melanoma associated with a giant congenital nevocellular nevus. *Plast Reconstr Surg* 1981; **67**: 782–90.

20 Padilla R, McConnell T, *et al.* Malignant melanoma arising in a giant congenital melanocytic nevus. *Cancer* 1988; **62**: 2589–94.

21 Swerdlow AJ, English JSC, *et al.* The risk of melanoma in patients with congenital nevi: a cohort study. *J Am Acad Dermatol* 1995; **32**: 595–9.

22 Fish J, Smith F, *et al.* Malignant melanoma in childhood. *Surgery* 1966; **59**: 309–15.

23 Everett M. The management of congenital pigmented nevi. *J Okla State Med Assoc* 1991; **84**: 213–18.

24 Rhodes AR, Mihm Jr MC. Origin of cutaneous melanoma in a congenital dysplastic nevus spilus. *Arch Dermatol* 1990; **126**: 500–5.

25 British Association of Dermatology. Melanoma study group guidelines. *Br J Dermatol* 2001; **145** (59): 12–137.

26 Vergnes P, Taieb A, *et al.* Repeated skin expansion for excision of congenital nevi in infancy and childhood. *Plast Reconstr Surg* 1993; **91**: 45–5.

27 Marchac D, Weston J. Abdominoplasty in infants for removal of giant congenital nevi: a report of three cases. *Plast Reconstr Surg* 1985; **75**: 155–8.

28 Kumagai N, Oshima H, *et al.* Treatment of giant congenital nevi with cryopreserved allogeneic skin and fresh autologous cultured epithelium. *Ann Plast Surg* 1997; **39**: 483–8.

29 Bauer B, Vicari F. An approach to excision of congenital giant pigmented nevi in infancy and early childhood. *Plast Reconstr Surg* 1988; **82**: 1012–21.

30 Johnson H. Permanent removal of pigmentation from giant hairy nevi by dermabrasion in early age. *Br J Plast Surg* 1977; **30**: 321.

31 Rompel R, Moser M, *et al.* Dermabrasion of congenital nevocellular nevi: experience in 215 patients. *Dermatology* 1997; **194**: 261–7,

32 De Raeve LE, De Coninck AL, *et al.* Neonatal curettage of giant congenital melanocytic nevi. *Arch Dermatol* 1996; **132**: 20–2.

33 Goldberg D, Stampien T. Q-switched ruby laser treatment of congenital nevi. *Arch Dermatol* 1995; **131**: 621–3.

14: The role of chemotherapy

Jacqueline C. Newby and Tim Eisen

Introduction

Malignant melanoma often presents as a potentially curable isolated primary lesion. However, if this lesion is > 4 mm thick, or has spread to involve local lymph nodes, then recurrence and dissemination of disease are common. Once distant metastases develop, multiple organ involvement leading to death is usual, with a median survival of only 6–9 months. Systemic treatments are used in oncology with the aims of prolonging life, inducing tumour regressions, improving symptoms of metastatic disease and, in the adjuvant setting, preventing relapse. This chapter discusses the extent to which these aims are realized with standard cytotoxic agents for the treatment of malignant melanoma. Combinations of cytotoxic agents with other treatment modalities are discussed elsewhere.

Adjuvant chemotherapy for malignant melanoma

Adjuvant therapy for malignant melanoma is a theoretically attractive treatment option. Only 2% of cases present with disseminated disease; long-term survival following resection of regional lymph node disease is only ~30% and even after resection of an isolated primary lesion is only 50% if that lesion is > 4 mm thick. In addition, the management options for disseminated disease are limited and long-term survival a rare occurrence. Hence from the 1970s, when the concept of adjuvant therapy for malignant disease became established, there have been studies of adjuvant therapy for patients with malignant melanoma.

Non-randomized and often small studies have suggested possible survival benefits for vindesine and dacarbazine (DTIC) as single agents and the combinations of carmustine, cisplatin with tamoxifen; vinblastine, procarbazine with actinomycin D; and cisplatin, vinblastine with DTIC as adjuvant treatments. The vindesine study is the most interesting of the non-randomized studies of adjuvant chemotherapy [1]. This study retrospectively compared survival in 87 patients with stage III malignant melanoma treated with adjuvant vindesine chemotherapy following lymph node resection with that of 82 concurrent control patients given no adjuvant therapy. The patients were taken from the centre's prospective database of all malignant melanoma patients referred to the unit. Adjuvant therapy was not offered by many of the referring hospitals and this was the reason for 'no treatment' in the majority of the control group. In a few cases, patients declined treatment. Adjuvant vindesine therapy was then examined as one of a number of potential prognostic factors for survival using Cox regression analysis. Vindesine treatment was a highly statistically significant factor for prolonged disease-free and overall survival in univariate analysis and remained so on multivariate analysis. The hazard ratio for overall survival in those treated with adjuvant vindesine was 0.52 ($P = 0.0095$) with 5-year survival rates of 49% in the treated arm and 28% in the untreated patients. Clearly, this needs further evaluation in a randomized fashion against a control arm.

Table 14.1 summarizes the results of randomized studies of adjuvant chemotherapy in malignant melanoma patients. In all of these studies the difference between the two arms is chemotherapy, though in some studies both arms receive 'immunotherapy' with Bacillus Calmette–Guérin (BCG) or *Corynebacterium parvum* in addition to the randomization to chemotherapy or no chemotherapy, without a 'no treatment' control arm. These studies generally contain small numbers of patients; only the World Health Organization (WHO) trial [6] included sufficient numbers of patients to detect a modest difference in survival between treatment arms. Also of note is the heterogeneity of patients included in these trials: all stages of disease are represented; even those studying 'high-risk stage I–II cases' differ significantly in the definition of high risk; and staging methods, particularly in the earlier studies, differed between trials.

Of the two positive randomized studies, Hansson *et al.* [8] showed improvements in both disease-free and overall survival in patients treated with either DTIC alone or a combination of DTIC, nitrosourea (CCNU) and vincristine following resection of stage I–II tumours compared to no treatment, but only included a total of 26 patients. A larger study [13] randomized 173 patients with resected stage III–IV disease between no treatment or a combination of carmustine (BCNU), vincristine and actinomycin D. Disease-free interval (DFI) was greater in the chemotherapy arms, but there was no improvement in overall survival, a debatable benefit of treatment in this setting.

The two most important negative adjuvant studies are the WHO and European Organization for Research on Treatment of Cancer (EORTC) studies. The WHO study [6] randomized 761 patients following resection of either stage II disease or high-risk (Clark level 3–5 or truncal location) stage I disease

Table 14.1 Randomized studies of adjuvant chemotherapy for malignant melanoma

Author	Number of patients	Disease stage	Treatment arms	Significant benefit of chemotherapy on DFS/OS
Wood *et al.* [2]	70	I–III	1 BCG 2 DTIC 3 DTIC + BCG	No
Fisher *et al.* [3]	181	High-risk I–II	1 None 2 BCG 3 BCG plus melanoma cells 4 Methyl-CCNU	No
Hill *et al.* [4]	174	I–III	1 None 2 DTIC	No
Jacquillat *et al.* [5]	117	I	1 None 2 Vinblastine, rofocromycine, methotrexate, DTIC 3 Intra-arterial DTIC	No
Veronesi *et al.* [6] (WHO)	761	High-risk I–II	1 None 2 DTIC 3 BCG 4 DTIC + BCG	No
Balch *et al.* [7]	136	III–IV	1 *C. parvum* 2 *C. parvum* + DTIC, cyclophosphamide	No
Hansson *et al.* [8]	26	High-risk I–II	1 None 2 Chemotherapy (DTIC or DTIC, CCNU, vincristine)	Yes
Karakousis & Emrich [9]	82	I–III	1 None 2 DTIC + estramustine 3 BCG	No
Tranum *et al.* [10]	3	I–II	1 None 2 Carmustine, hydroxyurea, DTIC	No
Lejeune *et al.* [11] (EORTC)	274	I	1 None 2 DTIC 3 Levamisole	No
Castel *et al.* [12]	82	High-risk I–II	1 BCG 2 BCG + chemotherapy	No
Karakousis & Blumenson [13]	173	III–IV	1 None 2 BCNU, actinomycin D, vincristine	DFS Yes OS No

Continued

Table 14.1 *Continued*

Author	Number of patients	Disease stage	Treatment arms	Significant benefit of chemotherapy on DFS/OS
Meisenberg *et al.* [14]	39	High-risk II	1 Adjuvant high dose chemotherapy with autologous bone marrow rescue (cyclophosphamide, cisplatin and carmustine) 2 High dose chemotherapy at relapse	No

Abbreviations: BCG, Bacillus Calmette–Guérin; CCNU, 1-(-2-chloroethyl)-3-cyclohexyl-l-nitrosurea; DFS, disease-free survival; DTIC, dacarbazine; OS, overall survival.

to either: chemotherapy alone (DTIC single agent); BCG alone; combined immunochemotherapy (BCG + DTIC); or no treatment. There were no differences in disease-free or overall survival between the four groups. Statistically, this study had 80% power to detect a 14% difference in survival with a 10% chance of type I error. In the other large adjuvant study [11], 325 patients with stage I melanoma were randomized to DTIC alone, levamisole or placebo following surgery. Two hundred and seventy-four evaluable patients showed no difference in disease-free interval or overall survival.

The overall conclusion to be drawn from these randomized studies is that to date there is no convincing evidence for a role for conventional cytotoxic agents alone (or in combination with BCG/*Corynebacterium parvum*) in the adjuvant treatment of malignant melanoma. The only study large enough to detect a modest improvement in survival is the WHO study which did not find such a benefit. Many of the studies listed did not use the most effective cytotoxic agent, DTIC, in the chemotherapy arms. Amalgamation of results from different studies is impossible because of the variation in patient mix, staging methods and chemotherapy agents used.

The reason for the lack of benefit for adjuvant treatment may lie in the very modest activity of currently available cytotoxic agents against malignant melanoma as discussed later in this chapter. In the absence of more effective cytotoxic agents for malignant melanoma, it is difficult to see a role for chemotherapy alone in the adjuvant setting, particularly as immunotherapy appears more promising in this respect (see Chapter 15).

Neoadjuvant chemotherapy, perhaps not surprisingly in view of the above discussion, has not received a great deal of attention. In one pilot study [15], 52 patients with locoregional recurrence of malignant melanoma were treated with combination chemotherapy using cisplatin, vinblastine and DTIC. Surgery was performed after 2–3 cycles of treatment and responders went on to complete a total of eight cycles postoperatively. A 10% pathological complete response rate was seen, together with a 38% partial response rate. Interestingly, two of the pathological complete responders were clinically assessed as having only partial response or stable disease. At a median follow-up of 4.5 years, disease-free survival was 38% which is not significantly different from that expected for this stage of disease following surgery alone. This study clearly documents the activity of chemotherapy in locoregional disease assessed pathologically. It is impossible to draw any conclusions about survival from such a study. Long-term survivors following neoadjuvant chemotherapy for very poor prognosis disease (including stage IV disease with multiple organ involvement) are reported [16] but randomized studies have not been carried out.

Chemotherapy for metastatic disease

Single agent chemotherapy

The best single agent for malignant melanoma to date is the alkylating agent DTIC, with consistent objective response rates in the 15–20% range in phase II studies now numbering several thousand patients. Other established agents with documented activity include nitrosureas, vinca alkaloids and platinum agents (both cisplatin and, more recently, carboplatin). Newer agents include temozolomide (an orally active analogue of DTIC), taxanes, treosulphan and the nitrosurea fotemustine which appears effective in the treatment of cerebral metastases, for which DTIC, which does not cross the blood–brain barrier, is ineffective. Table 14.2 summarizes the active single agents in metastatic melanoma. 'Active' agents are those with an objective response rate of > 10% in the absence of significant toxicity.

Given the above, is there currently a role for single agents other than DTIC in the treatment of metastatic melanoma? It is difficult to justify agents other than DTIC as first-line therapy on the available evidence except for the management of central nervous system (CNS) disease for which DTIC is ineffective, and for which fotemustine and temozolomide show promising activity. Fotemustine has recently been studied in a randomized study for the treatment of cerebral metastases with and without whole brain irradiation [40]. Fotemustine alone was as effective as the combined therapy in terms of tumour response, control of symptoms and overall survival.

Newer agents showing reasonable response rates in Phase II studies should either be compared in a randomized fashion to single agent DTIC or combined with DTIC and compared to single agent DTIC in the treatment of visceral

Table 14.2 Response rates to single agent chemotherapy in metastatic melanoma

Drug	Number of patients	ORR (%)	Reference(s)
BCNU	122	18	Lee *et al.* [17]
CCNU	270	13	Lee *et al.* [17]
TCNU	42	17	Nolte *et al.* [18]
PCNU	32	16	Earhart *et al.* [19]
Fotemustine	245	25	Jacquillat *et al.* [20], Schallreuter *et al.* [21], Falkson *et al.* [22], Petit *et al.* [23]
Vincristine	52	12	Lee *et al.* [17]
Vinblastine	62	13	Lee *et al.* [17]
Vindesine	273	14	Lee *et al.* [17]
Detorubicin	42	19	Chawla *et al.* [24]
Cisplatin	188	23	Lee *et al.* [17]
High dose cisplatin	38	22	Mortimer *et al.* [25]
Carboplatin	99	15	Evans *et al.* [26], Casper & Bajorin [27], Chang *et al.* [28]
Piritrexim	31	23	Feun *et al.* [29]
Mitozolomide	41	12	Gundersen *et al.* [30], Harding *et al.* [31]
Temozolomide	60	21	Bleehen *et al.* [32]
Docetaxel		14	Verweij *et al.* [33]
Docetaxel	77	9	Bedikian *et al.* [34], Einzig *et al.* [35]
Paclitaxel	71	24	Wiernik *et al.* [36], Legha *et al.* [37], Einzig *et al.* [38]
Treosulphan	14	21	Neuber *et al.* [39]

Abbreviations: BCNU, 1,3-bis(2-chloroethyl-1-nitrosurea; CCNU, 1-(-2-chloroethyl)-3-cyclohexyl-l-nitrosurea; ORR, objective response rate (complete + partial responses).

disease outside the CNS. A randomized Phase III study of temozolomide vs. single agent DTIC in 305 patients with advanced melanoma has recently been reported [41]. Objective response rates were similar (13.5 vs. 12.1%). Both DFI and overall survival (OS) were better with temozolomide treatment (DFI 1.9 vs. 1.5 months, $P = 0.01$; OS 7.9 vs. 5.7 months, $P = 0.06$). Of importance in this study was the assessment of quality of life (QOL) by the EORTC QLQ-C30 questionnaire. Again the results, currently reported in abstract form only, favoured temozolomide with better preservation of physical function. Other agents which might benefit from such an approach include fotemustine, paclitaxel, docetaxel and maybe treosulphan.

Following failure of first-line therapy with DTIC, no agent has shown consistent activity as salvage treatment, though responses have been documented with a variety of agents and combinations in small studies. At present, second-line chemotherapy for malignant melanoma should be confined to the context of clinical trials.

Combination chemotherapy

The best single agent chemotherapy for metastatic melanoma, DTIC, produces only 15–20% objective response rates with a low complete response rate and very few long-term survivors. A logical progression has been to combine chemotherapy agents with different mechanisms of actions and side-effect profiles to try to increase the response rates and survival, with acceptable toxicity. A large number of different two, three and four drug combinations have been used over the last 30 years, most, though not all of which have included DTIC. Some have also included agents which do not appear effective as a single agent, for example bleomycin. In the 1970s and 1980s, combinations mainly consisted of DTIC with a nitrosurea and vinca alkaloid. Comparison of combination regimens with single agents did not show any significant advantage for combination therapy in terms of response rates. In 1975 Moon *et al.* [42] showed single agent DTIC in either of two schedules to have higher response rates than a BCNU–vincristine combination (24 vs. 16%); a result confirmed in a separate study of 50 patients with response rates of 29 and 23% for first-line DTIC and BCNU–vincristine, respectively [43]. In 1976 Carter *et al.* [44] compared single agent DTIC with three combination regimens: DTIC, CCNU and vincristine; DTIC, CCNU and hydroxyurea; or DTIC, BCNU and vincristine. For 243 evaluable patients, overall response rates were 17% with no difference between the four treatment arms. An Eastern Cooperative Oncology Group (ECOG) study randomized 450 patients to either DTIC, CCNU or a combination of the two agents. Response rates were 14, 15 and 14%, respectively [45]. Luikart *et al.* [46] randomized 57 patients between DTIC alone or a combination of vinblastine, bleomycin and cisplatin (VBC). Response rates were 14 and 10%, respectively. No significant differences in overall or disease-free survival were seen, though there was a trend for longer survival in the DTIC treated patients.

In more recent years the focus has been on combinations including DTIC, vinca alkaloids, cisplatin and nitrosureas with or without tamoxifen as a biomodulator. These combinations include the most active single agents in this disease. The Dartmouth regimen is a representative example using DTIC, BCNU, cisplatin and tamoxifen. This was first described in 1984 [47] and has been studied at a number of institutions in Phase II studies. Response rates in such studies range from 20 to 60%, averaging approximately 30% (Table 14.3). The same combination of cytotoxic agents with megestrol acetate rather than tamoxifen has shown similar results in Phase II studies [58,59]. On the basis of such Phase II studies, many centres have adopted these combination regimens as standard therapy for metastatic disease. Unfortunately, the superiority of this regimen—or any other combination of cytotoxic agents—over single agent DTIC has not been confirmed by randomized studies. A recently published study randomized 240 patients between DTIC alone and

Table 14.3 Studies of the Dartmouth chemotherapy regimen for the treatment of metastatic melanoma

Author	Number of patients	Objective response rate (%)
Del Prete *et al.* [47]	20	55
McClay *et al.* [48]	20	50
Richards *et al.* [49]	20	55
Saba *et al.* [50]	14	29
Fierro *et al.* [51]	32	43
Reintgen & Saba [52]	47	46
Lattanzi *et al.* [53]	42	54 (with tamoxifen) 25 (without tamoxifen)†
Rusthoven *et al.* [54]	199	30 (with tamoxifen) 21 (without tamoxifen)†
Tan & Ang [55]	13	60
Margolin *et al.* [56]	79	15
Chapman *et al.** [57]	119	17

* data from randomized study
† difference not statistically significant

the Dartmouth regimen [57]. Response rates were not significantly different (9.9 vs. 16.8%, $P = 0.09$) and, perhaps more importantly, overall survival was no different between the two groups (6.3 vs. 7.7 months). In this study no complete responses were seen in either group.

Thus, combination chemotherapy for metastatic malignant melanoma has not been shown to offer any advantage over single agent DTIC either in terms of response rates or survival.

High-dose chemotherapy

In an attempt to improve on the disappointing results with conventional dose chemotherapy, high-dose regimens have been studied. There is circumstantial evidence for a dose–response effect with many cytotoxic agents in malignant melanoma. One study of combination chemotherapy including escalating dosage of DTIC showed increasing responses rates in line with the DTIC dosage [60]. A case report describes a patient with hepatic metastases who responded to intra-arterial therapy with DTIC [61]. The patient then failed to respond to systemic DTIC at relapse, but again responded to intrahepatic artery with the same agent. Melphalan does not have any activity when given systemically at conventional dosage [62], yet is the most common agent used in isolated limb perfusion for malignant melanoma at much higher dosage, with complete response rates of 50–60% (see Chapter 17).

Such data have led to a number of studies using high-dose chemotherapy with autologous bone marrow rescue in the management of malignant melanoma, both for metastatic disease and for adjuvant therapy of high-risk cases. So far these high-dose regimens using autologous bone marrow rescue have produced encouraging objective response rates including high proportions of complete responses (up to 81% with 25% complete responses in one study [63]) but none has yet shown a survival benefit for high-dose therapy. The toxicity of such regimens for patients with survival in the range of 6–9 months is unacceptable.

Marrow reconstitution with peripheral blood stem cells, which has now become standard practice following high-dose chemotherapy, may have the additional benefit of an immune antitumour mechanism in its own right. The concept of high-dose chemotherapy with allogeneic marrow or stem cell rescue to harness a potential graft-vs.-tumour effect is theoretically attractive. A preliminary study treated four patients with metastatic melanoma with allogeneic HLA-matched peripheral blood stem cells following pretreatment with cyclophosphamide and fludarabine [64]. Two of the patients showed 'tumour regression', one progressed rapidly and the fourth progressed following graft rejection. Further Phase I–II studies of allogeneic peripheral blood stem cell transplantation are in progress.

Optimizing current chemotherapy treatment for metastatic melanoma

If DTIC is the best agent that we have, are we getting the best out of it or are there ways in which its use could be modified or enhanced? Numerous Phase II studies have shown an overall response rate of ~20% including occasional complete responses (~5%); a median duration of response of 5–6 months and a median overall survival of 6–9 months with 5-year overall survival rates of ~2%. It is more effective against disease in skin, lymph nodes and lung than in other visceral sites and is ineffective against CNS disease. Doses and regimens vary but outpatient administration of a single dose of 850–1000 mg/m^2 repeated every 3 weeks is a common and practical protocol. The major side-effects are nausea and vomiting, which are much improved with the introduction of serotonin antagonists and steroids into routine antiemetic practice. Haematological toxicity is rarely a significant problem at this dosage. Flu-like symptoms, malaise and photosensitivity are commonly reported but rarely severe. Potentially fatal veno-occlusive disease of the liver has also been reported but is rare. No study has randomized DTIC against best supportive care for metastatic disease.

DTIC is metabolized to the active agent MTIC (5-(3-methyl-1-triazeno)imidazole-4-carboxamide) which methylates cellular molecules including DNA. Twelve different DNA lesions are produced by this metabolite, but the major cytotoxic effect is linked to production of the O^6-methyl guanine (O^6-MeG) moiety. The amount of this product varies greatly between individuals treated with DTIC and this may be responsible for some of the variation in response. There is clinical evidence in support of this as responses do correlate with O^6-MeG levels following DTIC therapy [65]. Analogues of DTIC are being developed to try to avoid this variability and to maximize the amount of O^6-MeG produced. Temozolomide is promising in this respect as it is not dependent on metabolic activation and hence eliminates some of the interpatient variability. As already discussed, temozolomide has produced superior survival rates and quality of life in a randomized trial against single agent DTIC [41]. Alkyltransferase enzymes degrade the methylated species and combinations of temozolomide with alkyltransferase inhibitors are currently in Phase I clinical trials. Oral activity and CNS penetration are additional advantages over DTIC.

For DTIC the optimal dose and regimen has not been established. No schedule has been shown to be superior to any other in a randomized study. Retrospective data suggest a small benefit of prolonged daily over shorter regimens and this is also the case with temozolomide. Current protocols have settled on a simple and practical 3-weekly outpatient intravenous bolus of 850–1000 mg/m^2. In the palliative setting, ease of administration and tolerability probably outweigh any minor advantage of a longer regimen.

Regional treatment is one way of giving a higher dose of a given agent to the area involved while reducing the risks of systemic toxicity. Isolated limb perfusion is one example of a regional treatment which has the potential to increase survival rates for a specific group of patients and is discussed elsewhere (see Chapter 17). Other regional routes for the administration of chemotherapy for malignant melanoma have been reported including intraperitoneal, intracarotid artery, intrahepatic artery and isolated pelvic perfusion. This approach may have a limited role for patients with single organ/region metastatic disease or for the management of a particularly symptomatic site in a patient with multiorgan involvement, but will not substantially increase the overall survival rate.

What sort of a patients will respond to DTIC? Many studies have confirmed that patients with skin, soft tissue nodal and lung metastases are more likely to get a response than those with other visceral sites of disease, and that those with CNS disease will not respond to DTIC. However, responses have been documented in patients with unfavourable disease sites (CNS excepted). *In vitro* assessment of tumour sensitivity to cytotoxic agents is possible and has been used in melanoma patients [66]. However, in a limited study comparing clinical outcome between a retrospective analysis of sensitivity which did not affect choice of chemotherapy and a prospective group of patients where the results of *in vitro* sensitivity testing were used to determine the choice of cytotoxic agent, no significant differences were seen despite encouraging specificity and sensitivity results for the tests. Current studies are measuring the O^6-MeG levels in peripheral blood cells following DTIC therapy to establish whether these could predict for response early in the course of therapy (e.g. 24 h after the first dose) rather than waiting 4–6 weeks for clinical response determination. At the present time, patients with CNS metastases from malignant melanoma should not be treated with DTIC. There are clinical studies of fotemustine and temozolomide therapy for these patients.

Does chemotherapy make patients feel better?

The discussion regarding the treatment of metastatic melanoma has so far focused on the ability of chemotherapeutic agents to produce 'objective tumour responses (> 50% reduction in the size of measurable disease). This does not necessarily translate directly into a benefit to the patient in terms of how he or she actually feels. It also disregards the group of patients for whom chemotherapy results in stable disease. In other malignancies, stable disease on treatment puts patients into an equivalent prognostic group regarding survival to those achieving partial response (e.g. hormone treatment of metastatic breast cancer) and in clinical practice, stable disease is usually counted as a positive result of treatment.

If chemotherapy resulted in a significant number of long-term survivors, quality of life on treatment would be a relatively unimportant factor. This is not the case for treatment of metastatic melanoma. In these circumstances, improvement in quality of life rather than tumour response should be the criterion of success for any treatment. This is often summed up in clinical practice as aiming to make patients feel 'as well as possible for as long as possible'.

Many studies have shown that DTIC responders live longer than non-responders. It is not clear whether this longer survival is a result of the treatment or of the disease itself. Randomized studies of DTIC against best supportive care for metastatic disease have not been performed, and it is quite possible that the longer survival and the response to DTIC therapy are both independent results of the biology of individual tumours.

Quality of life (QOL) is more difficult to measure than length of life. As most studies of chemotherapy for the treatment of metastatic melanoma are small Phase II trials, formal QOL assessments have generally not been included. Randomized Phase III studies have evaluated response rates, survival and toxicity but rarely QOL. It is well recognised that formal toxicity assessment does not reflect QOL as assessed by questionnaire methods. Often 'minor' grade 1–2 toxicities can have a far greater impact on how a patient feels than medically significant grade 3–4 toxicity.

A Swedish group have focused on QOL assessment in malignant melanoma patients [67]. They developed a disease-specific melanoma module to be used in conjunction with the EORTC core QOL questionnaire (then the

QLQ-C36, now replaced by the modified QLQ-C30) and validated this module in malignant melanoma patients. The group then applied these questionnaires to patients with advanced melanoma on chemotherapy in a longitudinal study [68]. A total of 95 patients were entered into this study, most as part of a randomized trial comparing two combination chemotherapy regimens (DTIC–vindesine ± cisplatin). Quality of life was assessed prechemotherapy and at defined time points during and after treatment. Time points during chemotherapy were chosen to reflect maximum and minimum periods of treatment-related toxicity. Other clinical endpoints were also assessed, including performance status, tumour response, survival and toxicity.

Only six patients completed the full 1-year assessment protocol, mainly because of disease progression. Many QOL measures, including overall QOL, deteriorated significantly up to 9 weeks of the study, i.e. during the course of treatment. This deterioration was still evident for some factors (physical functioning, fatigue and neurological symptoms) at 20 weeks, after completion of treatment. However, overall QOL had returned to pretreatment levels at this point. There was no correlation between QOL and more standard clinical outcome measurements except for between the neurological symptom item in the disease-specific module and WHO neurotoxicity. This would be expected where the QOL item was designed to reflect the known neurotoxicity of vindesine and cisplatin used in this trial, neither of which should be considered standard treatment. The lack of correlation with other clinical outcomes is in line with other QOL studies.

This paper is the first to attempt to assess QOL in patients receiving chemotherapy for metastatic melanoma. However, it cannot answer the question posed at the beginning of this section. Though performed in the context of a randomized study, the randomization was between two non-standard chemotherapy regimens and not 'standard' chemotherapy vs. no treatment. Much of the toxicity, reflected in the QOL assessment, was caused by non-standard cytotoxic agents used in the regimens. There was inevitably a very high non-compliance rate for the full 1-year protocol, but the missing data may in this context may be more important than the data collected.

The only other study to include QOL assessment in metastatic melanoma patients on chemotherapy is the recently reported Phase III randomized comparison between DTIC and temozolomide [41]. Quality of life was assessed by the EORTC QLQ-C30. The full study with details of QOL results has not been published yet. Patients receiving temozolomide therapy were less likely to report a deterioration in physical functioning than those receiving DTIC.

These studies do not directly address the question 'does chemotherapy make patients feel better?' This would require QOL assessment in the context of a randomized study of best chemotherapy against no treatment: such a study has not been carried out.

Conclusions

In the absence of evidence that chemotherapy improves QOL, or that it has any significant effect on survival, its use should be restricted to symptomatic metastatic disease. Improvement in those symptoms and overall QOL should be the main criteria on which the success of the chemotherapy treatment is judged on an individual basis. Treatment of asymptomatic patients is not justified as a routine on the current evidence and should be confined to clinical trials.

DTIC is the best single agent chemotherapy treatment for advanced melanoma (except for CNS disease) and should be considered the standard against which other agents and combinations should be evaluated in clinical trials. Temozolomide has several theoretical advantages and early clinical results of comparison with single agent DTIC appear favourable.

Optimization of currently available agents and regimens is not likely to produce dramatic improvements in the survival of patients with this relatively unresponsive disease, though it may make minor improvements to our overall management of these patients. Combination regimens, including DTIC with newer agents, may improve on current results regarding response rates and possibly survival. It will be important to include symptom control and/or QOL assessments in the evaluation of such regimens in addition to the formal assessment of tumour response.

However, completely innovative agents aside, the future of treatment for malignant melanoma is clearly not in the realms of cytotoxic agent(s) alone. Combinations of cytotoxic agents and biological therapies (see Chapter 15) are the current focus for research into the treatment of malignant melanoma and combinations of cytotoxic agents alone may not have a role if these fulfil their current promise.

To end on a slightly more optimistic note, the advent of cisplatin transformed the management of metastatic teratoma, now one of the most curable of malignant diseases, from an equally dismal situation in the 1970s and it is possible that such a cytotoxic agent for metastatic melanoma is already in development.

References

1 Retsas S, Quigley M, Pectasides D, Macrae K, Henry K. Clinical and histological involvement of regional lymph nodes in malignant melanoma: adjuvant vindesine improves survival. *Cancer* 1994; 73: 2119–30.

2 Wood WC, Cosimi AB, Carey RW, Kaufman SD. Randomized trial of adjuvant therapy for 'high risk' primary malignant melanoma. *Surgery* 1978; 83: 677–81.

3 Fisher RI, Terry WD, Hodes RJ, *et al.* Adjuvant immunotherapy or chemotherapy for malignant melanoma: preliminary report of the National Cancer Institute randomized clinical

trial. *Surg Clin North Am* 1981; **61**: 1267–77.

4 Hill GJ II, Moss SE, Golomb FM, *et al.* DTIC and combination therapy for melanoma: III. DTIC (NSC 45388) Surgical Adjuvant Study COG PROTOCOL 7040. *Cancer* 1981; **47**: 2556–62.

5 Jacquillat C, Banzet P, Meral J, *et al.* Clinical trials of chemotherapy and chemoimmunotherapy in primary malignant melanoma. *Recent Results Cancer Res* 1982; **80**: 254–8.

6 Veronesi U, Adamus J, Aubert C, *et al.* A randomized trial of adjuvant chemotherapy and immunotherapy in cutaneous melanoma. *N Engl J Med* 1982; **307**: 913–16.

7 Balch CM, Murray D, Presant C, Bartolucci AA. Ineffectiveness of adjuvant chemotherapy using DTIC and cyclophosphamide in patients with resectable metastatic melanoma. *Surgery* 1984; **95**: 454–9.

8 Hansson J, Ringborg U, Lagerlof B, Strander H. Adjuvant chemotherapy of malignant melanoma: a pilot study. *Am J Clin Oncol* 1985; **8**: 47–50.

9 Karakousis CP, Emrich LJ. Adjuvant treatment of malignant melanoma with DTIC + estracyt or BCG. *J Surg Oncol* 1987; **36**: 235–8.

10 Tranum B, Dixon D, Quagliana J, *et al.* Lack of benefit of adjunctive chemotherapy in Stage I malignant melanoma: a Southwest Oncology Group study. *Cancer Treat Rep* 1987; **71**: 643–4.

11 Lejeune FJ, Macher E, Kleeberg U, *et al.* An assessment of DTIC versus levamisole or placebo in the treatment of high risk stage I patients after surgical removal of a primary melanoma of the skin: a phase III adjuvant study. EORTC protocol 18761. *Eur J Cancer Clin Oncol* 1988; **24**: S81–90.

12 Castel T, Estape J, Vinolas N, *et al.* Adjuvant treatment in stage I and II malignant melanoma: a randomized trial between chemoimmunotherapy and immunotherapy. *Dermatologica* 1991; **183**: 25–30.

13 Karakousis C, Blumenson L. Adjuvant chemotherapy with a nitrosurea-based protocol in advanced malignant melanoma. *Eur J Cancer* 1993; **29A**: 1831–5.

14 Meisenberg BR, Ross M, Vredenburgh JJ, *et al.* Randomized trial of high-dose chemotherapy with autologous bone marrow support as adjuvant therapy for high-risk, multi-node positive malignant melanoma. *J Natl Cancer Inst* 1993; **85**: 1080–5.

15 Buzaid AC, Legha SS, Balch CM, *et al.* Pilot study of pre-operative chemotherapy with cisplatin, vinblastine, and dacarbazine in patients with local-regional recurrence of melanoma. *Cancer* 1994; **74**: 2476–82.

16 Sasson HN, Poo WJ, Bakas MH, Ariyan S. Prolonged survival in patients with advanced melanoma treated with neoadjuvant chemotherapy followed by resection. *Ann Plast Surg* 1996; **37**: 286–92.

17 Lee SM, Betticher DC, Thatcher N. Melanoma: chemotherapy. *Br Med Bull* 1995; **51**: 609–30.

18 Nolte H, Lindgaard-Nedsen E, Bloomquist E, *et al.* Phase II evaluation of tauromustine in disseminated malignant melanoma. *Proc Am Soc Clin Oncol* 1988; **7**: 249.

19 Earhart RH, Muggia FM, Golomb FM. Phase II trial of PCNU in advanced malignant melanoma: an Eastern Cooperative Oncology Group pilot study. *Invest New Drugs* 1985; **3**: 297–301.

20 Jacquillat C, Khayat D, Banzet P, *et al.* Chemotherapy by fotemustine in cerebral metastases of disseminated malignant melanoma. *Cancer Chemother Pharmacol* 1990; **25**: 263–6.

21 Schallreuter KU, Wenzel E, Brassow FW, Berger J, Breitbart EW, Teichmann W. Positive phase II study in the treatment of advanced malignant melanoma with fotemustine. *Cancer Chemother Pharmacol* 1991; **29**: 85–7.

22 Falkson CI, Falkson G, Falkson HC. Phase II trial of fotemustine in patients with metastatic malignant melanoma. *Invest New Drugs* 1994; **12**: 251–4.

23 Petit T, Borel C, Rixe O, *et al.* Complete remission seven years after treatment for metastatic malignant melanoma. *Cancer* 1996; **77**: 900–2.

24 Chawla SP, Legha SS, Benjamin RS. Detorubicin: an active anthracycline in untreated metastatic melanoma. *J Clin Oncol* 1985; **3**: 1529–34.

25 Mortimer JE, Schulman S, MacDonald JS,

Kopecky K, Goodman G. High-dose cisplatin in disseminated melanoma: a comparison of two schedules. *Cancer Chemother Pharmacol* 1990; **25**: 373–6.
26 Evans LM, Casper ES, Rosenbluth R. Phase II trial of carboplatin in advanced malignant melanoma. *Cancer Treat Rep* 1987; **71**: 171–2.
27 Casper ES, Bajorin D. Phase II trial of carboplatin in patients with advanced melanoma. *Invest New Drugs* 1990; **8**: 187–90.
28 Chang A, Hunt M, Parkinson DR, Hochster H, Smith TJ. Phase II trial of carboplatin in patients with metastatic malignant melanoma: a report from the Eastern Cooperative Oncology Group. *Am J Clin Oncol* 1993; **16**: 151–5.
29 Feun LG, Gonzalez R, Savaraj N, *et al.* Phase II trial of piritrexim in metastatic melanoma using intermittent low-dose administration. *J Clin Oncol* 1991; **9**: 464–7.
30 Gundersen S, Aamdal S, Fodstad O. Mitozolomide (NSC 353451), a new active drug in the treatment of malignant melanoma: Phase II trial in patients with advanced disease. *Br J Cancer* 1987; **55**: 433–5.
31 Harding M, Docherty V, Mackie R, Dorward A, Kaye S. Phase II studies of mitozolomide in melanoma, lung and ovarian cancer. *Eur J Cancer Clin Oncol* 1989; **25**: 785–8.
32 Bleehen NM, Newlands ES, Lee SM, *et al.* Cancer Research Campaign phase II trial of temozolomide in metastatic melanoma. *J Clin Oncol* 1995; **13**: 910–3.
33 Verweij J, Catimel G, Sulkes A, *et al.* Phase II studies of docetaxel in the treatment of various solid tumours: EORTC early clinical trials group and the EORTC soft tissue and bone sarcoma group. *Eur J Cancer* 1995; **31A** (Suppl 4): 21–4.
34 Bedikian AY, Weiss GR, Legha SS, *et al.* Phase II trial of docetaxel in patients with advanced cutaneous malignant melanoma previously untreated with chemotherapy. *J Clin Oncol* 1995; **13**: 2895–9.
35 Einzig AI, Svhuchter LM, Recio A, Coatsworth S, Rodriquez R, Wiernik PH. Phase II trial of docetaxel (Taxotere) in patients with metastatic melanoma previously untreated with cytotoxic chemotherapy. *Med Oncol* 1996; **13**: 111–7.
36 Wiernik PH, Schwartz EL, Einzig A, Strauman JJ, Lipton RB, Dutcher JP. Phase I trial of taxol given as a 24-hour infusion every 21 days: responses observed in metastatic melanoma. *J Clin Oncol* 1987; **5**: 1232–9.
37 Legha SS, Ring S, Papadopoulos N, Raber M, Benjamin RS. A phase II trial of taxol in metastatic melanoma. *Cancer* 1990; **65**: 2478–81.
38 Einzig AI, Hochster H, Wiernik PH, *et al.* A phase II study of taxol in patients with malignant melanoma. *Invest New Drugs* 1991; **9**: 59–64.
39 Neuber K, tom Dieck A, Blodorn-Schlicht N, Itschert G, Karnbach C. Treosulphan is an effective alkylating cytostatic for malignant melanoma *in vitro* and *in vivo*. *Melanoma Res* 1999; **9**: 125–32.
40 Mohr P, Mornex F, Thomas L, *et al.* Fotemustine chemotherapy with or without whole brain irradiation in patients with brain metastases of malignant melanoma. *Proc Am Soc Clin Oncol* Abstract 2050, 1999.
41 Middleton MR, Gore M, Tilgen W, *et al.* A randomized Phase III study of temozolomide versus dacarbazine in the treatment of patients with advanced metastatic melanoma. *Proc Am Soc Clin Oncol* Abstract 2069, 1999.
42 Moon JH, Gailani S, Cooper. MR, *et al.* Comparison of the combination of 1,3-bis(2-chloroethyl-1-nitrosurea (BCNU) and vincristine with two dose schedules of 5-(3,3-dimethyl-1-triazino) imidazole 4-carboxamide (DTIC) in the treatment of disseminated malignant melanoma. *Cancer* 1975; **35**: 368–71.
43 Bellett RE, Mastrelangelo MJ, Laucius JF, Bodurtha AJ. Randomized prospective trial of DTIC (NSC-45388) alone versus BCNU (NSC-409962) plus vincrisitne (NSC-67574) in the treatment of metastatic malignant melanoma. *Cancer Treat Rep* 1976; **60**: 595–600.
44 Carter RD, Krementz ET, Hill GJ II, *et al.* DTIC (NSC-45388) and combination therapy for melanoma. I. Studies with DTIC, BCNU (NSC-409962), CCNU (NSC-79037), vincristine (NSC-67574), and hydroxyurea (NSC-32065). *Cancer Treat Rep* 1976; **60**: 601–9.
45 Costanza ME, Nathanson L, Schoenfeld D, *et al.* Results with methyl-CCNU and

DTIC in metastatic melanoma. *Cancer* 1977; **40**: 1010–15.

46 Luikart SD, Kennealey GT, Kirkwood JM. Randomized phase III trial of vinblastine, bleomycin, and cis-dichlorodiamine-platinum versus dacarbazine in malignant melanoma. *J Clin Oncol* 1984; **2**: 164–8.

47 Del Prete SA, Maurer LH, O'Donnell J, Forcier RJ, LeMarbre P. Combination chemotherapy with cisplatin, carmustine, dacarbazine and tamoxifen in metastatic melanoma. *Cancer Treat Rep* 1984; **68**: 1403–5.

48 McClay EF, Mastrangelo MJ, Bellet RE, Berd D. Combination chemotherapy and hormonal therapy in the treatment of malignant melanoma. *Cancer Treat Reps* 1987; **71**: 465–9.

49 Richards JM, Gilewski TA, Ramming K, Mitchel B, Doane LL, Vogelzang NJ. Effective chemotherapy for melanoma after treatment with interleukin-2. *Cancer* 1992; **69**: 427–9.

50 Saba HI, Cruse CW, Wells KE, Klein CJ, Reintgen DS. Treatment of stage IV malignant melanoma with dacarbazine, carmustine, cisplatin and tamoxifen regimens: a University of South Florida and H. Lee Moffit Melanoma Center Study. *Ann Plast Surg* 1992; **28**: 65–9.

51 Fierro MT, Bertero M, Novelli M, *et al.* Therapy for metastatic melanoma: effective combination of dacarbazine, carmustine, cisplatin and tamoxifen. *Melanoma Res* 1993; **3**: 127–31.

52 Reintgen D, Saba H. Chemotherapy for stage 4 melanoma: a three-year experience with cisplatin, DTIC, BCNU, and tamoxifen. *Semin Surg Oncol* 1993; **9**: 251–5.

53 Lattanzi SC, Tosteson T, Chertoff J *et al.* Dacarbazine, cisplatin and carmustine, with or without tamoxifen, for metastatic melanoma: a 5 year follow-up. *Melanoma Res* 1995; **5**: 365–9.

54 Rusthoven JJ, Quirt IC, Iscoe NA, *et al.* Randomized, double-blind, placebo-controlled trial comparing the response rates of carmustine, dacarbazine and cisplatin with and without tamoxifen in patients with metastatic melanoma, National Cancer Institute of Canada Clinical Trials Group. *J Clin Oncol* 1996; **14**: 2083–90.

55 Tan EH, Ang PT. Combination chemotherapy (dacarbazine, carmustine, cisplatin and tamoxifen) in advanced melanoma. *Singapore Med J* 1996; **37**: 165–7.

56 Margolin KA, Liu PY, Flaherty LE, *et al.* Phase II study of carmustine, dacarbazine, cisplatin and tamoxifen in advanced melanoma: a Southwest Oncology Group study. *J Clin Oncol* 1998; **16**: 664–9.

57 Chapman P, Einhorn LH, Meyers M, *et al.* Phase III multicenter randomized trial of the Dartmouth regimen versus dacarbazine in patients with metastatic melanoma. *J Clin Oncol* 1999; **17**: 2745–51.

58 Nathanson L, Meelu MA, Losada R. Chemohormone therapy of metastatic melanoma with megestrol acetate plus dacarbazine, carmustine and cisplatin. *Cancer* 1994; **73**: 98–102.

59 Nathanson L, Garrison M. Megestrol melanoma study. *World J Surg* 1995; **19**: 337–42.

60 Lee SM, Margison GP, Woodcock AA, Thatcher N. Sequential administration of varying doses of dacarbazine and fotemustine in advanced malignant melanoma. *Br J Cancer* 1993; **67**: 1356–60.

61 Hoelzer KL, Harrison BR, Luedke DW, Mahanta B. Dose–response relationship to dacarbazine demonstrated in a patient with malignant melanoma. *Cancer Treatment Reports* 1986; **70**: 1211–2.

62 Hochster H, Strawderman MH, Harris JE, *et al.* Conventional dose melphalan is inactive in metastatic melanoma: results of an Eastern Cooperative Oncology Group Study (E1687). *Anticancer Drugs* 1999; **10**: 245–8.

63 Thatcher D, Lind M, Morgenstern G, *et al.* High-dose double alkylating agent chemotherapy with DTIC, melphalan or ifosfamide and marrow rescue for metastatic malignant melanoma. *Cancer* 1989; **63**: 1296–302.

64 Childs R, Clave E, Bahceci E, *et al.* Non-myeloablative allogeneic peripheral blood stem cell transplantation as adoptive allogeneic immunotherapy for metastatic melanoma and renal cell carcinoma. *Proc Am Soc Clin Oncol* Abstract 196, 1999.

65 Lee SM, Margison GP, Thatcher N, O'Connor P, Cooper D. Formation and loss of O6-methyl deoxyguanosine in human leukocyte DNA following

sequential DTIC and fotemustine chemotherapy. *Br J Cancer* 1994; **69**: 853–7.
66 Tveit KM, Gundersen S, Hoie J, Pihl A. Predictive chemosensitivity testing in malignant melanoma: reliable methodology—ineffective drugs. *Br J Cancer* 1988; **58**: 734–7.
67 Sigurdardottir V, Bolund C, Brandberg T, Sullivan M. The impact of generalized malignant melanoma on quality of life evaluated by the EORTC questionnaire technique. *Qual Life Res* 1993; **2** (3): 193–203.
68 Sigurdardottir V, Brandberg Y, Sullivan M. Criterion-based validation of the EORTC QLQ-C36 in advanced melanoma: the CIPS questionnaire and proxy raters. *Qual Life Res* 1996; **5**: 375–86.

15: What is the role of biological response modifiers in the treatment of melanoma?

Alexander M.M. Eggermont & Ulrich Keilholz

Introduction

Biological response modifiers (BRMs) have been used for many years for treatment of patients with melanoma, especially α-interferon (IFN-α) and interleukin 2 (IL-2). However, despite numerous studies, the role of BRMs remains controversial. Large randomized studies are currently underway to define the role of both these cytokines and ganglioside GM2 vaccine for the treatment of melanoma patients. In addition, numerous Phase II studies with specific vaccines (peptides, proteins, DNA) are currently being carried out with decisive Phase III trials to follow.

This chapter summarizes the current status on the three agents in Phase III studies: GM2, IFN-α, and IL-2.

Biological response modifiers as adjuvant therapy for high-risk melanoma

Aspecific immunotherapy with or without chemotherapy

The focus in the development of adjuvant therapy for high-risk melanoma has traditionally been on the modulation and activation of the immune system, because chemotherapy has been proven to be virtually without effect in stage IV melanoma. Aspecific immunostimulation by agents such as Bacillus Calmette–Guérin (BCG) or *Corynebacterium parvum* was investigated in the 1960s and 1970s. Studies were carried out in stage II and III melanoma patients of either chemotherapy alone, immunotherapy alone or immunochemotherapy combinations, compared to observation. A review on this topic has been published recently [1].

Eleven trial reports on the efficacy of adjuvant therapy with either chemotherapy (dacarbazine, DTIC; lomustine, CCNU; or carmustine, BCNU) alone or with BCG alone, or the combination of chemoimmunotherapy with BCG have been published; three negative trials on the use of

C. parvum alone or in combination with DTIC and one positive trial report on the use of *C. parvum* alone in comparison to BCG. On the use of yet another aspecific immunostimulant, levamisole, three negative and one partially positive trial report have been published. The sporadic positive results in mostly small and underpowered trials has been overwhelmingly outweighed by the negative outcome of a far larger number of trials. Among these trials there are two European Organization for Research on Treatment of Cancer Melanoma Cooperative Group (EORTC-MCG) trials, one on BCG and one on levamisole. It is of interest that the first trial launched by the EORTC-MCG, which compared vaccination with BCG to observation in patients with high-risk melanoma, was stopped under pressure of public opinion declaring such a trial 'unethical', as it had been 'proven' that BCG was beneficial to melanoma patients. Ever since the early days it should be considered a reasonable prerequisite that a treatment can be considered standard of care when *confirmed* proof of efficacy is present.

Vaccines in Phase III trials

Adjuvant specific (tumour cell vaccines) immunotherapy

Experience with vaccines that are supposed to induce a specific antimelanoma immunoresponse has been very limited so far in the treatment of melanoma. Three sizable active specific immunotherapy trials with whole tumour cell vaccines [2–4] did not show significant impact on disease-free survival (DFS) or overall survival (OS). A trial in the USA in 251 patients with a viral oncolysate of melanoma cells [5] and a very large trial in Australia with a viral oncolysate [6] were also negative.

Ganglioside GM2 vaccine

The expression of gangliosides, such as GM2, have been well described to differ from that of normal melanocytes and most normal tissues. Serological studies of melanoma have suggested a favourable prognosis for patients with pre-existing or vaccine-induced antibody titres against GM2. However, autologous antibodies against GM2 are infrequently detected in non-immunized patients. Livingston *et al.* [7] evaluated a series of autologous and allogeneic tumour vaccine regimens, and more recently purified ganglioside combined with immunological adjuvants. A randomized trial of GM2–BCG adjuvant therapy following surgery for American Joint Committee on Cancer (AJCC) stage III melanoma has been conducted in 122 patients at Memorial Sloan-Kettering (MSK) Cancer Center between 1987 and 1988 [7]. This trial demonstrated the induction of anti-GM2 IgM antibodies in most treated patients and the presence of natural antibodies against GM2 in a small subset of the control unvaccinated group of patients. Serological responses against GM2 were again demonstrated to be a favourable prognostic factor. In addition, the vaccinated group of patients has shown a borderline prolongation of relapse-free survival, confounded by the unanticipated presence of anti-GM2 antibodies among six patients in the control group. With the removal of these confounding results in patients who had prestudy serological reactivity to GM2, the impact of GM2–BCG vaccination upon relapse-free survival was significant ($P=0.02$).

Cytokines in Phase III trials

α-Interferon

Many trials with α-interferon (IFN-α) have been conducted and are discussed below.

γ-Interferon

Results of a Southwest Oncology Group (SWOG) trial on adjuvant therapy with γ-interferon (IFN-γ) were reported by Meyskens *et al.* [8] demonstrating a detrimental effect of adjuvant therapy with IFN-γ. Very recently the results of the EORTC 18771/DKG-80 (Deutsche Krebsgesellschaft) trials have been reported [9]. In the EORTC 18771/DKG-80 trial, DFS and OS in the IFN-γ arm were no different from the observation arm. Quite importantly, this trial also showed that the mistletoe extract, Iscador, which is a popular 'alternative medicine' preparation in central Europe precribed to many cancer patients, had no positive impact on DFS or OS when administered in the adjuvant setting in high-risk melanoma patients.

Interleukin 2

Interleukin 2 (IL-2) has modest activity in stage IV melanoma but so far has not been evaluated widely in the adjuvant setting in melanoma. In a Swiss–German Phase III trial in stage II melanoma patients using low doses of IL-2 and IFN-α, no impact on DFS or OS was observed [10].

All non-IFN-α immunotherapy trials are summarized in Table 15.1.

Table 15.1 Aspecific immunotherapy adjuvant therapy trials in stage II–III melanoma

Randomized Phase III trials	DFS/OS	Reference
BCG/C. parvum/levamisole ± chemotherapy		
Adjuvant chemotherapy		
(DTIC, CCNU, BCNU) or	–/–	
Aspecific immunotherapy		
(BCG, *C. parvum*, levamisole) or	–/–	Eggermont [1]
Combined chemoimmunotherapy	–/–	
Vaccines		
Tumour-specific vaccines		
BCG + allogeneic tumour cells	–/–	Morton *et al.* [2]; Terry *et al.* [3]
BCG + allogeneic tumour cells	–/–	Morton [4]
Viral oncolysate vaccines		
USA	–/–	Wallack *et al.* [5]
Australia	–/–	Hersey *et al.* [6]
Ganglioside GM2 vaccine		
GM2/BCG vs. BCG MSK trial	+/+	Livingston *et al.* [7]
Cytokines		
IFN-α (see Table 15.2)		
IFN-γ		
Southwest Oncology Group	–/–	Meyskens *et al.* [8]
EORTC 18771/DKG-80	–/–	Kleeberg *et al.* [9]
Interleukin 2		
IL-2 + IFN subcutaneously (Swiss–German trial)	–/–	Hauschild *et al.* [10]

Abbreviations: BCG, Bacillus Calmette–Guérin; BCNU, carmustine; CCNU, lomustine; DFS, disease-free survival; DKG, Deutsche Krebsgesellschaft; DTIC, dacarbazine; EORTC, European Organization for Research on Treatment of Cancer; IFN, interferon; IL-2, interleukin-2; MSK, Memorial Sloan-Kettering; OS, overall survival.

α-Interferon

Trials in stage III

Many trials with IFN have been performed in stage II–III melanoma patients over the last decade. Many trials have been underpowered, have suffered from the fact that mixed populations were studied (node-negative and node-positive patients in one and the same trial), and have investigated a variety of regimens. In an attempt to create some clarity, the patients in mixed stage II–III trials have been separated out into stages II and III in Table 15.2, which presents a summary of the results. Moreover, Table 15.2 divides trials into high-dose IFN (HDI) trials (doses of > 10 MU) and low-dose IFN (LDI) trials (doses < 5 MU).

Table 15.2 Phase III trials with IFN-α in stage II–III melanoma

	Number of patients	Treatment	DFS	OS
Stage II (A+B) or IIB				
High-dose IFN				
	122	NCCTG	–	–
	31	ECOG 1684	–	–
	163	ECOG 1690	–	–
Low-dose IFN				
	499	French trial	+	–
	311	Austrian trial	+	–
	99	Scottish trial	–	–
	340	EORTC 18871/DKG-80	–	–
Stage III				
High-dose IFN				
	160	NCCTG	–	–
	249	ECOG 1684	+	+
	479	ECOG 1690	+	–
Low-dose IFN				
	427	WHO-16	–	–
	490	EORTC/DKG	–	–

Abbreviations: DFS, disease-free survival; DKG, Deutsche Krebsgesellschaft; ECOG, Eastern Cooperative Oncology Group; EORTC, European Organization for Research on Treatment of Cancer; IFN, interferon; NCCTG, North Central Cancer Treatment Group; OS, overall survival; WHO, World Health Organization.

High-dose interferon

In only one rather small trial of 280 patients (Eastern Cooperative Oncology Group (ECOG) 1684), a significant benefit on DFS and OS has been observed after HDI treatment with IFN-2b for 1 year consisting of 4 weeks' daily intravenous administration of 20 MU/m^2, followed by 48 weeks of 10 MU/m^2 subcutaneously t.i.w. [11]. In the North Central Cancer Treatment Group (NCCTG) trial (262 patients) it was demonstrated that at the same high dose when administered intramuscularly t.i.w. for only 12 weeks, there was no significant impact on survival in this mixed population of stage II patients with primaries thicker than 1.7 mm and stage III melanoma patients [12]. Both HDI regimens were associated with significant toxicity in the range of grade III–IV toxicity in about 75% of the patients, requiring dose reductions and interruptions of the treatment regimens.

Low-dose interferon

Low-dose IFN treatment was evaluated in the WHO-16 trial. In this trial, 427 stage III melanoma patients were evaluated after randomization into either the observation arm or the LDI treatment arm (3 MU, subcutaneously t.i.w. for 3 years). Although a temporary effect on DFS was observed in the treatment arm, in the final analysis no DFS or OS benefit was observed in the WHO-16 study [13]. Another LDI (1 MU, subcutaneously, on alternative days for 1 year) regimen was evaluated in the EORTC 18871/DKG-80 trial, showing not even a trend for a benefit [9]. Unfortunately, the impact on OS by HDI therapy was not confirmed by the recently unblinded ECOG 1690 study, in spite of a significant benefit on DFS [14]. Low-dose IFN treatment at 3 MU for 2 years, in the ECOG 1690 trial did not demonstrate a benefit for either DFS or OS, just as in the WHO-16 trial.

Conclusions on stage III

Overall, it can be stated that observations have been inconsistent on the efficacy of IFN-α in the adjuvant setting for high-risk melanoma. Dose intensity as well as duration of treatment are not clearly defined and the efficacy of any regimen has yet to be demonstrated or confirmed by more than one trial. Table 15.2 summarizes the experience with IFN in adjuvant Phase III trials up to 1999.

Trials in stage II

In stage II patients with primary melanomas >1.5 mm clinically node-negative, three trials in Europe have completed accrual. These three trials are similar in dosage, all using IFN-2α at low doses of 3 MU for 6 months (Scottish trial), 12 months (Austrian trial) or 18 months (French trial). A preliminary report on the Scottish trial has not demonstrated a benefit in DFS or OS [1], whereas use for 12 months has been reported to result in a significant benefit on relapse rate [15]. The Austrian study has not reached maturity and so far no significant impact on OS has been observed. The French trial has reached maturity and a significantly prolonged DFS was observed in the IFN arm. The impact on OS failed to reach significance but demonstrated a favourable trend [16]. The NCCTG trial which evaluated the impact of HDI, intramuscularly t.i.w. for 3 months was negative both for DFS and OS in the stage II population of this mixed stage II–III trial [12]. Moreover, both ECOG 1684 and 1690 did not show a significant impact of HDI on DFS or OS in the stage IIB population of these trials [11–14]. In the ECOG 1690 trial in the LDI arm no effect of DFS or OS was observed on the stage IIB patients. Also in the EORTC/DKG-80 trial, the very low dose of 1 MU, subcutaneously t.i.w. for 1 year, no impact on DFS or OS in the stage II patients in this trial was observed. So, in summary, we can state that in stage II melanoma in only two trials an impact of IFN on DFS was observed whereas in three other low-dose trials as well as in three high-dose trials this has not been the case. A significant benefit on OS has not been reported in a single trial.

Impact of sentinel node staging and stage migration

The data on the impact of treatment with IFN are still unclear, especially whether the treatment will have any sizeble effect on OS. The EORTC-MCG has preferred to investigate a treatment option with considerable fewer side-effects in this stage II patient population which, as a consequence of the increasing use of sentinel node staging, will be transformed into a population with a much better prognosis and lower risk for relapse. Prognosis in sentinel node-negative patients is better than 95% survival at 4 years [17–19] and thus so excellent that it will no longer justify (even the evaluation of) toxic adjuvant therapy.

Hence, in trial EORTC 18961 in a population of 1300 patients the efficacy of vaccination with the ganglioside vaccine GM2-KLH/QS-21 will be compared to the outcome in patients receiving standard of care (observation) [1].

Current and future trials

The largest trial by far in high-risk melanoma patients (stage IIB–III) is the EORTC 18952 trial in 1300 patients. This trial evaluates the impact of intermediate doses of IFN where, after an induction period of 4 weeks, 5 days/week, 10 MU, subcutaneously, is followed by a maintenance period of 10 MU, subcutaneously t.i.w. for 1 year vs. 5 MU subcutaneously t.i.w. for 2 years, vs. observation. This trial was designed to explore the effects of intermediate doses of IFN, hoping to identify a well-tolerated regimen that would have an 'above threshold' activity, comparable to the HDI schedule of ECOG 1684, but without the HDI-associated toxicity. The negative outcome of ECOG 1690 has somewhat undercut this philosophy. This trial will be analysed in the autumn of the year 2000.

On the basis of the results with IFN in stage II patients and on the basis of the observation of a rebound in relapse rates in the IFN-treated patients in a number of trials (WHO-16 trial in stage III, French trial in stage II) the hypothesis has been raised that IFN needs to be administered for very long periods of time in order to be effective. This hypothesis is also based on the antiangiogenic mode of action of IFN, as demonstrated by Fidler and others [20,21].

The EORTC-MCG study will evaluate long-term therapy with IFN to standard of care (observation) in stage III melanoma. Long-term therapy has two prerequisites: low toxicity and easy administration. A well-tolerated dose of the pegylated form [22] of IFN-α (Peg-Intron) is being evaluated, as this agent needs only to be administered subcutaneously once a week, for a total treatment period of 5 years. This trial was activated in May 2001 (EORTC 18991). Roughly 50% of the total population of about 900 patients are expected to enter the trial as patients with microscopic metastatic involvement of regional lymph node(s) as a consequence of the steady increase in sentinel node mapping in Europe. The other 50% will be patients with clinically overt (palpable) regional node involvement. Side studies regarding the value of reverse transcription polymerase chain reaction (RT-PCR) of the sentinel node and other nodes in the regional node basin and of RT-PCR of blood samples will provide further insight into the biological importance and predictive value of such procedures. In this respect one must signal that the first report on the predictive value for relapse on the basis of RT-PCR on the sentinel node, by the group of Reintgen of the Lee Moffit Cancer Center, are very promising and convincing [19].

The ECOG is at present evaluating the GM2-KLH/QS-21 vaccine in stage IIB–III patients in the ECOG 1694 trial. In this trial 851 patients are randomized into either HDI (ECOG 1684 schedule) or the vaccine arm. Early results have shown a survival benefit for HDI compared to vaccine but these results require longer follow-up. In stage II patients the EORTC 18961 trial will evaluate in 1300 patients the impact of vaccination with GM2-KLH/QS-21 vs. standard of care (observation). The ECOG is evaluating in trial 1697 the impact of 4 weeks of IFN, 20 MU/m^2, intravenously, for 4 weeks vs. observation in 1420 patients. These huge numbers of patients are necessary because of the tremendous impact of sentinel node mapping and the excellent prognosis of sentinel node-negative patients. In the USA, two other very large adjuvant trials are ongoing. The Sunbelt trial evaluates the impact of sentinel node staging and the use of RT-PCR methods on sentinel node evaluation, and HDI (ECOG 1684 schedule) in a multiarm trial in 3000 patients [23]. Morton's polyvalent melanoma cell vaccine (PMV), a melanoma cell line–based vaccine that thus far has only been studied in non-controlled trials [24,25] is now being evaluated in a large multicentre trial in 750 stage III patients. BCG+PMV treatment will be compared to treatment with BCG alone.

Biological response modifiers as therapy for advanced melanoma

Various IL-2 regimens and combinations with IFN-α have been tested in patients with advanced melanoma during the past decade. The response rate reported with IL-2 as a single agent or in combination with IFN-α is from 10 to 41% with a small, but remarkable proportion of long-term responders. Subsequently, regimens combining IL-2, IFN-α and chemotherapy (chemoimmunotherapy) have been evaluated in Phase II trials suggesting improved response rates. Recent Phase III trials have investigated the role of chemoimmunotherapy for the treatment of advanced melanoma. Here the results of the clinical trials are discussed.

Single agent and combination immunotherapy

IL-2 as a single agent has yielded response rates of up to 24% in a number of Phase II trials [26–32]. The rationale of combining IL-2 and IFN-α is based on *in vitro* observations that IFN-α upregulates the expression of HLA class I molecules on tumour cells [33] and synergizes with IL-2 in activating immunological effector cells [34]. In larger Phase II studies (Table 15.3) [31,35–43], the objective response rates of the combination treatment of IL-2 and IFN-α was between 0 and 41%. However, the role of IFN-α in addition to IL-2 was never proven. The only randomized trial investigating IL-2 alone vs. IL-2+IFN-α was terminated because of low response rates in both treatment arms [31].

The published data concerning duration of responses and survival are too few to permit meaningful conclusions on long-term effects of IFN-α and IL-2 combinations. However, in most trials a proportion of patients is observed with durable remissions. In one cohort 17% of 65 patients survived for more than 3 years, and 11% for more than 5 years, of which 9% had no evidence of clinical disease at 5 years post treatment [37].

IL-2 has been tested in a variety of regimens. Initially, the maximal tolerable dose of IL-2 applicable under intensive care unit conditions was determined to be 600 000 IU/kg every 8 h for up to 5 days [35]. To investigate the role of treatment duration, two sequential studies were carried out with either a 5-day regimen of bolus IL-2 and IFN-α or a 3-day regimen. In this study, the 5-day regimen resulted in prohibitive cardiotoxicity and central nervous system toxicity. The 3-day regimen was associated with manageable toxicity. The response rate with the 5-day regimen was 41% and with the 3-day regimen only 20% [36]. West *et al.* [38] reported that continuous intravenous infusion of IL-2 is better tolerated than repeated bolus application and may be similarly effective. Addition of IFN-α to continuous intravenous infusion of IL-2 does not significantly increase toxicity and the response rates of this regimen range from 10 to 20% [38–40].

Based on the hypothesis that an initial high concentration of IL-2 is necessary to saturate the IL-2 receptors on non-activated T lymphocytes and a subsequent lower concentration may suffice to keep T lymphocytes activated, a decrescendo continuous infusion schedule has been developed. The IL-2 dose is increased fourfold as compared to the West protocol [38] over the initial 6 h, and subsequently tapered to a low maintenence dose. In two sequential studies, patients received 5 days of IFN-α followed either by continuous infusion of IL-2 at 18 MU/m^2/24 h for 5 days (West protocol) or the decrescendo

Table 15.3 Clinical trials of cytokine treatment in advanced melanoma

Reference	IL-2 administration and concomitant treatment	Number of patients	Response rate (%)	Duration (months)
IL-2 only				
Rosenberg *et al.* [26]	b.	42	24	2–>41
Thatcher *et al.* [27]	b.	31	3	NR
Parkinson *et al.* [28]	b.	46	22	4–>20
Whitehead *et al.* [29]	b.	42	10	NR
Dorval *et al.* [30]	c.i.v.	27	22	4–>45
Sparano *et al.* [31]*	b. (reduced dose)	44	5	10–>14
Legha *et al.* [32]	c.i.v.	33	22	NR
IL-2 ±IFN-α				
Rosenberg *et al.* [42]	b.+IFN-α	44	36	NR
Kruit *et al.* [39]	c.i.v. (reduced dose)+IFN-α	54	20	NR
Keilholz *et al.* [40]	c.i.v.+IFN-α	27	18	3–22
	Decrescendo+IFN-α	27	41	3–>36
Sparano *et al.* [31]*	b. (reduced dose)+IFN-α	41	10	2–15
Marincola *et al.* [43]	b.+IFN-α	82	24	NR
Kruit *et al.* [36]	b.+IFN-α (5 days)	17	41	2–37
	b.+IFN-α (3 days)	25	20	4–>10
EORTC-MCG [55]*	Decrescendo+IFN-α	66	18	3–>36
IL-2 ±chemotherapy				
Stoter *et al.* [44]	c.i.v.+DTIC 850 mg/m^2	24	25	2–13
Dillman *et al.* [45]	c.i.v.+LAK+DTIC 1,2 g/m^2	27	26	3–>24
Flaherty *et al.* [46]	c.i.v.+DTIC 1 g/m^2	32	22	2–>22
Demchak *et al.* [47]	b.+CDDP 150 mg/m^2	27	37	1–>30
Flaherty *et al.* [48]	s.c.+CDDP+DTIC	27	41	3–>20
Atkins *et al.* [49]	b.+tamoxifen+CDDP+DTIC	38	42	2–>20
Dummer *et al.* [50]	c.i.v.+DTIC 850 mg/m^2	57	25	NR
IL-2 ±IFN-α±chemotherapy				
Richards *et al.* [51]	b.+IFN-α+CDDP +DTIC+BCNU+tamoxifen	74	57	5–>10
Khayat *et al.* [52]	c.i.v.+IFN-α+CDDP±tamoxifen	39	54	3–>21
Buzaid & Legha [53]	b.+IFN-α+CDDP+DTIC	151	54	3–>24
Proebstle *et al.* [54]	Decrescendo+IFN-α+DTIC+CDDP	21	24	4–9†
EORTC-MCG [55]*	Decrescendo+IFN-α+CDDP	60	33	3–>36

Abbreviations: b., intravenous bolus; BCNU, carmustine; CDDP, cisplatin; c.i.v., continuous intravenous infusion; DTIC, dacarbazine; EORTC-MCG, European Organization for Research on Treatment of Cancer Melanoma Cooperative Group; IFN, interferon; LAK, lymphokine activated killer cells; s.c., subcutaneous.

* Randomized study.

† Very advanced disease patient population.

regimen (18 μm/m²/6 h, immediately followed by 18 MU/m²/12 h, 18 MU/m²/24 h and 4.5 MU/m²/24 h × 3). The toxicity of the decrescendo regimen was significantly lower. A response rate of 18% was observed with the continous IL-2 dose and 41% with the decrescendo regimen [41]. This schedule was therefore used for subsequent EORTC trials.

Combination with cytotoxic agents: chemoimmunotherapy

A number of Phase II trials investigated the efficacy of chemoimmunotherapy for advanced melanoma and response rates in excess of 50% have been reported by several groups (Table 15.3). Comparing the treatment regimens, it is evident that high response rates have been achieved, especially with regimens including the agents IL-2, IFN-α and cisplatin (CDDP).

Database on IL-2-containing treatments in melanoma

To develop solid hypotheses for designing Phase III trials, the EORTC collected a database on high-dose IL-2-based treatments with emphasis on long-term results of melanoma patients, who had received IL-2 alone, in combination with IFN-α, or with cytotoxic drugs from 11 European institutions and the MD Anderson Cancer Center in Houston [56]. The median survival of all patients was 10.5 months and the 2-and 5-year survival rates were 19.9 and 10.4%, respectively (Table 15.4).

This investigation defines serum lactate dehydrogenase (LDH), metastatic site and performance status as stratification factors for randomized trials in metastatic melanoma. The long-term survival rates observed in melanoma patients treated with IL-2- and IFN α containing regimens are notable in contrast to the reported 5-year survival rates of 2–6% achieved with chemotherapy, but need to be prospectively confirmed in randomized trials.

Comparative trials

Within the EORTC-MCG, the first prospectively randomized Phase III trial was carried out in 1993 in order to evaluate systematically the components of chemoimmunotherapy regimens for impact on survival, as well as on response and response duration of melanoma patients.

The first protocol was designed to evaluate IFN-α (10 MU/m², days 1–5) and IL-2 (decreasing intravenous infusions on days 4–9) with or without a single dose of cisplatin (100 mg/m² on day 1) [55].

The results are summarized in Table 15.5. The overall response rate was 18% for patients receiving IFN-α and IL-2, as expected for this advanced patient cohort, and increased to 35% with the addition of cisplatin. Disease

Table 15.4 Survival analyses for patients with advanced melanoma

Reference	Number of patients	Treatment	Survival rate at: Median survival	2 years (%)	5 years (%)
Balch 1982 [57]	198	Various	6.0	8	2
Ahmann 1989 [58]	503	Chemotherapy	—	9	2
Lakhani 1990 [59]	164	Chemotherapy	—	4	—
Sirott 1993* [60]	284	Various	7.4	—	—
Creagan 1990 [61]	191	Interferons	6.0	9	2
Barth 1995* [62]	1521	Various	7.5	14	6
EORTC report 1997 [55]		Response rate (%)			
IL-2 only	14.9	7.5	12	4	
IL-2+chemotherapy	23.0	9.9	13	8	
IL-2+IFN-α	20.8	10.5	24	14	
IL-2+chemotherapy+IFN-α	44.8	11.4	22	12	

*Patient collection not based on intent to treat.

Table 15.5 Results of treatment of the EORTC trial IFN-α/IL-2±cisplatin

	IFN-α/IL-2	IFN-α/IL-2+cisplatin
Number of patients	66	60
Complete remission	4	3
Partial remission	8	17
Objective response rate	18%	33%
Median time to progression	8 weeks	14 weeks
Median survival	9 months	9 months
Survival at 2 years	15%	15%

progression occurred on average after 53 days in patients treated with cytokines alone and after 92 days in patients treated with chemotherapy. Overall survival was identical in the two treatment groups; there was only a hint towards improved survival in the patient stratum with more advanced disease.

This trial shows that the addition of cisplatin to cytokine treatment offers palliation, because the response rates were doubled with the addition of a single dose of cisplatin and the progression-free survival was also doubled. However, the addition of cisplatin did not influence overall survival. The most obvious explanation would be that cisplatin yields only short-term responses. An alternative explanation is that subsequent treatment of patients progressing at any time after protocol treatment (which is 90% of the study population) may have blurred the survival analysis. Cisplatin was not to be given for patients failing treatment in this trial, but subsequent treatment with other cytotoxic agents or Phase I vaccination efforts may have had an impact.

There are no Phase II data available systematically evaluating the efficacy of reduced dose IL-2 regimens with less than 50% of the total dose of the West regimen or the decrescendo regimen. However, the role of reduced dose IL-2 in combination therapies has recently been evaluated in two trials. A randomized Phase II trial performed at the Royal Marsden Hospital, London, UK evaluated the effect of the addition of IFN-α and IL-2 to the BCNU, cisplatin, DTIC and tamoxifen (BCDT) chemotherapy regimen [63]. Patients were assigned to receive either chemotherapy alone on day 3 (BCDT), or concomitant subcutaneous administration of IL-2 (18×10^6 IU t.i.d. on day 1, 9×10^6 IU b.i.d. on days 2 and 3) and IFN-α (9×10^6 IU on days 1–3). In this study, the addition of cytokines to the chemotherapy regimen was associated with significant toxicity and resulted in an impaired response rate (23 with and 27% without cytokines, respectively) and an identical progression-free and overall survival.

The Association of German Dermatological Oncologists (ADO) recently provided data on an interim survival analysis from an ongoing randomized trial [64]. In this trial, patients with advanced melanoma were randomized to receive treatment with DTIC (850 mg/m^2 on day 1) and a prolonged regimen of IFN-α (3×10^6 IU b.i.d. on day 1, followed by 3×10^6 IU once daily on days 2–5, and 5×10^6 IU three times per week in weeks 2–4) with or without the following regimen of IL-2: 5×10^6 IU/m^2 intravenously over 3 h on day 3, followed by 10×10^6 IU/m^2 intravenously over 24 h, and 5×10^6 IU/m^2 subcutaneously on days 4–7. There was a lower response rate in patients treated with IL-2 as compared to patients who did not receive this IL-2 regimen (20 and 32%, respectively), and no effect on survival. As in the Royal Marsden trial, patients randomized to the IL-2 arm more frequently went off protocol treatment because of side-effects.

In 1995, a second trial, EORTC 18951, was initiated to determine the role of high-dose IL-2 for survival. The study evaluates a different schedule of cisplatin (30 mg/m^2 for 3 days) plus DTIC (250 mg/m^2 for 3 days) and IFN-α (10 MU/m^2 for 5 days) with or without the addition of high-dose IL-2 (decrescendo regimen). Full accrual was reached in March 2000, and initial results are expected at the end of 2000. A similar trial has been initiated more recently by the ECOG to define the value of cytokine treatment in addition to cisplatin, vindesine and DTIC for survival of patients with advanced melanoma.

Conclusions for IL-2 containing regimens in advanced melanoma

1 High-dose IL-2 is an active agent in the treatment of metastatic melanoma.
2 The contribution of IFN-α in conjunction with IL-2 is as yet unproven, although a beneficial effect on survival is suggested in the EORTC database.
3 Regimens with a total dosage of less than 50% of our decrescendo regimen

or the West protocol still possess considerable toxicity and have failed to impact on response rates and survival in two randomized studies.
4 The key trials to define the role of high-dose IL-2 are ongoing in the EORTC and the ECOG.

References

1 Eggermont AMM. The current Melanoma Cooperative Group adjuvant trial programme on malignant melanoma: prognosis versus efficacy, toxicity and costs. *Melanoma Res* 1997; 7 (Suppl 2): 127–31.
2 Morton DL, Holmes EC, Eilber FR, *et al.* Adjuvant immunotherapy: results of a randomized trial in patients with lymph node metastases, In: Terry WD, Rosenberg SA, eds. *Immunotherapy of Human Cancer.* New York: Elsevier North Holland, 1982: 245–9.
3 Terry WD, Hodes RJ, Rosenberg SA, *et al.* Treatment of stage I and II malignant melanoma with adjuvant immunotherapy or chemotherapy: preliminary analysis of a prospective randomized trial, In: Terry WD, Rosenberg SA, eds. *Immunotherapy of Human Cancer.* New York: Elsevier North Holland, 1982: 252–7.
4 Morton DL. Adjuvant immunotherapy of malignant melanoma: status of clinical trials at UCLA. *Int J Immunother* 1986; **2**: 31–6.
5 Wallack MK, Sivanandham M, Balch CM, *et al.* A phase III randomized, double-blind, multi-institutional trial of vaccinia melanoma oncolysate-active specific immunotherapy for patients with stage II melanoma. *Cancer* 1995; **75**: 34–42.
6 Hersey P, Coates P, Tyndall L. Is adjuvant therapy worthwhile? (Abstract). *Melanoma Res* 1997; 7 (Suppl.): 78.
7 Livingston PO, Wong GYC, Adluri S, *et al.* Improved survival in stage III melanoma patients with GM2 antibodies: a randomised trial of adjuvant vaccination with GM2 ganglioside. *J Clin Oncol* 1994; **12**: 1036–44.
8 Meyskens FL, Kopecky KJ, Taylor CW, *et al.* Randomized trial of adjuvant human γ-interferon versus observation in high risk cutaneous melanoma: a Southwest Oncology Group Study. *J Natl Cancer Inst* 1995; **87**: 1710–3.
9 Kleeberg U, Broecker EB, Chartier C, *et al.* EORTC 18871 adjuvant trial in high risk melanoma patients IFN-α vs. IFN-γ vs. Iscador vs. observation (Abstract). *Eur J Cancer* 1999; 35 (Suppl 4): 264.
10 Hauschild A, Burg G, Dummer R. Prospective randomized multicenter trial on the oupatient use of subcutaneous interleukin-2 and interferon-α2b in high risk melanoma patients (Abstract). *Melanoma Res* 1997; 7 (Suppl. 1): 401.
11 Kirkwood JM, Strawderman MH, Ernstoff MS, Smith TJ, Borden EC, Blum RH. Interferon-α2b adjuvant therapy of high-risk resected cutaneous melanoma: the Eastern Cooperative Oncology Group Trial EST 1684. *J Clin Oncol* 1996; **14**: 7–17.
12 Creagan ET, Dalton RJ, Ahmann DL, *et al.* Randomized surgical adjuvant clinical trial or recombinant interferon-α2a in selected patients with malignant melanoma. *J Clin Oncol* 1995; **13**: 2776–83.
13 Cascinelli N. Evaluation of efficacy of adjuvant rIFNa 2A in regional node metastases (Abstract). *Proc Am Soc Clin Oncol* 1995; **14**: 410.
14 Kirkwood JM, Ibrahim J, Sondak V, *et al.* Preliminary analysis of the E1690/S9111/C9190 Intergroup Postoperative Adjuvant Trial of high- and low-dose IFN-α2b (HDI and LDI) in high-risk primary or lymph node metastatic melanoma (Abstract). *Proc Am Soc Clin Oncol* 1999; **18**: 2072.
15 Pehamberger H, Soyer P, Steiner A, *et al.* Adjuvant interferon-α2a treatment in resected primary stage II cutaneous melanoma. *J Clin Oncol* 1998; **16**: 1425–9.
16 Grob JJ, Dreno B, Chastang C, *et al.* Randomised trial of interferon-α2a as adjuvant therapy in resected primary melanoma thicker than 1.5 mm without clinically detectable node metastases. *Lancet* 1998; **351**: 1905–10.

17 Gershenwald JE, Colomi MI, Thompson W, *et al.* Patterns of recurrence following a negative sentinel lymph node biopsy in 243 patients with stage I or II melanoma. *J Clin Oncol* 1998; **16**: 2253–60.
18 Gershenwald JE, Thompson W, Mansfield PE, *et al.* Multi-institutional melanoma lymphatic mapping experience: value of sentinel lymph node status in 612 stage I or stage II melanoma patients. *J Clin Oncol* 1999; **17**: 976–83.
19 Shivers SC, Wang X, Li W, *et al.* Molecular staging of malignant melanoma: correlation with clinical outcome. *J Am Med Assoc* 1998; **28** (16): 1410–15.
20 Singh RK, Gutman M, Bucana CD, Sanchez R, Llansa N, Fidler IJ. Interferons-α and β down-regulate the expression of basic fibroblast growth factor in human carcinomas. *Proc Natl Acad Sci USA* 1995; **92**: 4562–6.
21 Dinney CP, Bielenberg DR, Perrotte P, Reich R, Bucana CD, Fidler IJ. Inhibition of basic fibroblast growth factor expression, angiogenesis and growth of human bladder carcinoma in mice by systemic interferon-α administration. *Cancer Res* 1998; **58**: 808–14.
22 Nucci M, *et al.* The therapeutic value of poly (ethylene glycol)-modified proteins. *Adv Drug Deliv Rev* 1991; **6**: 133–51.
23 Ross MR. Prospective randomized trials in melanoma: defining contemporary surgical roles. *Cancer Treat Res* 1997; **90**: 1–27.
24 Morton DL, Foshag LJ, Hoon DSB, *et al.* Prolongation of survival in metastatic melanoma after active specific immunotherapy with a new polyvalent melanoma vaccine. *Ann Surg* 1992; **216**: 463–70.
25 Morton DL, Hoon DSB, Nizze JA, *et al.* Polyvalent melanoma vaccine improves survival of patients with metastatic melanoma. *Ann NY Acad Sci* 1993; **690**: 120–4.
26 Rosenberg SA, Lotze MT, Yang JC, *et al.* Experience with the use of high dose interleukin-2 in the treatment of 652 cancer patients. *Ann Surg* 1989; **210**: 474–85.
27 Thatcher N, Dazzi H, Gosh A, Johnson RJ. Recombinant IL-2 given intra-splenically and intravenously in advanced malignant melanoma: a phase I/II study. *Cancer Treat Res* 1989; **16** (Suppl. A): 49–52.
28 Parkinson DR, Abrams JS, Wiernik PH, *et al.* Interleukin-2 therapy in patients with metastatic malignant melanoma: a phase II study. *J Clin Oncol* 1990; **8**: 1650–6.
29 Whitehead RP, Kopecky KJ, Samson MK, *et al.* Phase II study of intravenous bolus recombinant interleukin-2 in advanced malignant melanoma: Southwest Oncology Group study. *J Natl Cancer Inst* 1991; **83**: 1250–1.
30 Dorval T, Mathiot C, Brandely M, *et al.* Lack of effect of tumour infiltrating lymphocytes in patients with metastatic melanoma who failed to respond to interleukin 2 [Correspondence]. *Eur J Cancer* 1991; **27** (Suppl. 2): 99.
31 Sparano JA, Fisher RI, Sunderland M, *et al.* Randomized phase III trial of treatment with high-dose interleukin-2 either alone or in combination with interferon-α2a in patients with advanced melanoma. *J Clin Oncol* 1993; **11**: 1969–77.
32 Legha SS, Gianan MA, Plager C, Eton OE, Papadopoulous NEJ. Evaluation of interleukin-2 administered by continuous infusion in patients with metastatic melanoma. *Cancer* 1996; **77**: 89–96.
33 Giacomini P, Aguzzi A, Pestka S, *et al.* Modulation by recombinant DNA leukocyte (α) and fibroblast (β) interferons of the expression and shedding of HLA and tumor-associated antigens by human melanoma cells. *J Immunol* 1984; **133**: 1649–55.
34 Zoller M. IFN-treatment of B166-F1 versus B16-F10: relative impact on non-adaptive and T-cell-mediated immune defense in metastatic spread. *Clin Exp Metastasis* 1988; **6**: 411–29.
35 Rosenberg SA, Lotze MT, Muul LM, *et al.* Observations on the systemic administration of autologous lymphokine-activated killer cells and recombinant interleukin-2 to patients with metastatic cancer. *N Engl J Med* 1985; **313**: 1485–92.
36 Kruit WHJ, Punt CJA, Goey SH, *et al.* Dose-efficacy study of two schedules of high-dose bolus administration of interleukin-2 and α-interferon in patients with metastatic melanoma. *Br J Cancer* 1996; **74**: 951–5.

37 Keilholz U, Scheibenbogen C, Sommer M, Pritsch M, Geueke AM. Prognostic factors for response and survival in patients with metastatic melanoma receiving immunotherapy. *Melanoma Res* 1996; **6**: 173–8.

38 West WH, Tauer KW, Yanelli JR, *et al.* Constant infusion recombinant interleukin-2 in adoptive immunotherapy of advanced cancer. *N Engl J Med* 1987; **316**: 898–905.

39 Kruit WH, Goey SH, Monson JR, *et al.* Clinical experience with the combined use of recombinant interleukin-2 (IL-2) and interferon-α2a (IFN-α) in metastatic melanoma. *Br J Haematol* 1991; **79** (Suppl. 1): 84–6.

40 Keilholz U, Scheibenbogen C, Tilgen W, *et al.* Interferon-α and interleukin-2 in the treatment of malignant melanoma: a comparison of two phase II trials. *Cancer* 1993; **72**: 607–14.

41 Dillman RO, Church C, Oldham RK, *et al.* Inpatient continuous-infusion interleukin-2 in 788 patients with cancer: the National Biotherapy Study Group experience. *Cancer* 1993; **71**: 2358–70.

42 Rosenberg SA, Lotze MT, Yang JC, *et al.* Combination therapy with interleukin-2 and α-interferon for the treatment of patients with advanced cancer. *J Clin Oncol* 1989; **7**: 1863–74.

43 Marincola FM, White DE, Wise AP, Rosenberg SA. Combination therapy with interferon-α2a and interleukin-2 for the treatment of metastatic cancer. *J Clin Oncol* 1995; **5**: 1110–22.

44 Stoter G, Shiloni E, Aamdal S, *et al.* Sequential administration of recombinant human interleukin-2 and dacarbazine in metastatic melanoma: a multicentre phase II study. *Eur J Cancer Clin Oncol* 1989; **25** (Suppl. 3): 41–3.

45 Dillman RO, Oldham RK, Barth NM, *et al.* Recombinant interleukin-2 and adoptive immunotherapy alternated with dacarbazine therapy in melanoma: a National Biotherapy Study Group trial. *J Natl Cancer Inst* 1990; **82**: 1345–9.

46 Flaherty LE, Redman BG, Chabot GG, *et al.* A phase I–II study of dacarbazine in combination with outpatient interleukin-2 in metastatic malignant melanoma. *Cancer* 1990; **65**: 2471–7.

47 Demchak PA, Mier JW, Robert NJ, *et al.* Interleukin-2 and high-dose cisplatin in patients with metastatic melanoma: a pilot study. *J Clin Oncol* 1991; **9**: 1821–30.

48 Flaherty LE, Robinson W, Redman BG, *et al.* A Phase II study of dacarbazine and cisplatin in combination with outpatient administered interleukin-2 in metastatic malignant melanoma. *Cancer* 1993; **71**: 3520–5.

49 Atkins MB, O'Boyle KR, Sosman JA, *et al.* Multi-institutional phase II trial of intensive combination chemotherapy for metastatic melanoma. *J Clin Oncol* 1994; **12**: 1553–60.

50 Dummer R, Gore ME, Hancock BW, *et al.* A multi-center phase II clinical trial using dacarbazine and continuous infusion of interleukin-2 in metastatic melanoma: clinical data and immunomonitoring. *Cancer* 1995; **75**: 945–8.

51 Richards JM, Mehta N, Ramming K, Skosey P. Sequential chemoimmunotherapy in the treatment of metastatic melanoma. *J Clin Oncol* 1992; **10**: 1338–43.

52 Khayat D, Borel C, Tourani JM, *et al.* Sequential chemoimmunotherapy with cisplatin interleukin-2, interferon-α2 for metastatic melanoma. *J Clin Oncol* 1993; **11**: 2173–80.

53 Buzaid AC, Legha SS. Combination of chemotherapy with interleukin-2 and interferon-α for the treatment of advanced melanoma. *Semin Oncol* 1994; **6** (Suppl 14): 23–8.

54 Proebstle ThM, Keilholz U, Scheibenbogen C, Sterry W, Hunstein W. A phase II study of DTIC, CDDP, α-interferon, and high dose IL-2 in 'poor risk'melanoma. *Eur J Cancer* 1996; **32**: 1530–3.

55 Keilholz U, Goey SH, Punt CJA, *et al.* IFN-α/IL-2 with or without cisplatinum in metastatic melanoma: a randomized trial of the EORTC Melanoma Cooperative Group. *J Clin Oncol* 1997; **15**: 2579–88.

56 Keilholz U, Conradt C, Legha S, *et al.* Results of IL-2-based treatment in advanced melanoma: a case-record based analysis of 631 patients. *J Clin Oncol* 1998; **16**: 1921–26.

57 Balch CM, Soong S, Shaw HM, Urist MM, McCarthy WH. An analysis of prognostic factors in 8500 patients with cutaneous melanoma. In: Balch CM,

Houghton AN, Milton GW, Sober AJ, Soong S, eds. *Cutaneous Melanoma, 2nd edition*. Philadelphia: Lippincott, 1992: 165–87.

58 Ahman DL, Creagan ET, Hahn RG, Edmonson JH, Bisel HF, Schaid DJ. Complete responses and long-term survivals after systemic chemotherapy for patients with advanced malignant melanoma. *Cancer* 1989; **63**: 224–7.

59 Lakhani S, Selby P, Bliss JM, Perren TJ, Gore ME, McElwain TJ. Chemotherapy for malignant melanoma: combinations and high doses produce more responses without survival benefit. *Br J Cancer* 1990; **61**: 330–4.

60 Sirott MN, Bajorin DF, Wong GJC *et al.* Prognostic factors in patients with metastatic melanoma: a multivariate analysis. *Cancer* 1993; **72**: 3091–8.

61 Creagan ET, Schaid DJ, Ahmann DL, Frytak S. Disseminated malignant melanoma and recombinant interferon: Analysis of seven consecutive phase II investigations. *J Invest. Dermatol* 1990; **95**: 188S–192S.

62 Barth A, Wanek LA, Morton DL. Prognostic factors in 1,521 melanoma patients with distant metastases. *J Am Coll Surg* 1995; **181**: 193–201.

63 Johnston SRD, Constenia DO, Moore J, *et al.* Randomized phase II trial of BCDT with or without interferon-α and interleukin-2 in patients with metastatic melanoma. *Br J Cancer* 1998; 77: 1280–6.

64 Hauschild A, Garbe C, Dummer R, Tilgen W. Dacarbazine plus interferon-α with and without interleukin-2 in advanced melanoma: a German–Swiss phase III multicenter trial. *Proc ASCO* 1998; **17**: 516a.

16: Will vaccines really work for melanoma?

Peter Hersey

Introduction

The past decade has seen a marked resurgence in interest in the use of cancer vaccines to treat cancers in general and particularly melanomas. This interest is the result of the convergence of improved understanding of immune responses against tumours, the development of molecular biological approaches to identify tumour antigens and the application of recombinant molecular biological techniques to produce pharmacological quantities of cytokines involved in immune responses. These developments, together with well developed clinical trial procedures, underlie a degree of cautious optimism that immunotherapy will find its rightful place in the treatment of melanoma and other cancers.

However, this view contrasts with that held by many oncologists who point to past, often fruitless, efforts over a number of decades and who, with the benefit of hindsight, advance the view that the tumour has evolved under selection pressure to be resistant to natural defence mechanisms including those of the immune system. The advances in molecular biology which, on the one hand, have given much optimism for development of immunotherapy have, on the other hand, given new insight into tumour biology and the many mechanisms that tumour cells appear to develop against immune responses. These findings support a more cautious assessment of the role of immunotherapy and one which accepts that its role may be limited to certain subgroups of patients.

In the following sections the current trials of immunotherapy will be reviewed together with developments which may help to point to the eventual place of this treatment modality in patients with melanoma.

Melanoma vaccines being tested in Phase III trials

The melanoma vaccines which have progressed through to Phase III trials are summarized in Table 16.1. It is important to note that only two studies have

Table 16.1 Randomized trials with melanoma vaccines

Investigator/clinical stage of trial*	Melanoma vaccine	Trial design	Protocol	Number of patients/status
Hersey *et al.* [1,2] and III	Vaccinia lysates of 2/98) one allogeneic melanoma cell	Control untreated	i.d. q2w × 4, then q3w × 6, then q4w × 18	700 (closed IIB) In progress
Wallack *et al.* [3] III	Vaccinia lysates of three allogeneic melanoma cells	Control vaccinia alone	i.d. q1w × 13, then q2w × 40	250 Non-significant trend
Livingston *et al.* [4] III	GM2 + Cyclo and BCG vaccine	Control BCG/Cyclo	4–5 × over 6 months	122 Non-significant trend
ECOG 1694 [5] Schering/Bristol Myers IIB and III	GM2-KLH/QS21	Control HDI	s.c. q1w × 4, then each 12 weeks for 2 years	851 (closed 11/99) In progress
EORTC 18961 [6] Bristol Myers IIA, IIB	GM2-KLH/QS21	Control untreated	s.c. q1w × 4, then each 12 weeks for 2 years 6 monthly in year 3	1300–1500 (projected)
NCI/Morton *et al.* [7] IIB and III	Three allogeneic melanoma cells + BCG vaccine	Control HDI or BCG alone	i.d. q2w × 3, then monthly × 12, then 3 monthly × 4, then 6 monthly × 6	825 projected In progress
NCI/Morton *et al.* [7] IV	Three allogeneic melanoma cells + BCG vaccine	Control HDI or BCG alone	i.d. q2w × 3, then monthly × 12, then 3 monthly × 4, then 6 monthly × 6	420 projected In progress
Ribi/Schering Mitchell *et al.* [8] IIB and III	Two allogeneic melanoma cells + Detox + IFN 5×10^6	Control HDI	s.c. q1w × 4, then q2w × 1, then monthly with repeat courses 6-monthly	233/400 accrued In progress
SWOG 9035/Ribi/ Corixa IIA [9]	Two allogeneic melanoma cells + Detox	Control untreated	s.c. q1w × 4, then q4w × 1, then q8w × 5, then 6-monthly to 2 years	689 (closed 11/96) In progress
Avax/Berd *et al.* [9, 10] III	Cyclophosphamide Autol mel/DNP/BCG	Control HDI	s.c. q1w × 6 booster at 6 months	400 (25 sites) Projected
Bystryn [12] III	Shed antigens from 4 melanoma +alum	Placebo (Alb) +alum	i.d. q3w × 4 then monthly × 3, then to 5 years	36 Significant DFS Non-significant survival

* American Joint Committee on Cancer (AJCC) stages III and IV refer to patients with lymph node metastases and disseminated metastases, respectively. Stage IIA,B refers to localized melanoma > 1.5 and > 4.00 mm thick, respectively.

Abbreviations: Autol mel, autologous melanoma cells; BCG, Bacillus Calmette–Guérin; Cyclo, cyclophosphamide; DFS, disease-free survival; DNP, dinitrophenyl; ECOG, Eastern Cooperative Oncology Group; EORTC, European Organization for Research on Treatment of Cancer; i.d. intradermal; IFN, interferon; HDI, high-dose IFN-α2b; KLH, keyhole limpet haemocyanin; NCI, US National Cancer Institute; q*x*w, every *x* weeks; s.c. subcutaneous, SWOG, Southwest Oncology Group.

been completed: that by Wallack *et al.* [3]; and by Livingston *et al.* [4]. There was a non-significant trend in favour of the vaccine treatment in both studies but the patient numbers were relatively small and their power to exclude clinically significant benefits therefore low. Several large trials are now closed to patient accrual and results should be available over the next 1–2 years. These include the author's studies with vaccinia viral melanoma cell lysates (VMCL) [1,2], the Eastern Cooperative Oncology Group (ECOG) 1694 study on GM2 ganglioside vaccine [5] and the Southwest Oncology Group (SWOG) 9035 study with Melacine/Detox in stage IIA patients [9].

When these results are available we will be better able to answer whether vaccines will work in treatment of melanomas. Some indication that they may be of benefit comes from studies on patients with stage IV metastatic disease. Morton *et al.* [7] reported apparent improvements in the survival of patients with stage IV disease treated with a mixed allogeneic whole-cell vaccine. Although the study was non-comparative, the patient numbers were relatively large. A high number of patients (26%) survived for 5 years, which is unusual for this disease. These results have prompted a trial of CancerVax in patients with resected stage IV disease, which is now well advanced. Mitchell *et al.* [8] used vaccines prepared from a pool of ultrasonicated melanoma cells and a novel adjuvant, Detox. Treatment with this vaccine was reported to induce equivalent or higher response rates to those seen with chemotherapy with dacarbazine (DTIC) alone, and was associated with longer remission periods [8]. This particular vaccine, referred to as Melacine, is now produced commercially by Ribi Immunochemical and Corixa, and is licensed for use in Canada. The US National Cancer Institute (NCI) sponsored a controlled trial with this vaccine in patients with stage IV disease comparing Melacine with the Dartmouth chemotherapy regime [tamoxifen, dacarbazine, cisplatin (Cis-DPP) and carmustine (BCNU)]. There was no significant difference in survival of the patients in the two groups: the vaccine-treated patients fared no worse than those treated with chemotherapy. Both may have also been equally ineffective.

Berd *et al.* [10] attempted to increase the effectiveness of melanoma vaccines by coupling a chemical hapten, dinitrofluorobenzene (DNFB), to autologous melanoma cells. The immune response to DNFB on the tumour cells is believed to induce a strong response to the adjacent tumour antigens, analogous to the helper effect of viral antigens in vaccinia VMCL. These investigators showed that the DNFB-coupled melanoma cells induced a strong inflammatory response to distant metastases in 26 of 46 patients, and that 21 of 24 patients had histological evidence of a marked $CD8^+$ T-cell infiltrate [10]. Information about the clinical response rate is preliminary, but partial responses were seen in 5 of 46 patients. Subsequent adjuvant studies in patients with bulky lymph node metastases were also encouraging [11].

These studies therefore provide encouraging but not conclusive evidence that melanoma vaccines may be of benefit in the treatment of melanomas. Whether this promise is substantiated by Phase III trials should be known over the next few years. It is also true that most of the ideas involved in these trials were generated in the 1980s and are not based on the more up-to-date information that has accumulated during the 1990s. It is therefore of interest to scrutinize these studies to see, with the benefit of hindsight, whether there are major flaws in the design of the vaccine or administration protocol.

Vaccines based on induction of antibody responses against gangliosides on melanoma

Adoptive transfer studies in animal models have indicated that lymphocytes rather than antibodies are responsible for tumour rejection [13]. Nevertheless, two large randomized studies are based on the premise that antibody responses have an important role against melanoma. These include the ECOG 1694 [5] and the European Organization for Research on Treatment for Cancer (EORTC) 18961 trials [6], which aim to stimulate antibody response to the GM2 ganglioside expressed on most melanomas. There are relatively few animal studies to support this approach except the study by Zhang *et al.* [14] on antibodies to the GD2 ganglioside. Immunization of mice with GD2–KLH–QS21 was found to reduce the incidence of liver metastases from subcutaneous transplants of the EL4 lymphoma. However, passive infusion of MAb to GD2 were only effective in reducing metastases if given shortly after injection of the tumour and had no effect on the growth of tumour at the inoculation site. Therefore in this model the antibody appeared to act by limiting blood-borne metastases.

The main evidence in melanoma patients for the possible benefit of GM2 antibodies is the association of the latter with improved survival in patients with resected stage IIb or III disease [4,15,16]. This does not prove that the antibodies are directly responsible and may be merely an indicator of more relevant mechanisms. It seems unlikely that antibodies to GM2 would have direct effect on solid tumours because of poor penetration into the tumour and the presence of molecules on the tumour cells, such as CD55 [decay antibody-accelerating factor (DAF)] and CD59 (protectin), which degrade complement and inhibit complement-mediated lysis [17,18]. It is nevertheless possible that the antibodies to GM2 may clear melanoma cells from the circulation and thereby reduce the risk of metastases. This view would be supported by a number of studies showing that melanoma cells can be detected in the circulation of patients with resected stage II and III disease and that this is associated with an adverse prognosis [19,20]. This potential role of antibody to the gangliosides has not been studied and the protocols do not have particular design features to take this role into account. The use of the ganglioside vaccines is therefore controversial and the results of the trials will be awaited with great interest.

Similar vaccines have been prepared against GD3, GD2 and fucosylated GM1 [21] and immunization of 31 patients with vaccines against both GM2 and GD2 was reported to be well tolerated [22]. The use of anti-idiotype antibodies to induce immune responses is an interesting approach designed to circumvent the low immunogenicity of the gangliosides. Forty-seven patients were immunized with an anti-idiotype against GD2. One patient had a complete response and 18 patients had stabilization of their disease. Adjuvant studies were in progress on 44 of the patients [23].

Melanoma antigens recognized by T cells: are some antigens better than others in inducing tumour rejection?

The introduction of gene transfection and limiting dilution techniques [24,25] to screen cDNA libraries with T cells and the use of serological screening of expression libraries (SEREX) with antisera from patients [26] has led to the identification of a large number of melanoma antigens recognized by T cells, as summarized in Table 16.2. However, it is not yet clear which of these antigens are able to induce immune responses which cause regression of melanomas. Factors which are known to influence the development of effective T-cell responses are: the density of the antigen on melanoma; avidity of the T cells for the antigen; and the frequency of the T cells that can respond to the antigen [36].

Table 16.2 Melanoma antigens recognized by T cells

Antigen category		Reference*
Tumour specific antigens [Cancer testis (CT) antigens]	(TSA) MAGE 1–4, 6, 9–12. MAGE C1 BAGE, GAGE, DAM, LAGE NY-ESO-1 SSX2 (Hom-mel-40) SCP1, CT7 *N*-acetylglucosaminyl transferase	Fleischhauer *et al.* [27] Lethe *et al.* [28] Jaeger *et al.* [29] Tureci *et al.* [30]
Differentiation antigens	Tyrosinase, MART-1, gp100 Tyrosinase-related protein TRP1, TRP2	Parkhurst *et al.* [31] Lupetti *et al.* [32]
Individual specific mutated genes	N ras CDK4, Caspase 8, β-Catenin MUM-1, MUM-2	van Elsas *et al.* [33] Chiari *et al.* [34]
Overexpressed genes	p15, PRAME, CD63	Smith *et al.* [35]

* Additional references to these antigens are given elsewhere [24–26].

Table 16.3 Melanoma peptide vaccine trials

Reference	Peptide	Adjuvant	Number of patients	Clinical response*
Marchand *et al.* [37] Ludwig Institute	MAGE-1, 3A.1	Nothing	25	7
	MAGE-3A.1	MPL & QS21		
	MAGE-3A.2	Nothing		
	MAGE-3 protein	MPL & QS21		
Rosenberg *et al.* [38]	MART-1	IFA	23	
	gp100 154, 209, 280	IFA	28	
Rosenberg *et al.* [38]	gp100 209 2M	IFA	11	3 mixed
		IFA, IL-2	31	13–1 CR, 12 PR
Maeurer *et al.* [39]	MART-1, gp100, Tyrosinase 368	MF59 or Local IL-12		
Jaeger *et al.* [40,41]	MART-1, gp100, Tyrosinase 1, 368	GM-CSF (3 pt)	10	3–1 CR, 2 PR
Weber *et al.* [42]	MAGE-3A.1	IFA	18	NA
Weber *et al.* [43]	MART-1	IFA	25	NA
Cebon *et al.* [44]	MART-1	IL-12	20	1 CR, 1PR
Scheibenbogan *et al.* [45]	Tyrosinase 234, 368, 206, 192	GM-CSF	18	1 MR, 2 SD
Hersey *et al.* [46]	MART-1, 26 2L	Montanide ISA720	16	2 SD
	Tyrosinase, MAGE-3A.2			
	Gp100 209, 2M; 280, 9V	PPD ± GM-CSF		

* CR, PR and MR, complete, partial and mixed responses, respectively.
Abbreviations: IFA, incomplete Freund's adjuvant; IL, interleukin; MF59, oil-(squalene)-in-water emulsion with muramyldipeptide from bacterial cell walls; Montanide ISA720, water in (metabolisable) oil emulsion; MPL, monophosphoryl lipid A (modified LPS); NA, not available; PPD, purified protein derivative; QS21, carbohydrate extract of Quillaja Saponaria.

Some indication of the importance of some of the antigens may be derived from the Phase I–II studies on melanoma peptide vaccines or dendritic cell vaccines plus peptides, which are summarized in Tables 16.3 and 16.4. When the peptides are given alone it appears that those from the differentiation antigens are relatively ineffective [38–40] unless they are given with cytokines, such as GM-CSF [41], IL-2 [38] or IL-12 [44]. Responses were seen in patients immunized with these peptides on dendritic cells [53] and adoptive transfer of TIL against gp100-mediated tumour regression. In studies by Rosenberg *et al.* [38] responses to gp100 209 2M were mainly seen in patients also receiving IL-2. A

Table 16.4 Dendritic cell vaccines against melanoma

Reference	Source of antigen	Route	Number	Response†
Nestle *et al.* [47]	Melanoma tumour lysates or peptides* + KLH helper protein	Lymph nodes	16	2 CR, 3 PR
Hu *et al.* [48]	MAGE-1	i.d. and i.v.	3	–
Chakraborty *et al.* [49]	Melanoma lysates	i.d.	15	1 PR
Lotze *et al.* [50]	gp100, MART-1, Tyrosinase	i.v.	?	?
Thurner *et al.* [51]	MAGE-3A.1 i.v. × 3	s.c. and i.d. × 3	11	6 PR or mixed
Gajewsky [52]	MAGE-3 MART-1	s.c. +IL-12 s.c.	15	1 PR, 3 MR

* Peptides were Tyrosinase, gp100, MART-1 for HLA-A2 patients and MAGE-1A.1 for HLA-A1 patients.
† CR, PR and MR, complete, partial and mixed responses, respectively.
Abbreviations: IL-12, interleukin-12; i.d., intradermally; i.v., intravenous; s.c., subcutaneously.

randomized trial is now in progress to establish whether the clinical effects were caused by IL-2 alone or the combination with the peptides. Jaeger *et al.* [41] reported that addition of GM-CSF to the immunization had marked effects on immunological and clinical responses. These authors also reported that differentiation antigens could be lost during immunotherapy with peptides [53].

Impressive responses were seen in some studies where patients were immunized with HLA-A1 restricted peptides from MAGE-3, a member of the tumour-specific antigen (TSA), cancer testis (CT) antigen family [37]. This was supported by responses in patients immunized with this peptide on dendritic cells [51]. It is possible that these clinical responses may reflect higher avidity of the T cells for this class of antigen than to the differentiation antigens. The main limitation of the TSA–CT family may be the low frequency of T cells available to respond to the CT antigens [54]. Other potential advantages of the TSAs are their higher expression in metastatic lesions compared to primary melanoma (Table 16.5) perhaps because of demethylation associated with malignancy [65]. Coordinate expression of several of the family has been noticed, such as MAGE genes, LAGE and NY-ESO-1 [66], which would increase the number of T cells responding to the melanoma cells. It is not yet clear whether the antigens are lost during immune responses against the tumour, as reported for the differentiation antigens [53].

Table 16.5 Expression of TSA in melanoma

	Melanoma tissue			
	Percentage cell lines [55]	Primary	Percentage metastases	HLA restriction
MAGE-1* [56–58]	53	16	48	A1, A3, B37, Cw1601
MAGE-2	89	41	70	A3, B37
MAGE-3 [59–62]	94	36	76	A1,A2, A3, A24, B37, B44, DR11, DR13
MAGE-4A	55	11	22	
MAGE-6 [63]	89	?	?	
MAGE-12	89	?	?	
MAGE-C1 [36]		37	53	
BAGE			22	Cw1601
GAGE [63]			24	Cw6
LAGE [28]			50	
SSX-2 [30]			43	
NY-ESO-1 [29]			20–40	A2, A31
DAM [27]				A2
Glucosaminyl transferase V [24]			50	A2

* MAGE 9,10,11 are expressed only weakly in melanoma [56].

Advantages and limitations of individual specific antigens and autologous vaccines

As shown in Table 16.2, a number of antigens that are specific for individual patients have been described. A number of animal studies [13,24,25,36] have shown that individual specific antigens were much more effective in inducing regression of tumours than antigens common to tumours. It is quite possible that the same may apply in melanomas; it was reported that immune responses against the MUM-2 antigens were associated with long periods of remission in the patient concerned [31]. It is generally thought that the main reason for the effectiveness of individual neoantigens is that they may generate highly avid T-cell responses [36]. However, their strength as tumour rejection antigens is still dependent on the density of expression on melanoma cells and the frequency of responding T cells. The main limitation of immunization with individual specific antigens is the practical difficulty of obtaining a supply of such antigens. Until molecular biological approaches are developed to identify such antigens in individual patients, the only source is from the patient's own tumour, which limits this approach to patients with bulky tumours. Given that sentinel node biopsy techniques are leading to early resection of tumours involving lymph nodes, the number of patients that can be treated with autologous vaccines now and in the future is low. As indicated in Table 16.1, trials based on this approach are being conducted by Avax/Berd *et al.* and results are awaited with much interest [10,11].

Is one allogeneic melanoma cell vaccine likely to be superior to another?

It may be inferred from the information in Table 16.2 that allogeneic cell vaccines can only induce responses to differentiation antigens or to the tumour-specific antigens (TSA). It can also be assumed that all of the allogeneic vaccines will contain melanoma differentiation antigens to varying degrees and that major differences in responses to these antigens would not be expected. Any differences would therefore depend on their content of TSA or CT antigens such as MAGE and GAGE, etc. Information on this point is not freely available. In the case of the MM200 melanoma cell used in the author's vaccine study, it is known to express MAGE-1 and MAGE-3 but typing has not been carried out for the other members of the CT family. From Table 16.5 it may be seen that the MAGE family have high levels of expression in melanoma lines and it is quite likely that most allogeneic melanoma vaccines will contain some of these antigens. It is also clear that as more studies are carried out the major histocompatibility complex (MHC) restriction of the MAGE family is wide and includes helper CD4 T-cell epitopes [58,59]. Most patients would therefore have a response to one or more of the various epitopes on these molecules.

It would appear unlikely that there are major differences between the allogeneic vaccines based on their content of TSA or differentiation antigens. If differences do appear it is more likely they are a result of the adjuvant used with the vaccine or the dose, timing and frequency of administration of the injections. Are there other limitations from use of allogeneic vaccines? Space does not permit a full discussion of this topic, which is reviewed by Mitchell [67]. One possibility is that immunization with alloantigens may predominate over responses to tumour antigens. Another is that too many foreign antigens may occupy antigen-presenting cells and exclude low-frequency tumour antigens.

How important are differences in dose, timing and duration of vaccine administration?

In experimental models, large antigen doses were shown to result in antibody rather than cell-mediated responses [68]. This is one reason for use of small amounts of antigen rather than large amounts. The other is to select high avidity T cells. The VMCL vaccines in the author's studies [1] contain approximately 100 μg protein per vial (5×10^6 lysed cell equivalents), which is likely to be substantially less than that used in the other allogeneic cell vaccinia trials, e.g. the CVax vaccine of Morton *et al.* contains three lines and approximately 25×10^6 whole cells per injection [7]. The Ribi/Mitchell Melacine vaccine contains fragments from two lines to a total dose of 20×10^6 melanoma cells. This dose was based on dose–response precursor T-cell studies [69]. Avax/Berd uses approximately $20–25 \times 10^6$ autologous melanoma coupled with dinitrophenyl (DNP) [10,11]. Wallack *et al.* [3] prepared vaccinia viral lysates from four melanoma cells and adjusted each dose to 2 mg protein. Bystryn [12] gave 40 μg of protein with each dose.

The timing of vaccines administration has also varied substantially between studies. Two objectives underlie the timing of injections: to generate high numbers of cytotoxic T cells (CTL) to clear residual melanoma cells from tissues and circulation; and to obtain high numbers of circulating memory cells which can be reactivated should they be exposed to melanoma antigens again. Given that the lives of CTL are relatively short, it seems reasonable to have an initial period of frequent immunization and follow this with repeat immunizations at less frequent intervals to maintain high memory T-cell numbers. Whether any of the administration protocols achieve these aims is unknown but a wide variation exists between the studies, as shown in Table 16.1. Wallack *et al.* [3] administered their vaccine at multiple sites weekly for 12 weeks then fortnightly to 1 year. The author's study administered VMCL intradermally each 2 weeks for four doses then 3-weekly for six doses and monthly thereafter to 2 years. Morton *et al.* [7] administered CVax each 2 weeks for four doses then at increasing intervals up to 5 years. Melacine (Ribi/Mitchell) vaccines were given subcutaneously, weekly for four injections then one at an interval of 4 weeks and then 8-weekly to 4 years. Bystryn [12] gave injections intradermally at 3-weekly intervals for four injections then 4-weekly for three injections and at fixed intervals to 5 years. Berd *et al.* [10,11] gave injections each week for 6 weeks and repeated this after an interval of 4 weeks. A booster was given at 6 months.

The other possible variables are the adjuvant or helper molecules used to enhance responses to the vaccines. The author's study relied on the response to vaccinia to 'help' responses to melanoma antigens. This effect was evident in the first 3 months but may not have been as effective with repeated immunizations [46,70]. Morton *et al.* admixed the first two doses with Bacillus Calmette–Guérin (BCG) to provide help and Bystryn used alum as the adjuvant. Ribi/Mitchell employed a more advanced adjuvant which included detoxified lipopolysaccharide (LPS), bacterial cell walls and squalene (oil-in-water) emulsion [67]. Berd *et al.* gave the initial vaccine in each 6-week course in BCG. Each 6-week course was preceded by intravenous cyclophosphamide [10].

There are therefore substantial differences between the different studies in these practical aspects which may well have an important influence on the effectiveness of immunotherapy.

Why is immunotherapy not more effective?

It is clear from the above that considerable effort has gone into development of melanoma vaccines. It can be expected that the next few years will see further description of tumour rejection antigens and measures to optimize levels of immunity. A realistic assessment at present would conclude that only few patients receive benefit from this treatment approach. Two broad categories of explanations can be advanced to explain this: the immune system either fails to recognize the tumour antigens; or mounts an ineffective adaptive non-lytic response. The possible reasons for this are shown in Table 16.6 and involve release of factors from the tumour cells or from infiltrating leukocytes. This situation is similar to that involved in vaccination against parasitic diseases and may be viewed as the problem of converting anergic or TH2, TC2 responses to TH1, TC1 responses against the tumour.

These problems do not seem insurmountable and recent studies on *ex vivo* production and maturation of dendritic cells suggests that CTL responses can be generated by injection of dendritic cells produced by this approach [47,47]. Histamine also appears to reduce the immunosuppressive effect of tumour infiltrating macrophages and concomitant administration of IL-2 may overcome anergy in T cells against the melanoma antigens. Vascular endothelial growth factor (VEGF) and transforming growth factor-β (TGF-β) appear to inhibit antigen presentation and, perhaps more importantly, to down-regulate adhesion molecules such as VCAM-1 and intercellular adhesion molecule-1 (ICAM-1) involved in migration of lymphocytes into the tumour [82]. Clinical

Table 16.6 Mechanisms involved in inhibition of immune responses to melanoma

Mechanism	Factors involved	Reference
Inhibition of antigen presentation	VEGF, IL-10	[71,72]
Inhibition of cytokine production	IL-10, TGF-β, α-MSH	[73–75]
Tolerance/anergy of T cells	Hydrogen peroxide, TGF-β	[74,76]
	α-MSH	[77]
Shift of TH_1TC_1 to TH_2TC_2	IL-10, TGF-β, FasL	[78,79]
Inhibition of migration of	PGE_2, tumour matrix	[80,81]
leukocytes from blood vessels	VEGF	[82]
Tumour-mediated destruction of T cells	FasL	[83]
Resistance of tumour cells to killing	IL-10, immunoselection of HLA	[84,85]
	and antigen loss variants	[53,86]

Abbreviation: VEGF, vascular endothelial growth factor.

trials of VEGF-specific tyrosine kinase inhibitors [87] or with MAbs to VEGF [71] are in progress and may provide valuable reagents to augment immunotherapy.

A more serious problem relates to changes that occur in the melanoma cell under the selection pressure of the immune system and other growth control mechanisms. The loss of human leucocyte antigens (HLAs) on melanoma cells has been well publicized [84] but the frequency with which it occurs is debated [88]. It is also well documented that antigens related to differentiation molecules may be downregulated or lost during immunotherapy [53]. In some instances the immune system has adapted to this loss by recognition of less dominant antigens associated with other MHC antigens [89].

A less obvious mechanism of resistance of melanoma cells to immunotherapy deserves further attention, namely their resistance to apoptosis. This follows from studies which showed that a member of the tumour necrosis factor (TNF) family—TNF-related apoptosis-inducing ligand (TRAIL)—appeared to be the main mechanism by which CD4 T cells mediate the killing of melanomas. Importantly, we found that melanoma cells that were resistant to TRAIL were also resistant to killing by CD4 T cells [90,91]. This did not apply to killing by CD8 T cells but immunohistological studies show that regression of primary melanoma is usually associated with CD4 T-cell infiltrates and not CD8 T-cell infiltrates [92]. It is also of much interest to find that sensitivity to TRAIL is predictive of sensitivity to certain chemotherapeutic agents, perhaps because of the involvement of TRAIL-dependent apoptosis in killing by the chemotherapeutic agents. Circumstantial evidence for the importance of TRAIL or other TNF family members in immunotherapy comes from studies in animal models, which show that expression of Flice inhibitory protein (FLIP) protects tumour cells from T-cell immunity and results in selection of tumour cells with high FLIP levels [93,94]. The same results were seen in perforin knockout mice. FLIP is known to block FasL- and TRAIL-mediated killing of tumour cells but not perforin granzyme killing [93]. The results suggest that the TNF family may be much more important in the control of tumour growth than at first thought. Melanoma cells in surgical specimens were shown to have high FLIP levels [95] so that it is reasonable to infer that TRAIL may be a major mediator of regression induced by the immune system. This conclusion further implies that understanding mechanisms of resistance to TRAIL may provide much needed insights into the resistance of most melanomas to immunotherapy.

Conclusions

Studies on patients with stage IV melanoma show that a small proportion of melanomas undergo regression during immunotherapy with relatively crude autologous or allogeneic vaccines. Large randomized trials in an adjuvant setting are now in progress in stage II, III and IV melanomas which should provide a measure of their effectiveness in improving patients' survival. Major differences in the antigenic content of the allogeneic vaccines seem unlikely but administration protocols and dosage of the vaccines differ widely between the studies. While these studies are maturing, a number of Phase I–II studies with purified melanoma antigens are in progress which promise to define the principal rejection antigens in melanoma and the adjuvants/cytokines which maximize responses to these antigens.

The challenge over the next decade will be to incorporate information about tumour-derived immunosuppressive factors into protocols that counteract these properties of tumour cells. Understanding the basis of resistance of melanoma cells to TRAIL-induced apoptosis may also provide much needed new insights into the resistance of melanoma to immunotherapy and provide therapeutic approaches which will increase the proportion of patients who respond to this important treatment modality. Until these advances are made we must answer the question 'will vaccines really work for melanoma?' by saying 'yes, in some patients—but we cannot identify which patients'.

References

1 Hersey P, Edwards A, Coates A, Shaw H, McCarthy W, Milton G. Evidence that treatment with vaccinia melanoma cell lysates (VMCL) may improve survival of patients with stage II melanoma. *Cancer Immunol Immunother* 1987; **25**: 257–65.

2 Hersey P, Coates A, McCarthy WH. Interim analysis of a randomized trial of immunotherapy with vaccinia melanoma cell lysates (VMCL) following surgical removal of high risk melanoma. *Proc Am Assoc Cancer Res* 1996; **37**: 489.

3 Wallack MK, Sivanandham M, Balch CM, *et al.* Surgical adjuvant active specific immunotherapy for patients with stage III melanoma: the final analysis of data from a phase III, randomized, double-blind, multicenter vaccinia melanoma oncolysate trial. *J Am Coll Surg* 1998; **187**: 69–77.

4 Livingston PO, Wong GY, Adluri S, *et al.* Improved survival in stage III melanoma patients with GM2 antibodies: a randomized trial of adjuvant vaccination with GM2. *J Clin Oncol* 1994; **12** (5): 1036–44.

5 Chapman PB, Morrissey D, Ibrahim J, *et al.* Eastern Cooperative Oncology Group phase II randomized adjuvant trial of GM2-KLH + QS21 (GMK) vaccine ± α2b (HD IFN) in melanoma (MEL). *Proc ASCO* 1999; **18**: 538a.

6 Eggermont AM. Strategy of the EORTC-MCG trial programme for adjuvant treatment of moderate-risk and high-risk melanoma. *Eur J Cancer* 1998; **34** (Suppl. 3): 22–6.

7 Morton DL, Foshag LJ, Hoon DSB, *et al.* Prolongation of survival in metastatic melanoma after active specific immunotherapy with a new polyvalent melanoma vaccine. *Ann Surg* 1992; **216** (4): 463–82.

8 Mitchell MS, Harel W, Kempf RA, *et al.* Active-specific immunotherapy for melanoma. *J Clin Oncol* 1990; **8** (5): 856–69.

9 Sondak VK. Multi-institutional melanoma vaccine trial. *Ann Surg Oncol* 1996; **3**: 588–9.

10 Berd D, Murphy G, Maguire HC Jr, Mastrangelo MJ. Immunization with haptenized, autologous tumour cells induces inflammation of human melanoma metastases. *Cancer Res* 1991; **51**: 2731–4.

11 Berd D, Maguire HC, Schuchter LM, *et al.* Autologous hapten-modified melanoma vaccine as postsurgical adjuvant treatment after resection of nodal metastases. *J Clin Oncol* 1997; **15** (6): 2359–70.
12 Bystryn J-C, Oratz R, Shapiro RL, *et al.* Double-blind, placebo-controlled, trial of a shed, polyvalent, melanoma vaccine in stage III melanoma. *Proc ASCO* 1999; **18**: 434a.
13 Hellstrom I, Hellstrom KE. Tumour immunology: an overview. In: Bystryn J-C, Ferrone S, Livingston P, eds. *Specific Immunotherapy of Cancer with Vaccines.* New York: Academy of Sciences, 1993.
14 Zhang H, Zhang S, Cheung N-KV, Ragupathi G, Livingston PO. Antibodies against GD2 ganglioside can eradicate syngeneic cancer micrometastases. *Cancer Res* 1998; **58**: 2844–9.
15 Jones PC, Sze LL, Liu PY. Prolonged survival for melanoma patients with elevated IgM antibody to oncofetal antigen. *J Natl Cancer Inst* 1981; **66**: 249–54.
16 Takahashi H, Johnson TD, Nishinaka Y, Morton DL, Irie RF. IgM anti-ganglioside antibodies induced by melanoma cell vaccine correlate with survival of melanoma patients. *J Invest Dermatol* 1999; **112**: 205–9.
17 Cheung NK, Walter EI, Smith-Mensah WH, Ratnoff WD, Tykocinski ML, Medof ME. Decay-accelerating factor protects human tumour cells from complement-mediated cytotoxicity *in vitro*. *J Clin Invest* 1988; **81**: 1122–8.
18 Brasoveanu LI, Altomonte M, Fonsatti E, *et al.* Levels of cell membrane CD59 regulate the extent of complement-mediated lysis of human melanoma cells. *Lab Invest* 1996; **74**: 33–42.
19 Curry BJ, Myers K, Hersey P. MART-1 is expressed less frequently on circulating melanoma cells in patients who develop distant compared to locoregional metastases. *J Clin Oncol* 1999; **17**: 2562–72.
20 Ghossein RA, Coit D, Brennan M, *et al.* Prognostic significance of peripheral blood and bone marrow tyrosinase messenger RNA in malignant melanoma. *Clin Cancer Res* 1998; **4**: 419–28.
21 Livingston P. Ganglioside vaccines with emphasis on GM2. *Semin Oncol* 1998; **25**: 636–45.
22 Israel RJ, Chapman PB, Hamilton WB, Zhan C, Morrissey D. Phase I–II dose-ranging clinical trials of the ganglioside conjugate cancer vaccines GM2-KLH/QS-21 (GMK) and GM2-KLH/GD2-KLH/QS-21 (MGV) [Abstract]. *Proc ASCO* 1999; **18**: 437a.
23 Foon KA, Sen G, Hutchins L, *et al.* Antibody responses in melanoma patients immunized with an anti-idiotype antibody mimicking disialoganglioside GD2. *Clin Cancer Res* 1998; **4**: 1117–24.
24 Boon T, van der Bruggen P. Human tumour antigens recognized by T lymphocytes. *J Exp Med* 1996; **183**: 725–9.
25 Rosenberg SA. A new era for cancer immunotherapy based on the genes that encode cancer antigens. *Immunity* 1999; **10**: 281–7.
26 Old LJ, Chen Y-T. New paths in human cancer serology. *J Exp Med* 1998; **187**: 1163–7.
27 Fleischhauer K, Gattinoni L, Dalerba P, *et al.* The DAM gene family encodes a new group of tumour-specific antigens recognized by human leukocyte antigen A2-restricted cytotoxic T lymphocytes. *Cancer Res* 1998; **58**: 2969–72.
28 Lethe B, Lucas S, Michaux L, *et al.* LAGE-1, a new gene with tumour specificity. *Int J Cancer* 1998; **76**: 903–8.
29 Jaeger E, Chen Y-T, Drijfhout JW, *et al.* Simultaneous humoral and cellular immune response against cancer-testis antigen NY-ESO-1: definition of human histocompatibility leukocyte antigen (HLA) -A2-binding peptide epitopes. *J Exp Med* 1998; **187**: 265–70.
30 Tureci O, Chen YT, Sahin U, *et al.* Expression of SSX genes in human tumours. *Int J Cancer* 1998; **77**: 19–23.
31 Parkhurst MR, Fitzgerald EB, Southwood S, Sette A, Rosenberg SA, Kawakami Y. Identification of a shared HLA-A*0201-restricted T-cell epitope from the melanoma antigen Tyrosinase-related protein 2 (TRP2). *Cancer Res* 1998; **58**: 4895–901.
32 Lupetti R, Pisarra P, Verrecchia A, *et al.* Translation of a retained intron in tyrosinase-related protein (TRP) 2 mRNA generates a new cytotoxic T lymphocyte

(CTL) -defined and shared human melanoma antigen not expressed in normal cells of the melanocytic lineage. *J Exp Med* 1998; **188**: 1005–16.
33 van Elsas A, Scheibenbogen C, van der Minne C, Zerp SF, Keilholz U, Schrier PI. UV-induced N-ras mutations are T-cell targets in human melanoma. *Melanoma Res* 1997; 7 (Suppl 2): 107–13.
34 Chiari R, Foury F, De Plaen E, Baurain JF, Thonnard J, Coulie PG. Two antigens recognized by autologous cytolytic T lymphocytes on a melanoma result from a single point mutation in an essential housekeeping gene. *Cancer Res* 1999; **59**: 5785–92.
35 Smith M, Bleijs R, Radford K, Hersey P. Immunogenicity of CD63 in a patient with melanoma. *Melanoma Res* 1997; **7**: 5161–8.
36 Gilboa E. The makings of a tumour rejection antigen. *Immunity* 1999; **11**: 263–70.
37 Marchand M, van Baren N, Weynants P, *et al.* Tumour regressions observed in patients with metastatic melanoma treated with an antigenic peptide encoded by gene MAGE-3 and presented by HLA-A1. *Int J Cancer* 1999; **80**: 219–30.
38 Rosenberg SA, Yang JC, Schwartzentruber DJ, *et al.* Immunologic and therapeutic evaluation of a synthetic peptide vaccine for the treatment of patients with metastatic melanoma. *Nat Med* 1998; **4**: 321–7.
39 Maeurer MJ, Storkus WJ, Kirkwood JM, Lotze MT. New treatment options for patients with melanoma: review of melanoma-derived T-cell epitope-based peptide vaccine. *Melanoma Res* 1996; **6**: 11–24.
40 Jaeger E, Bernhard H, Romero P, *et al.* Generation of cytotoxic T-cell responses with synthetic melanoma-associated peptides *in vivo*: implications for tumour vaccines with melanoma-associated antigens. *Int J Cancer* 1996; **66**: 162–9.
41 Jaeger E, Ringhoffer M, Dienes HP, *et al.* Granulocyte-macrophage-colony-stimulating factor enhances immune responses to melanoma-associated peptides *in vivo*. *Int J Cancer* 1996; **67**: 54–62.
42 Weber JS, Hua FL, Spears L, Marty V, Kuniyoshi C, Celis E. A phase I trial of an HLA-A1 restricted MAGE-3 epitope peptide with incomplete Freund's adjuvant in patients with resected high-risk melanoma. *J Immunother* 1999; **22**: 431–40.
43 Wang F, Bade E, Kuniyoshi C, *et al.* Phase I trial of a MART-1 peptide vaccine with incomplete Freund's adjuvant for resected high-risk melanoma. *Clin Cancer Res* 1999; **5**: 2756–65.
44 Cebon JS, Jaeger E, Gibbs P, *et al.* Phase I studies of immunization with Melan-A and IL-12 in HLA A2+ positive patients with stage III and IV malignant melanoma. *Proc ASCO* 1999; **18**: 434a.
45 Scheibenbogen C, Schmittel A, Keilholz U, *et al.* Vaccination with tyrosinase peptides and GM-CSF in metastatic melanoma: a phase II trial. *Proc ASCO* 1999; **18**: 436a.
46 Hersey P, Edwards A, D'Alessandro G, MacDonald M. Phase II study of vaccinia melanoma cell lysates (VMCL) as adjuvant to surgical treatment of stage II melanoma. *Cancer Immunol Immunother* 1986; **22**: 221–31.
47 Nestle FO, Alijagic S, Gilliet M, *et al.* Vaccination of melanoma patients with peptide- or tumour lysate-pulsed dendritic cells. *Nat Med* 1998; **4**: 328–32.
48 Hu X, Chakraborty NG, Sporn JR, Kurtzman SH, Ergin MT, Mukherji B. Enhancement of cytolytic T lymphocyte precursor frequency in melanoma patients following immunization with the MAGE-1 peptide loaded antigen presenting cell-based vaccine. *Cancer Res* 1996; **56**: 2479–83.
49 Chakraborty N, Tortora A, Sporn J, *et al.* Melanoma cell lysate loaded autologous antigen presenting cell (APC) as a vaccine in melanoma. *Proc Am Assoc Cancer Res* 1997; **38**: 400.
50 Lotze MT, Storkus WJ, Falo L, *et al.* Dendritic cells (DCs) and the immunotherapy of melanoma. *Melanoma Res* 1997; 7 (Suppl 1), 4.
51 Thurner B, Haendle I, Roder C, *et al.* Vaccination with Mage-3A1 peptide-pulsed mature, monocyte-derived dendritic cells expands specific cytotoxic T cells and induces regression of some metastases in advanced stage IV melanoma. *J Exp Med* 1999; **190**: 1669–78.
52 Gajewski TF, Fallarino F, Vogelzang N, Posner MC, Ashikari A, Sherman ML. Effective melanoma antigen vaccination

without dendritic cells (DC): a phase I study of immunization with Mage3 or Melan-A peptide-pulsed autologous PBMC plus RhIL-12. *Proc ASCO* 1999; **18**: 539a.

53 Jaeger E, Ringhoffer M, Altmannsberger M, *et al.* Immunoselection *in vivo*: independent loss of MHC class I and melanocyte differentiation antigen expression in metastatic melanoma. *Int J Cancer* 1997; **71**: 142–7.

54 Chaux P, Vantomme V, Coulie P, Boon T, van der Bruggen P. Estimation of the frequencies of anti-MAGE-3 cytolytic T-lymphocyte precursors in blood from individuals without cancer. *Int J Cancer* 1998; **77**: 538–42.

55 Zakut R, Topalian SL, Kawakami Y, Mancini M, Eliyahu S, Rosenberg SA. Differential expression of MAGE-1, -2 and -3 messenger RNA in transformed and normal human cell lines. *Cancer Res* 1993; **53**: 5–8.

56 De Plaen E, Arden K, Traversari C, *et al.* Structure, chromosomal localization, and expression of 12 genes of the MAGE family. *Immunogenetics* 1994; **40**: 360–9.

57 McIntyre CA, Rees RC, Platts KE, *et al.* Identification of peptide epitopes of MAGE-1-2-3 that demonstrate HLA-A3-specific binding. *Cancer Immunol Immunother* 1996; **42**: 246–50.

58 van der Bruggen P, Szikora J-P, Boel P, *et al.* Autologous cytolytic T lymphocytes recognize a MAGE-1 nonapeptide on melanomas expressing HLA-Cw*1601*. *Eur J Immunol* 1994; **24**: 2134–40.

59 Chaux P, Vantomme V, Stroobant V, *et al.* Identification of MAGE-3 epitopes presented by HLA-DR molecules to CD4 (+) T lymphocytes. *J Exp Med* 1999; **189**: 767–78.

60 Manici S, Sturniolo T, Imro MA, *et al.* Melanoma cells present a MAGE-3 epitope to CD4 (+) cytotoxic T cells in association with histocompatibility leukocyte antigen DR11. *J Exp Med* 1999; **189**: 871–6.

61 Oiso M, Eura M, Katsura F, *et al.* A newly identified MAGE-3-derived epitope recognized by HLA-A24-restricted cytotoxic T lymphocytes. *Int J Cancer* 1999; **81**: 387–94.

62 Valmori D, Gileadi U, Servis C, *et al.* Modulation of proteasomal activity required for the generation of a cytotoxic T lymphocyte-defined peptide derived from the tumour antigen MAGE-3. *J Exp Med* 1999; **189**: 895–906.

63 Zorn E, Hercend TA MAGE-6-encoded peptide is recognized by expanded lymphocytes infiltrating a spontaneously regressing human primary melanoma lesion. *Eur J Immunol* 1999; **29**: 602–7.

64 Van den Eynde B, Peeters O, De Backer O, Gaugler B, Lucas S, Boon T. A new family of genes coding for an antigen recognized by autologous cytolytic T lymphocytes on a human melanoma. *J Exp Med* 1995; **182**: 689–98.

65 Brasseur F, Rimoldi D, Lienard D, *et al.* Expression of MAGE genes in primary and metastatic cutaneous melanoma. *Int J Cancer* 1995; **63**: 375–80.

66 Dalerba P, Ricci A, Russo V, *et al.* High homogeneity of MAGE, BAGE, GAGE, tyrosinase and Melan-A/MART-1 gene expression in clusters of multiple simultaneous metastases of human melanoma: implications for protocol design of therapeutic antigen-specific vaccination strategies. *Int J Cancer* 1998; **77**: 200–4.

67 Mitchell MS. Active specific immunotherapy of cancer: therapeutic vaccines ('Theraccines') for the treatment of disseminated malignancies. In: Mitchell, MS, ed. *Biological Approaches to Cancer Treatment*. New York:. McGraw-Hill, 1993: 326–51.

68 Parish CR. Immune deviation: a historical perspective. *Immunol Cell Biol* 1996; **74**: 449–56.

69 Mitchell MS. Attempts to optimize active specific immunotherapy for melanoma. *Int Rev Immunol* 1991; **7**: 331–47.

70 Hersey P. Vaccinia viral lysates in treatment of melanoma. In: Mitchell, MS, ed. *Biological Approaches to Cancer Treatment*. New York: McGraw-Hill, 1993: 302–25.

71 Gabrilovich DI, Ishida T, Nadaf S, Ohm JE, Carbone DP. Antibodies to vascular endothelial growth factor enhance the efficacy of cancer immunotherapy by improving endogenous dendritic cell function. *Clin Cancer Res* 1999; **5**: 2963–70.

72 De Waal Malefyt R, Haanen J, Spits H, *et al.* Interleukin 10 (IL-10) and viral IL-10 strongly reduce antigen-specific human

T cell proliferation by diminishing the antigen-presenting capacity of monocytes via downregulation of class II major histocompatibility complex expression. *J Exp Med* 1991; **174**: 915–24.

73 Fiorentino DF, Bond MW, Mosmann TR. Two types of mouse T helper cell. IV. Th2 clones secrete a factor that inhibits cytokine production by Th1 clones. *J Exp Med* 1989; **170**: 2081–95.

74 Bodmer S, Strommer K, Frei K, *et al.* Immunosuppression and transforming growth factor-β in glioblastoma. *J Immunol* 1989; **143**: 3222–9.

75 Liu PY, Johansson O. Immunohistochemical evidence of α-, β- and γ- 3-melanocyte stimulating hormone expression in cutaneous malignant melanoma of nodular type. *J Dermatol* 1995; **10**: 203–12.

76 Kono K, Salazar-Onfray F, Petersson M, *et al.* Hydrogen peroxide secreted by tumour-derived macrophages down-modulates signal-transducing zeta molecules and inhibits tumour-specific T cell- and natural killer cell-mediated cytotoxicity. *Eur J Immunol* 1996; **26**: 1308–13.

77 Grabbe S, Bhardwaj RS, Mahnke K, Simon MM, Schwarz T, Luger TA. α-Melanocyte-stimulating hormone induces hapten-specific tolerance in mice. *J Immunol* 1996; **156**: 473–8.

78 Maeda H, Shiraishi A. TGF-β contributes to the shift toward Th2-type responses through direct and IL-10 mediated pathways in tumour-bearing mice. *J Immunol* 1996; **156**: 73–8.

79 Zhang QJ, Brunner T, Carter L, *et al.* Unequal death in T helper cell (Th) 1 and Th2 effectors: Th1, but not Th2, effectors undergo rapid Fas/FasL-mediated apoptosis. *J Exp Med* 1997; **185**: 1837–49.

80 Oppenheimer-Marks N, Kavanaugh AF, Lipsky PE. Inhibition of the transendothelial migration of human T lymphocytes by prostaglandin E2. *J Immunol* 1994; **152**: 5703.

81 Wick M, Dubey P, Koeppen H, *et al.* Antigenic cancer cells grow progressively in immune hosts without evidence for T cell exhaustion or systemic anergy. *J Exp Med* 1997; **186**: 229–38.

82 Griffioen AW, Damen CA, Mayo KH, *et al.* Angiogenesis inhibitors overcome tumour induced endothelial cell anergy. *Int J Cancer* 1999; **80**: 315–19.

83 Strand S, Hofmann WJ, Hug H, *et al.* Lymphocyte apoptosis induced by CD95 (APO-1/Fas) ligand-expressing tumour cells: a mechanism of immune evasion? *Nat Med* 1996; **2**: 1361.

84 Ferrone S, Marincola FM. Loss of HLA class I antigens by melanoma cells: molecular mechanisms, functional significance and clinical relevance. *Immunol Today* 1995; **16**: 487–94.

85 Matsuda M, Salazar F, Petersson M, *et al.* Interleukin 10 pretreatment protects target cells from tumour- and allo-specific cytotoxic T cells and downregulates HLA class I expression. *J Exp Med* 1994; **180**: 2371–6.

86 Restifo NP, Marincola FM, Kawakami Y, Taubenberger J, Yannelli JR, Rosenberg SA. Loss of functional β_2-microglobulin in metastatic melanomas from five patients receiving immunotherapy. *J Natl Cancer Inst* 1996; **88**: 100.

87 Shaheen RM. Antiangiogenic therapy targeting the tyrosine kinase receptor for vascular endothelial growth factor receptor inhibits the growth of colon cancer liver metastasis and induces tumour and endothelial cell apoptosis. *Cancer Res* 1999; **59**: 5412–16.

88 Cormier JN, Hijazi YM, Abati A, *et al.* Heterogeneous expression of melanoma-associated antigens and HLA-A2 in metastatic melanoma *in vivo*. *Int J Cancer* 1998; **75**: 517–24.

89 Ikeda H, Lethe B, Lehmann F, *et al.* Characterization of an antigen that is recognized on a melanoma showing partial HLA loss by CTL expressing an NK inhibitory receptor. *Immunity* 1997; **6**: 199–208.

90 Thomas WD, Hersey P. TNF-related apoptosis-inducing ligand (TRAIL) induces apoptosis in Fas ligand-resistant melanoma cells and mediates CD4 T cell killing of target cells. *J Immunol* 1998; **161**: 2195–200.

91 Zhang XD, Franco A, Myers K, Gray C, Nguyen T, Hersey P. Relation of TNF-related apoptosis-inducing ligand (TRAIL) receptor and FLICE-inhibitory protein expression to TRAIL-induced apoptosis of melanoma. *Cancer Res* 1999; **59**: 2747–53.

92 Tefany FJ, Barnetson RS, Halliday GM,

McCarthy SW, McCarthy WH. Immunocytochemical analysis of the cellular infiltrate in primary regressing and non-regressing malignant melanoma. *J Invest Dermatol* 1991; **97**: 197–202.
93 French LE, Tschopp J. Inhibition of death receptor signaling by FLICE-inhibitory protein as a mechanism for immune escape of tumours. *J Exp Med* 1999; **190**: 891–3.
94 Medema JP, de Jong J, van Hall T, Melief CJM, Offringa R. Immune escape of tumours *in vivo* by expression of cellular FLICE-inhibitory protein. *J Exp Med* 1999; **190**: 1033–8.
95 Irmler M, Thome M, Hahne M, *et al.* Inhibition of death receptor signals by cellular FLIP. *Nature* 1997; **388**: 190–5.

17: Who should we consider for isolated limb perfusion?

Ferdy J. Lejeune and Danielle Liénard

Introduction

A limb heavily affected by a cancer condition—in-transit melanoma metastases, locally spreading skin carcinoma—is an appalling clinical situation, sometimes leading to palliative amputation. The idea came to Creech *et al.* from New Orleans [1], to isolate the affected limb and to connect it to a heart–lung machine, in order to deliver a high concentration of cytostatics within a closed circuit, while avoiding systemic toxicity (Fig. 17.1). Besides nitrogen mustard which was the first drug, melphalan or phenylalanine mustard (PAM) was quickly established as an effective agent in that setting, although it was poorly effective when given systemically. Regional efficiency will depend upon the chosen drug and its concentration: a concentration-dependent antitumour effect is a prerequisite. The lack of systemic toxicity will depend on: the quality of surgical isolation; the dissection of the vessels; the ligation of the collateral vessels; and efficacy and location of the tourniquet.

In malignant melanoma, the only indication for isolated limb perfusion (ILP) is in-transit metastasis confined to a limb, in such an anatomical condition that surgical vascular isolation can be performed.

In-transit melanoma metastasis

High-risk primary melanoma (>1.5 mm) of the limbs is prone to develop in-transit metastasis within 5 years in 6–10% of cases [2]. These metastases are lymph-borne. They are the consequence of the penetration of the tumour cells into the dermal lymph channels, followed by lymph flotation, adhesion to endothelial cells, extravasation and invasion of the adjacent tissues. The term 'in-transit' is classically reserved for metastasis developing in the subcutis or in the skin between the primary and the regional lymph basin. The term 'satellitosis' is assigned to dermo-epidermal metastases all around the primary site within a diameter of 5 cm. They originate from tiny dermal lymphatics, where the lymph flow is not necessarily stable, so that they can occur at any point

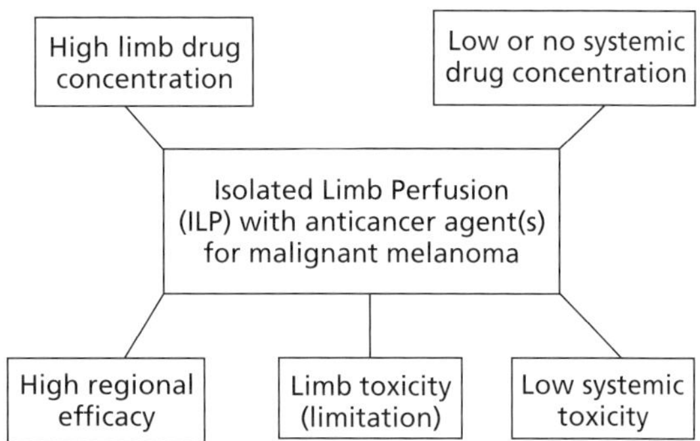

Fig. 17.1 Isolated limb perfusion.

'around the clock'. Larger lymph channels, especially collectors, have a centripedal flow directing the cell transit, carrying the metastases towards the draining lymph nodes. However, the distinction between satellitosis and in-transit metastasis has little biological significance, as the two patterns result from essentially the same stepwise events. Furthermore, it is not clear if some in-transit metastases are not preregional lymph node deposits as demonstrated by the evidence that some sentinel nodes have been found in the transit region [3].

Available treatments

Table 17.1 summarizes the routine management of in-transit metastasis. It shows that ILP is indicated when other less aggressive modalities have failed. In addition, when the clinical situation permits it, some patients may benefit from an active specific immunotherapy with peptides (see Prospects section p. 236).

Technical considerations

Isolated limb perfusion is a sophisticated procedure which should be performed by expert surgeons in adequately equipped operating theatres. The surgeons should be trained in oncological and vascular surgery and have access to heart–lung technology.

For lower limb perfusion—the most common indication—the recommended way is to perform an extensive iliac lymph node dissection and to ligate the collateral vessels. The cannulae will be inserted through veno- and arteriotomies above the inguinal ligament. The tip of the cannula should be in the common femoral artery, to allow optimal drug delivery. A tourniquet is applied around the root of the limb and twisted around a pin inserted into the iliac crest, in order to expose the whole root of the limb [2–4]. It is possible to use femoral or popliteal access for more distant disease; however, iliac ILP is

Table 17.1 Available treatment for in-transit melanoma metastases

Indication	Treatment
First appearence of several in-transit metastases	Surgical resection and histological confirmation
Recurrence of in-transit metastases in confined area	Surgical resection if not numerous CO_2 laser evaporation if numerous or cryotherapy if superficial Specific immunotherapy with peptides (only available in clinical trials)
Recurrence of in-transit metastases widespread and/or bulky	Isolated limb perfusion

preferred because of the staging provided by the iliac lymph node dissection, and because access is via the vascular area excluded from that to be treated.

Upper limb ILP is performed through axillary dissection and the vessels are best cannulated through a division of the pectoralis major muscle.

The extracorporeal circulation set-up consists of tubing, oxygenator (including heat exchanger and reservoir) and modular pump for the arterial line. Venous blood is recovered by gravity. The extracorporeal circulation should be monitored by a certified pump technician.

A critical issue is the leakage to the systemic circulation. A prerequisite for good isolation perfusion is the continuous monitoring of the leakage by using radiolabelled albumin and γ probe recording over the heart [5]. The main cause of leakage is too high a pump flow. Continuous leakage monitoring allows for the finding, at any moment, of the best equilibrium between the two compartments (perfusate and systemic circulation) by fine tuning of the pump.

Therapeutic isolated limb perfusion

The rationale for ILP is the view that in-transit metastases are not just 'satellites' or confined to a restricted area, but represent a contamination of a large portion of the lymph channel network. In the first instance, and especially in the primary onset of in-transit metastasis, surgical excision of the metastasis is recommended. It can be therapeutic in some cases and will allow a histological diagnosis. If a recurrence and/or new in-transit metastasis appears shortly after the first event (a few weeks) it can be expected that a large area of the lymphatic network is affected by the micrometastasis; this is a typical situation for therapeutic ILP. The metastases should not be excised prior to ILP because they will allow the evaluation of the efficacy of the treatment. Moreover, a randomized trial addressing the issue of prophylactic ILP with melphalan after removal of all in-transit metastases, showed no difference in survival rates [6].

Gold standard of therapeutic isolated limb perfusion

What drug regimen to use?

The gold standard is melphalan given at a dosage producing a perfusate concentration 10–30-fold the area under the curve (AUC) of systemic administration. There is a 50% chance of complete remission and 25% chance of partial remission [4]. It does not appear that the addition of actinomycin D increases efficacy although it does increase local toxicity [7]. Other drugs used alone, such as platinum or dacarbazine, do not reach the 50% response rate obtained by melphalan [4]. As shown in Table 17.2, response rates are not given for some regimens because excision of the in-transit metastasis was performed at the time of ILP.

New approaches to isolated limb perfusion

Recently, two new combinations based on synergism have been proposed (Table 17.2):

1 tumour necrosis factor (TNF) combined with melphalan (TM-ILP) or with melphalan and γ-interferon (IFN-γ), (TIM-ILP); and

2 systemic dacarbazine followed by a nitrosourea in the perfusate.

Table 17.2 Drugs used in isolated limb perfusion for melanoma in-transit metastasis

Name	Properties	ORR (%)*	Percentage of CR†	Regional toxicity
Single agents				
Melphalan (PAM)	Bifunctional alkylating agents	70–80	30–65	Skin and soft tissues
Cisplatin	Alkylating agent	Unknown	Unknown	Skin and soft tissues
Dacarbazine	Alkylating agent	Unknown	Unknown	None
Combinations				
Actinomycin D + melphalan	Antibiotic	70–80	Unknown	Skin and soft tissues
Dacarbazine‡ + fotemustine	Nitrosourea	Unknown	50	Late inflammation, necrosis
TNF + melphalan + IFN-γ	Antivascular effect	90	69	Skin and soft tissues
	Alkylating agent cytokine	100	78	

* Overal response rate (ORR).
† Complete reponse (CR) of unresected metastases.
‡ Dacarbazine given 4 h before fotemustine.

The first approach is based on dual targeting: TNF specifically destroys tumour-associated microvasculature by inducing apoptosis in angiogenic endothelial cells, while melphalan produces apoptosis of tumour cells [8]. Combined (or not) with IFN-γ, this regimen obtained the highest response rates ever seen: overall response of 90–100% and complete response of 70–80% [9]. While this regimen has been registered by the European pharmaceutical authorities (CPMP) for inextirpable soft tissue sarcoma, it has not been registered for melanoma because of the lack of randomized trial data comparing combined treatments with melphalan alone. However, comparison of TIM or TM-ILP with historical matched series treated by melphalan alone, show that the latter provided only 52% complete response as compared to 68–78% in combination with TNF [9].

Resistance to nitrosourea is a result of the enzyme alkyl transferase (AT) which demethylates alkylated DNA. Dacarbazine and temozolomide inactivate AT, thereby sensitizing melanomas to the nitrosourea fotemustine. It was reported [10] that the administration of dacarbazine systemically 4h before ILP with fotemustine gave a response rate of 50%, equal to melphalan. A Phase I–II study on this schedule is currently being conducted by the European Organization for Research on Treatment of Cancer Melanoma Cooperative Group (EORTC-MCG).

Follow-up after therapeutic isolated limb perfusion

Most sensitive in-transit melanoma metastases are the superficial 'epidermotropic' metastases which are often seen to dry off after a few weeks. Subcutaneous metastases are usually less responsive and slower to regress. It can sometimes take a few months before necrosis is seen. If a good but partial response is seen for multiple tumours, ILP should be repeated. Otherwise, destruction of the remaining tumours, 6–8 weeks after ILP, with laser or cryotherapy, or even scalpel, is a good option.

There is one area of the lower limb where drug penetration is almost always lower, the proximal and external aspect of the thigh, because it is vascularized by the vessels from the ischiatic artery and they are closed by the tourniquet. Irradiation of this region is a useful option, especially when in-transit metastases are already developed in this area.

ILP could be considered as an induction therapy and would ideally be followed by maintenance therapy. However, there is no established efficient adjuvant therapy after ILP although, in some selected cases, the administration of dacarbazine and/or temozolomide and/or fotemustine can induce useful response, even in the long term.

Survival after therapeutic isolated limb perfusion

No randomized trials have been conducted to compare survival after ILP to repeated local removal of in-transit metastases. However, one randomized Phase II study was conducted to compare TIM-ILP to TM-ILP, and survival after the two TNF-containing modalities were compared to historical data from patients treated with melphalan alone (Table 17.3). All survival curves were similar, leading to a median survival of 2.5 years [9]. In other words, obtaining either 80% complete response or 50% complete response with a different regimen does not influence survival. The benefit from regional therapy is limited to the region, with an expected improved quality of life.

Adjuvant isolated limb perfusion

Given the high response rate obtained after therapeutic ILP with melphalan, this treatment was advocated for prophylaxis of regional recurrences of either high-risk primary melanoma of the limbs or after removal of all detectable in-transit metastases.

The first randomized trial for excised melanoma in-transit (MD Anderson IIIA) was conducted by the Scandinavian Melanoma Group. A trend for a better regional disease-free interval was seen but there was no effect on survival [6].

A prematurely closed randomized trial was conducted with a mixture of high-risk primary cases and in-transit metastases. Although the authors

Table 17.3 Survival after isolated limb perfusion in melanoma

		Survival		
Stage	Drugs	5 years (%)	10 years (%)	Reference
I–II high-risk primary melanoma	Melphalan	80	65	Schraffordt Koops *et al.* [2]
III with in-transit metastases				
AJCC N2 b	Melphalan ± actinomycin D	35–70	28–50	Schraffordt Koops *et al.* [4]
AJCC N2 c	Melphalan ± actinomycin-D	29–40	23–34	Schraffordt Koops *et al.* [4]
	TNF + melphalan ± IFN-γ	(3 years)	50%	Liénard *et al.* [9]

Abbreviations: AJCC, American Joint Committee on Cancer; IFN-γ, γ–interferon; TNF, tumour necrosis factor.

claimed a benefit of survival, the data did not support it; too low a number of patients, mixed stages, tumours removed or not removed [11].

The first and probably last large-scale trial addressing the issue of prophylactic ILP for primary high risk (>1.5 mm thickness) melanomas was conducted jointly by the EORTC-MCG, the WHO Melanoma Programme and the North American Perfusion Group/Eastern Cooperative Oncology Group (ECOG) [2]. There were 852 evaluable patients. Randomization was made between wide excision or wide excision + ILP with melphalan. The decision to perform or not an elective lymph node dissection (ELND) was left to the institution policy; the balance between the two subgroups was good. Results showed that ILP made a significant reduction of in-transit metastases at first site of recurrence (3.3% after ILP and 6.6.% in control). In patients who were not submitted to ELND, there was also a reduction of regional lymph node metastases as an indirect consequence of the reduction of the in-transit metastases (12.6 vs. 16.7%). However, time to distant metastasis and overall survival were equal, whether or not ILP had been performed. Thus, it is concluded that melphalan ILP, either as an adjuvant after resection of metastases, or as prophylactic treatment (in high-risk primary melanoma) is not recommended.

Prospects

Isolated limb perfusion is a regional therapy with high therapeutic efficiency but confined to the treated area. In other words, it has no significant impact on survival from a disease which produces early distant micrometastasis. In addition, significant local relapse rates were reported in the therapeutic setting (Table 17.4).

Table 17.4 Local recurrence rate after isolated limb perfusion in melanoma

Stage	Drugs	Local/regional recurrence (%)	Reference
I–II high-risk primary melanoma	Melphalan*		Schraffordt Koops *et al.* [2]
		3.3	Schraffordt Koops *et al.* [2]
	No ILP	6	
III with in-transit metastases			
AJCC N2b/N2c	Melphalan + actinomycin D	38 (after resection post-ILP)	Baas *et al.* [7]
	Melphalan	45 (after resection post-ILP)	Hafstrom *et al.* [6]
	Melphalan + TNF	59 (no resection post-ILP)	Liénard *et al.* [9]

* Adjuvant isolated limb perfusion.

A simple alternative to ILP has been proposed: isolated hypoxic limb infusions with transcutaneous catheters. Preliminary results are encouraging [12], but it seems that efficacy of this treatment is restricted to distal leg metastases.

Efficient adjuvant treatments are not yet available, but melanoma is an immunogenic tumour for which cytotoxic T lymphocytes specific for histocompatibility complex (HLA) Class 1 presented peptides were found [13]. It is now possible to immunize patients with peptides. Specific active immunotherapy with HLA-A1 peptides was shown to induce 30% response, especially on in-transit metastases [14]. On-going studies will show if adjuvant specific immunotherapy is active after ILP.

References

1 Creech O, Ryan R, Krementz ET. Treatment of malignant melanoma by isolation perfusion technique. *J Am Med Assoc* 1959; **169**: 339–43.

2 Schraffordt Koops H.S, Vaglini M, Suciu S, *et al*. Prophylactic isolated limb perfusion for localized, high-risk limb melanoma: results of a multicenter randomized phase III trial. *J Clin Oncol* 1998; **16**: 2906–12.

3 Thompson JF, Uren RF, Shaw HM, *et al*. Location of sentinel lymph nodes in patients with cutaneous melanoma: new insights into lymphatic anatomy. *J Am Coll Surg* 1999; **189**: 195–204.

4 Schraffordt Koops H, Kroon B, *et al*. Management of local recurrence, satellites, and in-transit metastases of the limbs with isolation perfusion. In: Lejeune FJ, Prabir K, Chaudhuri TK. *Malignant Melanoma: Medical and Surgical Management*. New York: McGraw-Hill, 1994: 221–32.

5 Hoekstra H, Naujocks T, Schaffordt Koops H, *et al*. Continuous leakage monitoring during hyperthermic isolated regional perfusion of the lower limb: techniques and results. *Reg Cancer Treat* 1992; **4**: 301–4.

6 Hafstrom L, Rudenstam CM, Blomquist E, *et al*. Regional hyperthermic perfusion with melphalan after surgery for recurrent malignant melanoma of the extremities, Swedish Melanoma Study Group. *J Clin Oncol* 1991; **9**: 2091–4.

7 Baas PC, Schraffordt Koops H, Hoekstra HJ, Oosteruis JW, Vander Weele LT, Oldhoff J. Isolated regional perfusion in the treatment of local recurrence, satellitosis and in-transit metastases of extremity melanoma. *Reg Cancer Treat* 1988; **1**: 33–6.

8 Lejeune FJ, Ruegg C, Liénard D. Clinical applications of TNF-α in cancer. *Curr Opin Immunol* 1998; **10**: 573–80.

9 Liénard D, Eggermont AMM, Schraffordt Koops H, *et al*. Isolated limb perfusion with tumour necrosis factor α and melphalan with or without interferon γ for the treatment of in-transit melanoma metastases: a multicentre randomized phase II study. *Melanoma Res* 1999; **9**: 491–502.

10 Pontes L, Lopes M, Ribeiro M, Santos JG, Azevedo MC. Isolated limb perfusion with fotemustine after chemosensitization with dacarbazine in melanoma. *Melanoma Res* 1997; **7**: 417–19.

11 Ghussen F, Kruger I, Groth W, Stutzer H. The role of regional hyperthermic cytostatic perfusion in the treatment of extremity melanoma. *Cancer* 1988; **61**: 654–9.

12 Thompson JF, Kam P, Waugh RC, Harman CR. Isolated limb infusion with cytotoxic agents: a simple alternative to isolated limb perfusion. *Semin Surg Oncol* 1998; **14**: 238–47.

13 Romero P. Cytolytic T lymphocyte responses of cancer patients to tumor-associated antigens. *Springer Semin Immunopathol* 1996; **18**: 185–98.

14 Marchand M, van Baren N, Weynants P, *et al*. Tumor regressions observed in patients with metastatic melanoma treated with an antigenic peptide encoded by gene MAGE-3 and presented by HLA-A1. *Int J Cancer* 1999; **80**: 219–30.

18: Novel strategies for the treatment of melanoma

Sewa S. Legha

Introduction

Approximately 30% of all patients with primary melanoma subsequently develop metastatic disease which is ultimately fatal in 90–95% of patients. The treatment options for metastatic melanoma may include surgery, chemotherapy, biological therapy or various combinations of these treatment choices. Most of such patients can and often do avail themselves of chemotherapy, either as single drug therapy with dacarbazine (DTIC) or combinations of DTIC with other drugs (cisplatin, vinblastine, vindesine), or a nitrosourea (BCNU, CCNU, fotemustine). Although the probability of achieving a response to chemotherapy ranges from 20 to 40%, chemotherapy is rarely successful in eradicating metastatic disease completely.

Biological therapy using α-interferon (IFN-α) and interleukin 2 (IL-2) has been introduced more recently and each of these drugs can produce tumour regressions in 15–20% of patients with metastatic disease. Both agents have shown independent antitumour activity and are not cross-resistant with each other or with chemotherapy. Furthermore, complete tumour regression is achieved in approximately 5% of the patients, and nearly one half of these responses are longlasting, with documented patient survival for 5–10+ years [1].

Combined use of chemotherapy and biotherapy (biochemotherapy) has recently emerged as the most effective treatment for metastatic melanoma [2,3]. Biochemotherapy regimens, which incorporate combinations of multiple cytotoxic drugs, have resulted in objective response rates of approximately 50%, among which 15–20% are complete regressions. The achievement of a complete regression with biochemotherapy offers metastatic melanoma patients a 50% probability of long-term control of their disease and therefore has a definite curative potential.

Unfortunately, 90% of the patients with metastatic melanoma do not benefit to a substantial degree from the standard treatment approaches currently available and therefore are in need of alternative therapies. It is for this group that the new experimental treatment approaches or investigational drugs are the only hope for extending their survival. In this chapter, two promising new treatment approaches—angiogenesis modulation and gene therapy—which are currently in the developmental phase, will be discussed. Both are based on the contemporary understanding of the tumour biology which will be described first.

The new biology of cancer and targeted antitumour therapies

A better understanding of tumour biology has created new opportunities for the development and testing of new treatments for cancer. It has become quite clear that growth of the primary tumour and of the metastases is dependent on the development of tumour-associated blood vessels, a process known as angiogenesis or neovascularization. Angiogenesis is a multistep sequential process involving the recruitment and proliferation of endothelial cells, their subsequent migration to the tumour mass, morphogenesis into a tubular form and maturation into a network of new blood vessels [4].

A number of growth factors are known to stimulate the endothelial cell growth which is counterbalanced by a number of natural inhibitors in the body. Two of the best known angiogenic growth factors—vascular endothelial growth factor (VEGF) and basic fibroblast growth factor (bFGF)—are secreted by many tumours and appear to be most important in maintaining the growth of the capillary endothelial cells and indirectly that of the tumour. The VEGFs mediate angiogenic signals to the vascular endothelium via high affinity receptor tyrosine kinases. To date three receptors for the VEGFs have been identified and designated VEGFR1–3. Two naturally occurring angiogenesis inhibitors include angiostatin and endostatin, which are small fragments of larger, more familiar molecules, plasminogen and collagen, respectively. These proteins can block angiogenesis, inhibit tumour growth and metastasis and, in animals, have been shown to cause regression of primary tumours [4,5].

The development of tumours is characterized by evidence for an 'angiogenesis switch' by which tumours acquire the ability to form a neovasculature. Once the angiogenic switch is activated, tumour cells begin to secrete high levels of molecules such as VEGF which stimulate the proliferation of adjacent endothelial cells. Such angiogenic growth factors and their receptors are potential targets for angiogenesis inhibitors, e.g. antibodies against VEGF. The molecular basis for the angiogenic switch may be the acquisition of activated oncogenes, such as activated *ras* that induce the transcription of angiogenic growth factors. Drugs that target these oncogenic pathways, such as farnesyl transferase inhibitors, block *ras* signalling and may exert their antitumour effects through such antiangiogenic mechanisms. The endothelial cells respond to angiogenic factors via the transmembrane receptors. Specific inhibitors of such receptors have been developed, e.g. SU-5416 which blocks one of the VEGF receptors, VEGFR-2. After exposure to growth factors, endothelial cells express high levels of an extracellular matrix protein receptor, $\alpha v\beta 3$ integrin. In animal models, administration of antibodies to this integrin causes apoptotic endothelial cell death making it a potential therapeutic agent.

A number of proteolytic enzymes have been identified in the tumour microenvironment. These enzymes—matrix metalloproteinases (MMPs)—degrade the proteins of the extracellular matrix which facilitates endothelial cell growth and angiogenesis in tumours at the primary and metastatic sites [6]. MMPs are secreted both from tumour cells and the endothelial cells and probably also by the host stromal cells, including the inflammatory cells such as macrophages. A number of recently synthesized MMP inhibitors (MMPIs) block angiogenesis, tumour growth and ability of tumour cells to metastasize by vascular invasion.

Complete inhibition of angiogenesis can be predicted to have few side-effects in cancer patients. The turnover of the endothelial cells in normal adult tissues is very slow except during pregnancy and during the cyclical reproductive functions of ovulation and menstruation. Therefore angiogenesis is primarily confined to the growing tumours and to certain benign conditions of wound healing, inflammatory arthritis, ischaemic heart disease and retinopathy of diabetes. Besides toxicity, a major problem associated with the use of cytotoxic chemotherapy is the development of drug resistance in the tumour cells. This process is related to the genetic instability inherent in malignant tumours. As angiogenesis is partly dependent on the genetically stable normal stromal tissue surrounding the tumour, angiogenesis inhibitors are less susceptible to acquired drug resistance.

Clinical experience with angiogenesis modulators

Increasing understanding of the biology of angiogenesis has led to the development of several novel antiangiogenic drugs which are currently in various phases of clinical development (Table 18.1). A number of these agents (approximately 30 in number) are in clinical trials; some of them, especially the MMPIs, are undergoing Phase III studies [6–9]. The parameters to assess the antitumour effects of these agents are still somewhat controversial, in that the commonly used endpoint of tumour regression or objective response may not be achievable with these drugs. Instead, prolonged stablity or lack of tumour progression is more likely to be the expected biological effect of many of these drugs which are inherently cytostatic and not cytotoxic. Consequently, a number of these agents have progressed from Phase I studies

Table 18.1 Angiogenesis inhibitors in clinical development

Class of drug	Mechanism of action	Drug source
VEGF receptor inhibitors		
Anti-VEGF antibody	Neutralizing antibody against VEGF	Genentech, SanFrancisco, CA
SU-5416	Small molecule, blocks VEGF receptor	Sugen, Inc., Redwood City, CA
IFN-α	Inhibits release of endothelial growth factor	Commercially available
Drugs that prevent new blood vessels from invading surrounding tissue		
Marimastat	Synthetic MMPI	British Biotech, Annapolis, MD
AG-3340	Synthetic MMPI	Agouron, La Jolla, CA
Bay 12-9566	Synthetic MMPI	Bayer, West Haven, CT
Interrupts functions of dividing endothelial cells		
TNP-470 (AGM-1470)	Inhibits endothelial cell growth	TAP Pharm Inc., Deerfield, IL
Targeted antivascular therapy		
Anti-integrin antibody, LM609 or vitaxin	Causes endothelial apoptosis by blocking AvB3 integrin	Scripps Research Institute, La Jolla, CA
ZD-0101 (CM-101)	Bacterial toxin selectivity toxic to endothelial cells in new blood vessels	Zeneca Pharmaceuticals, Wilmington, DE
Endogenous angiogenesis inhibitors		
Angiostatin, endostatin	Unknown, generated by MMPs from proteolysis of plasminogen and collagen	Entremed Inc., Rockville, MD
Miscellaneous, unknown mechanisms	Pentosan, thalidomide, CAI, IL-12, squalamine platelet factor-4	Various

Abbreviations: IFN-α, α-interferon; IL-12, interleukin-12; MMP, matrix metalloprotease; MMPI, matrix metalloprotease inhibitor; VEGF, vascular endothelial growth factor

straight to Phase III trials, where increased survival will be used as the key parameter of their efficacy. Whether these drugs may be more efficacious when used as adjuvant therapies will soon be tested. However, this will require large randomized controlled trials, testing their use alone as well as in combination with standard cytotoxic agents.

The early results of clinical trials with angiogenesis modulators in several advanced solid tumours have shown a lack of obvious antitumour activity with single agents, suggesting the need to test these drugs in combination with the commonly used cytotoxic agents which are generally used in the initial phases of treatment. Nevertheless, occasional tumour regressions have been observed, lending support for further testing, using novel strategies to quantify the probable cytostatic effects of these agents which may ultimately translate into increased survival [7].

Despite the increasing understanding of the complex regulation of angiogenesis, the definitive mode of action of some of the antiangiogenic drugs currently in clinical trials (e.g. thalidomide, squalamine, suramin and IFN-α) remains unknown. Thalidomide is currently undergoing Phase II trials in a number of solid tumours, including prostate cancer, breast cancer, lung cancer, brain tumours and malignant melanoma [8,9]. Objective tumour regressions have been observed in preliminary trials in renal cell carcinoma [9] and in glioblastoma multiforme. Consequently, thalidomide has recently been combined with other drugs active in the respective tumours, such as carboplatin in recurrent glioblastoma and DTIC in metastatic melanoma.

Gene therapy

Gene therapy is most suitable where a single defective gene can be replaced with a functional copy of that gene. In that regard, cancer is not a particularly suitable target for the classical approach of gene replacement therapy as cancer is generally associated with a multiplicity of gene alterations, many of them still unknown. Moreover it would be necessary to deliver therapeutic genes to every cancer cell, which is beyond the capability of the currently used vectors. The prevailing rationale used by many investigators is the possibility of bystander effects, defined as cytotoxic effects produced by the transduced cancer cells on the non-transduced cancer cells. The major treatment strategies [10] that have been used in clinical trials of gene therapy include:

1 the use of various immunotherapeutic agents in the form of cytokines and recombinant vaccines;
2 the use of vectors to deliver pro-drugs;
3 the replacement of non-functioning tumour suppressor genes or inactivation of oncogenes; and
4 gene therapy with antisense oligonucleotides.

Augumentation of antitumour immunity

A number of gene therapy studies have focused on enhancing the immunogenicity of the tumour or modifying the host response to the tumour. The gene therapy approaches aimed at augmentation of antitumour immunity take into account the various steps of tumour antigen presentation and the required elements of the host immune response. The currently ongoing immunogene therapy protocols utilize various cytokines involved in normal immune response to exogenous antigens. The cytokines involved in the T-cell response, such as IFN-γ and IL-12, help drive the T-cell response towards cell-mediated immunity, whereas IL-4 and IL-10 drive the response towards humoral response to antigens.

In addition, a better understanding of the role of costimulatory molecules and various cytokines in the immune response to the tumour antigens have been incorporated into several clinical gene therapy trials. In experimental animals it has been shown that the transduced cytokines induce local recruitment of the leucocytes which then secrete secondary cytokines, creating a favourable environment for tumour rejection and allowing the development of both CD4 and CD8 T-cell dependent systemic immunity. IL-2 is the cytokine used most often for gene transfer experiments and has been transduced into a number of mouse tumours where it can successfully lead to local tumour growth inhibition mediated by cytotoxic T cells, natural killer cells and macrophages. Haematopoietic growth factors, such as G-CSF and GM-CSF, have also been transduced into tumour cells. When G-CSF was transduced into a mouse tumour, a massive infiltration of neutrophils led to rapid tumour destruction. GM-CSF activity is largely dependent on upregulation of dendritic cell survival and function with subsequent priming of cytotoxic T lymphocyte responses. Overall, the cytokines released by the transduced tumour cells trigger an inflammatory response which has frequently translated into tumour regression.

Another approach to delivery of immunogenic therapies involves transduction of cytokine genes directly into intact cancer lesions *in vivo*. This approach requires vectors other than retroviral ones so that stable integration in proliferating cells can be avoided. These vectors include adenoviral and vaccinia vectors used to transduce mouse tumours with IL-2 and IL-12 genes. This approach has resulted in efficient gene transduction, local tumour growth inhibition and systemic immunity.

Human clinical trials

After successfully transducing cytokine genes into human tumour cell lines, clinical trials have been initiated using either autologous tumour cell vaccines transduced with a variety of cytokines or a plasmid DNA expression vector containing IL-2 gene [11]. Several of these trials have utilized direct intralesional injections into intact tumours with occasional observation of successful tumour regression in tumours such as metastatic melanoma [11]. Overall, the immunogenic therapy of cancer is still in its infancy and much remains to be learned, but the fact that clinical responses have been observed in some of these trials serves as a proof of the principle which has encouraged the continuing further refinements of these approaches for better clinical outcomes.

Pro-drug gene therapy

In this approach, a novel gene is transferred into a cell and this gene then produces an enzyme that metabolizes a relatively non-toxic drug into a substance toxic to the cell [10]. This approach is most useful when the novel gene has specificity for the tumour cells with relative sparing of the normal cells. In addition, the gene transfer must occur in all tumour cells for a successful control of the tumour. One of the common systems utilized is based on the use of a pro-drug metabolizing gene, such as the herpes simplex thymidine kinase (HSVtk) which is used in conjunction with systemic administration of the pro-drug ganciclovir which is converted by the enzyme into a toxic metabolite, ganciclovir triphosphate. The toxic metabolite can easily diffuse across cell membranes and have cytotoxic effects, by inhibition of DNA synthesis, on the surrounding tumour cells by the phenomenon of bystander effect.

Another pro-drug gene therapy system has utilized an *Escherichia coli* cytosine deaminase gene transfer followed by systemic administration of 5-fluorocytosine (5-FC) which yields 5-fluorouracil (5-FU) as a toxic metabolite. The early preclinical studies were performed using a retroviral gene transfer vector which was relatively inefficient in transduction of tumour cells because of its dependence on active cell division. As a result of these shortcomings, the adenovirus was investigated as a more efficient vector system for pro-drug gene transfer.

A number of clinical trials are currently testing pro-drug gene therapy. Most of these trials involve central nervous system malignancies, which are inoculated by the stereotactic intratumoral injection for gene transfer followed by systemic administration of the pro-drug. At present it is too early to comment definitively on the efficacy of pro-drug gene therapy approaches in human malignancies. The data so far available indicate that both retrovirus- and adenovirus-mediated pro-drug therapies can be safely administered to humans and some suggestive evidence of biological effects is encouraging. In future trials the adenovirus which has been shown to be a more efficient vector will become the vector of choice for these strategies.

Tumour suppressor gene replacement and antioncogene strategies

Gene replacement therapy, initially applied to diseases with a single well-characterized deficiency, has potential applications to the treatment of cancer which is a multigenic disease where correction of all or many of the genetic abnormalities would be necessary to make a clinically significant impact on cancer cell growth. Some of the dominant gene families contributing to cancer causation include tumour suppressor genes, such as p53, and oncogenes, such as *ras*. Mutations or inactivation of p53 is the most common genetic defect in all common human cancers. Consequently, p53 replacement represents an important target for gene replacement therapy [12].

Early clinical trials of p53 replacement therapy using a retroviral vector containing wild-type p53 yielded very low levels of gene expression. More recently, vectors derived from adenoviruses have been used and have resulted in much higher levels of gene expression. The first p53 gene therapy clinical trial used an intratumoral injection of the vector in patients with non-small cell lung cancer and has shown clear biological activity, with three of nine patients showing evidence of tumour regression in the Phase I study [10].

More recently, a two-arm study involving adenovirus-mediated transfer of the p53 gene was started in patients with lung cancer where it is being tested alone and in combination with cisplatin. This product has shown therapeutic efficacy against a wide range of human tumour types containing non-functional p53 and it appears to have enhanced the antitumour activity of many chemotherapeutic drugs. Partial responses have been observed in lung cancer using the adenoviral p53 (Ad-p53). More recently, Ad-p53 has also been administered systemically in animal models and this approach is heading towards systemic gene replacement therapy in various human tumours.

Recently, ONYX Pharmaceuticals has developed a mutant adenovirus, dL-1520, which replicates in p53-deficient cells but not in normal cells, therefore having the general property of being cancer-specific [13]. This virus, now referred to as ONYX-015, has recently entered Phase I clinical trials in patients with recurrent head and neck cancer. The virus was injected directly into tumour masses where it has shown an excellent safety profile. In an ongoing Phase II trial, a combination of ONYX-015 with cisplatin has produced remarkable responses suggestive of additative antitumour activity [13].

Gene therapy with antisense oligonucleotides

Antisense therapy targets specific messenger RNA molecules to inhibit their translation into protein. Critical to the success of this approach is the selection of the appropriate protein target. Promising results have been reported for antisense oligonucleotides directed at key regulatory proteins in tumour cells, such as protein kinase C. The upregulation of the antiapoptotic protein bcl-2 is a very common alteration in human cancer and is associated with resistance to chemotherapy and radiotherapy. Inhibition of bcl-2 with a new agent, G-3139, appears to effectively lower bcl-2 expression in tissues, resulting in enhanced antitumour activity when used in combination with a cytotoxic agent, dacarbazine, against human melanoma grown in SCID mice [14]. On the basis of these experimental data a clinical trial of G-3139 in combination with dacarbazine against metastatic melanoma has been started recently [15].

Conclusions

Advances in molecular biology during the past 20 years have allowed us to identify genes that go awry in cancer and offer the opportunity to understand the molecular mechanisms underlying the disease. Many of these genes control signal transduction, cell cycle regulation, apoptosis and angiogenesis. The understanding of the molecular targets for anticancer drug development offers a great potential for developing cancer-specific therapies in the future [16]. However, a number of these mechanism-based cancer therapies are in early development and have not yet shown consistent evidence of antitumour activity. Furthermore, the new categories of drugs may prevent further growth of the tumour and its metastases and transform cancer into a chronic disease without necessarily causing regression of established tumours. It appears that a number of new molecular therapies will be better utilized in combination with the currently available cytotoxic agents in efforts to show enhanced survival in Phase III trials.

References

1 Legha S. Durable complete responses in metastatic melanoma treated with interleukin-2 in combination with interferon-α and chemotherapy. *Semin Oncol* 1997; **24** (Suppl 4): 39–43.

2 Legha S, Ring S, Bedikian A, *et al.* Treatment of metastatic melanoma with combined chemotherapy containing cisplatin, vinblastine and dacarbazine (CVD) and biotherapy using interleukin-2 and interferon. *Ann Oncol* 1996; **7**: 827–35.

3 Legha S, Ring S, Eton O, *et al.* Development of a biochemotherapy regimen with concurrent administration of cisplatin, vinblastine, dacarbazine, interferon-α, and interleukin-2 for patients with metastatic melanoma. *J Clin Oncol* 1998; **16**: 1752–9.

4 Klagsbrun M. Angiogenesis and cancer: AACR special conference in cancer research. *Cancer Res* 1999; **59**: 487–90.

5 Veikkola T, Karkkainen M, Claesson-Welsh L, *et al.* Regulation of angiogenesis via vascular endothelial growth factor receptors. *Cancer Res* 2000; **60**: 203–12.

6 Nelson A, Fingleton B, Rothenberg M, *et al.* Matrix metalloproteinases: biologic activity and clinical implications. *J Clin Oncol* 2000; **18**: 1135–49.

7 Kudelka A, Levy T, Verschraegen C, *et al.* A phase I study of TNP-470 administered to patients with advanced squamous cell cancer of the cervix. *Clin Cancer Res* 1997; **3**: 1501–5.

8 Fine H, Figg W, Jaeckle K, *et al.* Phase II trial of the antiangiogenic agent thalidomide in patients with recurrent high-grade gliomas. *J Clin Oncol* 2000; **18**: 708–15.

9 Eisen T, Boshoff C, Vaughan L, *et al.* Antiangiogenic treatment of metastatic melanoma, renal cell, ovary and breast cancer with thalidomide (Abstract 1699). *Proc Am Soc Clin Oncol* 1998; **17**: 441.

10 Roth J, Molldrem J, Smythe W. The current status of cancer gene therapy trials. *PPO Updates in Principles and Practice of Oncology*, Vol. 13 (11); 1999: 1–15.

11 Galanis E, Hersh E, Stopeck A, *et al.* Immunotherapy of advanced malignancy by direct gene transfer of an interleukin-2 DNA/DMRIE/DOPE Lipid Complex: phase I/II experience. *J Clin Oncol* 1999; **17**: 3313–23.

12 Baselga J. New horizons: gene therapy for cancer. *Anticancer Drugs* 1999; **10** (Suppl. 1): 39–42.

13 McCormick F. Cancer therapy based on p53. *Cancer J Sci Am* 1999; **5** (3): 139–43.

14 Jansen B, Schlagbauer-Wadl H, Brown B,

et al. bcl-2 Antisense therapy chemosensitizes human melanoma in SCID mice. *Nat Med* 1998; **4** (2): 232–4.

15 Jansen B, Wacheck V, Heere-Ress E, *et al.* A Phase I–II study with dacarbazine and BCL-2 antisense oligonucleotide G 3139 (Genta) as a chemosensitizer in patients with advanced malignant melanoma (Abstract 2049). *Proc Am Soc Clin Oncol* 1999; **18**: 531

16 Gibbs J. Mechanism-based target identification and drug discovery in cancer research. *Science* 2000; **287**: 1969–73.

19: Who should follow up melanoma patients and for how long?

Judy Evans

Introduction

The incidence of melanoma continues to rise in Western Europe [1,2]. Public education campaigns have raised awareness of melanoma and the importance of sun avoidance. Melanoma is now discussed every summer in the media, travel agents distribute sun safety information leaflets to holiday-makers and the meteorological office forecasts sun intensity figures daily.

There is evidence that, as a result of this increased public knowledge, melanoma is being detected earlier and there is a rise in incidence of 'thin' lesions with resultant change to the previously increasing mortality rates [3,4]. There is broad agreement among histopathologists concerning the main prognostic features of melanoma, but controversy remains. Some patients with lesions of apparent good prognosis, such as *in situ* or 'horizontal' growth phase melanoma, relapse. There is conversely a general debate concerning the metastatic potential of very thin lesions. It has been suggested that a proportion of good prognosis melanomas, which are increasingly frequently removed [5], may not have the potential to metastasize and therefore could be left untreated. Such a consideration is clearly only theoretical as no one suggests that such a policy should be put in to practice or even that a trial to answer this question should be performed. The early detection of new primaries therefore remains a universal aim. Although there remains some discussion about the significance of changes to mortality and incidence rates being made as a result of screening clinics, etc., progress does appear to be occurring.

In the past, few questioned the value of following up patients with cancer. It was assumed that follow-up should be performed simply because a diagnosis of malignant disease had been made. It was generally accepted that follow-up should be for 10 years as this was the most likely period during which relapse would occur, although there were anecdotal reports, particularly regarding patients with melanoma, where recurrence had occurred after a longer period. In more recent years the role of follow-up has been questioned in a number of cancers and it is particularly pertinent to challenge its role in patients with non-invasive melanoma where recurrence is very unlikely. It could be argued that in these patients follow-up has nothing to offer. However, patients can benefit from follow-up in a variety of ways which may have nothing to do with the early detection of relapse. For instance, patients with a genetic predisposition or who are young with a susceptible skin phenotype, could gain a survival advantage from the early detection of a second primary. Some patients have a greater need for information about their disease which can only be satisfied by repeated consultations or they may quite simply find a clinic attendance reassuring. There is also a group of patients who require reinforcement concerning the importance of sun avoidance which could have an important impact on their family's risk, particularly if young children are involved.

In the past, the responsibility for follow-up rested with the specialist doctor. The development of specialist non-medical clinical staff, such as nurse practitioners, has allowed for follow-up and education to be spread more widely. This expansion in services is part of the development of multidisciplinary teams and novel therapeutic and management strategies. These changes have resulted in greater psychological support and an increase in palliative care expertise for melanoma patients as well as greater opportunities for patients to enter clinical trials.

The increasing awareness of financial pressures in all aspects of medical care has increased the tendency to challenge traditional views on follow-up. It is important that policies regarding the frequency of outpatient attendances and the nature of any investigations are continually kept under review and audited.

Breaking the news

Patients who have suspicious lesions excised should always be given a follow-up appointment to receive the histology result. This appointment should be with a consultant who is a member of the local multidisciplinary melanoma team if there was a high enough clinical suspicion of melanoma at the time of the excision. When a melanoma is diagnosed when there had only been a low clinical suspicion of melanoma, the result comes as a shock to both the patient and the doctor who performed the excision. Frequently, such lesions are removed by GPs. It is very important that before the GP meets the patient to give the result, he or she makes an urgent appointment with the appropriate local melanoma specialist so that at the consultation the patient can be given the precise date and time of his or her hospital appointment. This helps remove any anxiety from the patient that there will be a delay in definitive treatment or that the appointment might get 'lost' in the system.

It is extremely important that the patient sees a specialist as soon as possible after the diagnosis so that a detailed explanation of the disease, the patient situation, the treatment options and prognosis can be discussed. Time should be made for patients to express their emotions and fears and appropriate reassurance given. It can also be helpful for the specialist to know exactly what the patient has been told. Similarly, it is vital that the specialist communicates as soon as possible with the GP, not simply the patient's disease status and prognosis, but what the patient has been told regarding investigations, future treatment, follow-up and prognosis.

Why follow-up?

True follow-up begins after recovery from the primary therapeutic procedure. Visits to the outpatient department may be necessary for dressings to wounds and removal of sutures. Final histology results, e.g. from a second surgical procedure, are generally given to the patient during the prefollow-up stage. The first true follow-up appointment is given some weeks after complete wound healing.

Follow-up clinics serve a number of purposes:

1 to educate the patient about the disease;

2 to teach self-examination techniques for recurrence and second primaries;

3 to check that self-examination is being performed regularly;

4 to allow the clinician to check for recurrence;

5 to organize additional non-medical help where necessary, particularly psychological support;

6 to organize further treatment if recurrences occur;

7 to facilitate onward referral if palliative treatment is required;

8 to maintain contact and support for the patient and his or her family, whether or not there is evidence of recurrence;

9 to allow patients access to clinical trials and to keep them up-to-date with new developments; and

10 to gather information about the patient where he or she is part of an existing trial or audit project.

The detection of metastases is an extremely important function of follow-up, particularly the detection of recurrence while it is still in a surgically treatable or even curable stage, e.g. local regional lymph node recurrence. Self-examination and its teaching are directed towards this end, although there are few data on the effectiveness of self-examination. Patients who present with lymph node recurrence limited to one node without extracapsular spread have a better prognosis [6] than those with more nodes and it seems likely therefore that patients whose nodal recurrences are detected by the follow-up clinic will do better than they would have done otherwise; this is the rationale for follow-up. However, the data to support this are lacking.

It is an ideal that all melanoma patients should have a follow-up appointment with a consultant whose primary interest is melanoma and who has ample time to answer all the patients' questions and address their anxieties. In reality, such a situation is unlikely to be universally achieved in most health care systems. However, it is possible to staff clinics appropriately with health care workers who are adequately trained to help fulfil all the requirements of follow-up. Specialist nurses are particularly important in this regard as they are often very well equipped to give information and support patients.

All clinical staff, whatever their training background, must have a thorough understanding of the biology of melanoma and the patterns of spread. They must be competent at examining lymph node basins and able to perform a thorough skin survey for other suspicious lesions. In the author's clinics, two nurse practitioners have been trained to perform these examinations and now form an integral part of the follow-up clinic. The nurse practitioner with an enthusiasm for the task is, in the author's experience, much more effective as a member of the follow-up team than a newly appointed junior doctor who requires instruction, needs time to gain experience and may not necessarily have a particular interest in melanoma.

Joint clinics between plastic surgeons, dermatologists, oncologists and specialist melanoma nurses are very useful. This clinic should have a 'see and treat' facility where suspicious lesions, which could potentially be second primaries, can be removed and sent for diagnosis without the necessity for a further clinic attendance. It is important to have ready access to the palliative care team at a time when the patient is attending the melanoma clinic.

Cancer care in the UK is changing and the principles of multidisciplinary team working are coming into practice and becoming the norm. Furthermore, regular multidisciplinary meetings to discuss patients and review the radiology and pathology findings must take place even if the diagnosis and treatment seem routine.

Self-examination

Self-examination for malignant nodes should not be taught until the patient has completely recovered from the primary surgical procedure. This is because of the lymphadenopathy that can be caused by complications, such as a minor wound breakdown. Detection of such inflammatory glands causes undue anxiety and it is therefore preferable to start teaching self-examination approximately 6–10 weeks after all surgical wounds are fully healed. The patient has to know where nodes are to be found and what to look for although nodes, particularly those in the inguinal area, are often brought to the patient's attention as a result of discomfort.

A thin patient can begin to feel a lymph node when it is 0.5–1 cm in diameter. Practical descriptions, such as 'imagine you are feeling a sugared almond through a blanket', can be helpful. Patients must understand that they are looking for a lump which is firm to hard, with a smooth edge and in the subcutaneous or deeper tissues. Patients also need to be told that lumps may be mobile but can become stuck to surrounding tissues. In the event of a lump being detected, patients should be instructed to re-examine themselves and if the mass is still present they should call the melanoma clinic or seek an urgent appointment with their GP.

Patients need to be shown the most likely nodal basin that drains the area of their primary tumour. They should be told about examining contralateral lymph nodes to check whether anything detected is a normal feature for that field, i.e. it is present on both sides. It is helpful to demonstrate the position of the femoral artery and demonstrate its pulsation so that it will not be confused with a lymph node. The best positions to self-examine lymph node basins are as follow.

1 *Axilla*. The patient is in an upright position, the arm flexed at the elbow and hand held on hip. The hollow between 'back wall' and 'front wall' of the armpit should be pointed out and the patient instructed to feel towards the apex of the axilla.

2 *Groin*. The patient lies almost flat (with one or two pillows), the leg to be examined is flexed at the knee and externally rotated so that the heel rests on or close to the opposite knee. The boundaries of the femoral triangle should be demonstrated.

3 *Neck*. The patient should be in an upright position. Examination should be directed towards the anterior part of the neck from clavicles to mandible, posteriorly from the area of the ear to the root of the neck and the supraclavicular fossi are identified and palpated. It is unhelpful to describe anatomical triangles but useful to point out normal structures, such as submandibular glands and thyroid cartilage.

Self-examination for second primaries follows the same advice as given for the detection of melanomas in public education awareness campaigns. Patients who have already had a melanoma may be more aware than the general public but can be frightened to seek advice. Patients with multiple moles or other skin lesions may benefit considerably from keeping photographs of their naevi at home so they can monitor any change in their lesions. They can also be given photographs of early melanomas so that a comparison can be made.

Duration of follow-up

The question of length of follow-up still causes much discussion. Kroon & Nieweg [7], in a consensus document on melanoma management in the Netherlands, state that 5 years is, in principle, sufficient for patients with lesions ≤ 1.5 mm and recommend 10 years follow-up if the primary is thicker than 1.5 mm. In the UK, the Melanoma Study Group guidelines recommend 3-monthly follow-up for 3 years [8]. At 3 years, patients with melanomas < 1 mm maybe discharged but others should be followed 6-monthly for a further 2 years.

Basseres *et al.* [9] suggest there is no agreement about surveillance after the resection of stage I melanomas, whereas Sylaidis *et al.* [10] have suggested that the frequency of follow up should be related to the risk of developing a treatable recurrence to follow-up. However, there is general agreement that melanoma patients with the dysplastic naevus syndrome should be followed up for life because these patients are at increased risk of developing second primaries.

Most recommendations suggest frequent visits in the early years after the primary diagnosis with more prolonged intervals thereafter. Frequent early visits coincide with the teaching of self-examination, maximum patient anxiety and the highest risk of recurrence. It seems likely that frequent visits during high risk of recurrence periods results in the early detection of metastases and that treatment is consequently more effective because tumour burdens are small. Basseres *et al.* [9] argues that clinic intervals should be related to the time taken for any metastases to become clinically detectable. Therefore, the clinic visits should never be more than 4 months apart and, when longer intervals are considered safe, follow-up should stop altogether. Two different trends in follow-up have emerged as a result of such differences of opinion.

1 The development of shared-care protocols between hospital and primary care.

2 The timing of follow-up matched to the risk of recurrence.

Both approaches rely on increasing patient and GP awareness to recognize operable interval recurrences.

Shared-care protocol

The author has developed a shared-care protocol approach, initially because of an ongoing study on the reduction of excision margins. Patients initially had to be followed up very closely to detect any possible increase in local recurrence rates as a result of this therapy. GPs who did not wish to participate in a shared-care protocol had their patients seen in the hospital-based melanoma clinic. Clinic visits now alternate between hospital and GP who checks that the patient is self-examining effectively and the GP examines the patient for evidence of recurrent disease. Knowledge of how to self-examine is not enough; it should be part of a patient's normal behaviour pattern. For instance, self-examination can be linked to a regular personal hygiene ritual, such as the shaving of legs in women. This type of linkage allows self-examination to become a lifetime habit and the clinician can then be reasonably confident that it is continuing as clinic visits become less frequent.

Follow-up protocols based on risk of recurrence

Sylaidis *et al.* (personal communication) have developed a protocol with the view that the frequency of outpatient follow-up should reflect the patient's annual risk of treatable recurrence: the higher the risk, the more frequent the follow-up. During high-risk periods it is calculated that up to half of the recurrences will be detected within intervals of 4 months. Sylaidis *et al.* [10] regard only local and regional recurrences as 'treatable'. This is because patients who have surgical excision of such recurrences have a 1 in 3 chance of remaining disease-free for a further 5 years.

This group of workers therefore recommend that intermediate-risk melanoma patients be kept under clinical review for approximately 5 years and that, although patients with thick melanomas are also discharged after this period of time, lifelong patient-led surveillance should continue. They argue that long-term survivors have treatable recurrences at a rate of 2.5% per annum and therefore from year 6 onwards only 1 in 8 long-term survivors will relapse with a treatable recurrence and therefore it is reasonable to discharge them from the clinic.

Conclusions

It is important to regard a melanoma service as a cooperative exercise. There must be good communication and collaboration of consultants with GPs who must be educated to a sufficient level that they are able to teach self-examination and provide appropriate follow-up between clinic visits if they are to be involved in this. Clinics can be organized around the specialist senior doctor but long-term, non-medical staff can be adequately trained to help with follow-up. Clinical nurse specialists and nurse practitioners are well suited this task and have a particularly important role in the management of the social and psychological consequences of a diagnosis of melanoma and the patient education issues that ensue.

Multidisciplinary team working is essential and the outpatient clinics need to reflect this. It may not always be necessary for all disciplines to be present at routine melanoma follow-up clinics, but organizing a clinic in an adjacent area to another discipline or at convenient times for other disciplines may be very useful. For example, to have a plastic surgery clinic adjacent to a dermatology clinic, both of which occur at the same time as the oncologist's outpatient clinic has obvious practical benefits. Many patients will require readmission at some time for either lymph node clearance or excision of non-nodal metastases and it is important for patients to feel that, under such circumstances, they have continuity of care. It should be possible even in district hospitals for patients who relapse with, for example, intestinal metastases, to be treated briefly in a general surgical ward but then transferred to the melanoma team who have previously cared for them.

It cannot be stressed too strongly that when self-examination becomes a major part of clinical practice there must be open access for the patient to a member of the melanoma team. Patients should be encouraged to attend the ward or outpatient clinic if they feel they have discovered a recurrence to seek advice from medical staff or a nurse practitioner. In this regard, an interchange of nursing staff between clinics and wards can be very useful and this can give follow-up expertise to a ward. The result of such an arrangement can be that a patient who discovers a metastasis on a Saturday morning is able to see a member of the melanoma team over the weekend on the ward, rather than having to wait for a formal clinic appointment during the working week.

Individualization of follow-up is very important. Some patients need more reassurance than others and have to be seen more frequently. Similarly, others may find self-examination difficult and should not be pressed to do this but given extra outpatient appointments. Those performing follow-up need to be properly trained in the task of diagnosing recurrences and second primaries. They also must be enthusiastic educators and interested in the long-term psychological support often needed by patients and their families.

References

1 Mackie RM, *et al.* Cutaneous malignant melanoma in Scotland: incidence, survival and mortality, 1979–94. *Br Med J* 1997; **315**: 7116.

2 Parkin D, Muir C, Whelan SEA. *Cancer Incidence in Five Continents.* IARC Scientific Publications 1992; **6**: 120 .

3 Giles GG, *et al.* Has mortality from melanoma stopped rising in Australia? Analysis of trends between 1931 and 1994. *Br Med J* 1996; **312**: 1121–5.

4 Melia J, *et al.* Cancer Research Campaign health education programme to promote the early detection of cutaneous malignant melanoma. *Br J Dermatol* 1995; **132**: 405–413.

5 Burton RC, *et al.* An analysis of a melanoma epidemic. *Int J Cancer* 1993; **55**: 765–70.

6 Balch CM, *et al.* An analysis of prognostic factors in 4000 patients with cutaneous melanoma. In: *Cutanteous Melanoma.* Balch CM, Milton GW, eds. Philadelphia: Lippincott, 1985; 321–51.

7 Kroon BB, Nieweg OE. Management of malignant melanoma. *Ann Chir Gynaecol* 2000; **89** (3): 242–50.

8 Newton Bishop J, *et al.* UK guidelines for the management of cutaneous melanoma. *Br J Plast Surg* 2001; in press.

9 Basseres N, *et al.* Cost-effectiveness of surveillance of stage I melanoma: a

retrospective appraisal based on a 10-year experience in a dermatology department in France. *Dermatology* 1995; **191** (3): 199–203.

10 Sylaidis P, *et al.* Follow-up requirements for thick cutaneous melanoma. *Br J Plast Surg* 1997; **50** (5): 349–53.

20: What is the role for radiotherapy in melanoma?

Andrew G. Goodman

Introduction

In 1936, Patterson [1] labelled melanoma a radio-resistant tumour and wrote that radiotherapy for melanoma was futile. In 1939, Ellis [2] wrote that, treated with adequate dosage, melanoma responds like other tumours. Sixty years later there remains the same polarization of opinion. The *Oxford Textbook of Oncology*, published in 1995 [3], makes no mention of radiotherapy in its chapter on melanoma. On the other hand, the 1997 edition of de Vita *et al.* [4] envisages a clear role for radiation therapy even though significant areas of controversy remain.

Of all interventions in medicine, radiotherapy requires an assiduous assessment of risks and benefits, not least because many of the side-effects of treatment are delayed, progressive and not predicted or predictable from side-effects seen at the time of treatment, when treatment schedules could be modified. This is particularly important in relation to fractionation of radiotherapy. Because melanoma has been considered to show a disappointing response to conventionally fractionated radiotherapy (treatment 5 days a week, 1.8–2.67 Gy per fraction), much of the radiotherapy literature relates to hypofractionated treatment, delivering a small number of treatments with a high dose each time, treating once, twice or three times per week. For equivalent antitumour effects, high doses per fraction produce more late effects than low doses per fraction. If the risk of the long-term toxicity is increased, then the chance of benefit needs to be clear.

Hypofractionated radiotherapy in melanoma

A number of clinical studies have analysed response rates in irradiated melanoma from the point of view of fraction size [5–11]. Virtually all of the studies are retrospective and contain a great degree of heterogeneity of treatment regimens and subjects. Often, series have not reported results in terms of total dose or overall treatment time. None the less, such studies appear to show higher response rates with larger doses per fraction. Both Overgaard [6] and Hornsey [5] observed increasing response rates with increasing dose per fraction when giving palliative radiotherapy to lymph node masses and cutaneous deposits. Hornsey [5] found responses in 21% (6/28) patients at 2–3 Gy, 55% (16/29) with 3–4 Gy and 54% (20/37) with 4–8 Gy. Overgaard [6] reported 35% (6/17) at <4 Gy, 70% (14/20) with 4–7 Gy, and 100% (12/12) with 8 Gy. In another study, Overgaard *et al.* [7] found the complete response rate to be doubled (57 vs. 24%) using large doses per fraction. Harwood & Cummings [8], reporting data on the Toronto regimen (24 Gy in three treatments on days 0, 7 and 21), found local control in 82% (18/22) of patients with microscopic residual disease after surgery for nodal recurrence and in 53% (17/32) of those with gross residual or recurrent tumour. In a small randomized trial using data from 35 tumours in 14 patients, Overgaard *et al.* [9] compared 40 Gy in eight fractions in 4 weeks with 27 Gy in three fractions in 1.5 weeks. They found a high complete response rate in both groups, suggesting no advantage for escalating dose per treatment above 5 Gy.

However, there does remain some doubt about this conclusion. In terms of complete response, Harwood *et al.* [10] and Rounsaville *et al.* [11] found no difference with doses above and below 4 Gy. They reported rates of 14 vs. 11% and 8 vs. 8%, respectively. Lobo *et al.* [12] reported a 52% complete response rate using conventional size fractions of between 1.8 and 3 Gy. In particular, while many of their patients received 30 Gy in 10 fractions, they noted complete or partial responses in 84% (16/19) patients given 40 Gy or more in fractions of 1.8–2.5 Gy. Trott *et al.* [13] used local control and recurrence rates rather than response rates as an endpoint and noted that shorter overall treatment time rather than number of fractions or dose per fraction was important. They found 45% (20/44) of tumours controlled at 2 years. Patients were treated with a variety of regimens. Half of those controlled were treated with 2.25 or 2.7 Gy per fraction. More recently, Fenig *et al.* [14] have reported no significant difference with doses per fraction above or below 3 Gy when used for palliation (overall response rate 52 vs. 35%), nor when used as adjuvant treatment after nodal recurrence.

These data have often been combined with radiobiological observations to justify the use of high doses per fraction. A number of observers found cell survival curves with a broad shoulder but relatively low (sensitive) D_0 values [15,16]. This was the laboratory basis for believing that hypofractionated treatment would somehow surmount the cell's ability to repair sublethal damage. Hornsey [5] estimated by extrapolation the size of this threshold, calculating that 2.75 Gy per treatment was required to overcome the shoulder of the curve. Other work, notably by Rofstadt [17], has suggested that melanoma has a very heterogeneous response to radiation.

In the only randomized trial of conventional vs. hypofractionated treatment, the RTOG [18] compared 50 Gy in 20 fractions over 4 weeks with 32 Gy in four fractions over 4 weeks, in patients with nodal or skin and soft tissue metastases. This trial found a complete response rate of 24% and an overall response rate of just under 60% in both groups with no statistical difference between them. The study is notable for delivering both schedules in the same overall treatment time. As hypofractionated regimens tend to have shorter overall treatment times as well as large doses per fraction, only by keeping overall time constant can we examine the effects of fraction size alone.

Are there conclusions to be drawn about dose per fraction for melanoma? Unfortunately, the data from RTOG 83-05, although randomized and representing one of the larger reported series, do not put the issue beyond doubt. Trials of radiotherapy in melanoma will therefore continue to need to address this issue.

Role of radiotherapy in melanoma

Palliative treatment

There is little doubt that radiotherapy is a useful treatment in the palliation of symptoms from melanoma. A number of authors have reported results in relation to the treatment of bone, brain, subcutaneous and lymph node metastases [19–33].

Bone metastases

For bone deposits, response rates—often defined subjectively—of the order of 50–65% have been reported. Rounsaville *et al.* [11] reported marked regression or elimination of pain in 24 of 28 bony sites treated but were unable to derive any conclusions about dose or fractionation. Others have reported responses of 50 [19] and 67% [20,21], respectively. It is of interest that Katz [22] found no relation to dose per fraction for response of bone disease, nor did Lobo *et al.* [12]. Kirova *et al.* [21] noted no difference using either 3 or 4 Gy per fraction. However, many bone lesions will be adequately palliated with a single treatment of 8 Gy [23].

Brain metastases

Cerebral metastases are common in melanoma, both at multiple sites and as solitary deposits. Hilaris *et al.* [19] reported at 67% response rate for whole brain irradiation. Kirova *et al.* [21], 36 years later, reported a 57% improvement in neurological condition. These rates are similar to those achieved with cerebral metastases from other tumours. Kirova *et al.* used either 20 Gy in five fractions over 1 week or 30 Gy in 10 fractions over 2 weeks, both standard fractionation schemes for treatment in the UK. Ziegler & Cooper [24] showed no advantage in using 30 Gy in five or six fractions over 2.5–3 weeks compared to 30 Gy in 10 fractions in terms of median survival, though toxicity was increased with higher dose per fraction.

Melanoma is one of the tumours particularly associated with solitary cerebral metastasis. These may be treated surgically or with single fraction stereotactic radiotherapy (stereotactic radiosurgery; SRS), usually with a dose of 15–18 Gy. Several series have found that SRS compares favourably with resection. Loeffler *et al.* [25] reported permanent local control in excess of 80% with SRS in a wide range of cerebral metastases. Melanoma responded as well as other cancers in this series. Lavine *et al.* [26] reported on 45 patients in whom 59 sites were treated with gamma knife radiosurgery. They reported 78% improvement or stabilization of neurological function. Although median survival after treatment was 8 months, only two of their 45 patients died as a result of progressive neurological disease.

The issue of whether whole brain radiotherapy should be given after either surgical resection or SRS is an important one. Skibber *et al.* [27] considered 34 patients who had solitary metastases resected. Twelve were treated with surgery alone and 22 had postoperative radiotherapy. Intracerebral recurrence was seen in 75% of the non-irradiated group, but in only 23% of those receiving radiotherapy. This had an impact on median survival, which was 6 months in those not irradiated compared to 18 months in those receiving treatment. This group did not have extracranial disease. Hagen *et al.* [28] treated patients with solitary metastases, some of whom had extracranial disease. Radiotherapy extended the median time to central nervous system recurrence from 6 to 27 months and reduced the likelihood of dying from central nervous system disease from 85 to 24% but median survival was not affected.

Chidel *et al.* [29] analysed 135 patients treated for cerebral metastases (various histologies including melanoma) with SRS with or without whole brain irradiation. There was little difference in overall survival. However, local control at 2 years and prevention of new sites developing within the brain were better in those having immediate whole brain irradiation. Sneed *et al.* [30] found similar results. While there was no difference in survival or local freedom from progression, there was a significant difference in freedom from progression within the brain as a whole (at 1 year relapse within the brain was 70% without whole brain irradiation, 28% with). When successful salvage of brain relapse was included there was little difference from adding whole brain irradiation. Seung *et al.* [31] suggests that results with SRS from melanoma mirror other histologies. Lavine *et al.*'s series [26] confirms that for melanoma, SRS without whole brain irradiation reduces the risk of death from neurological disease. Mori *et al.* [32] examined 60 patients with 118 lesions treated by

SRS; 51 patients had whole brain irradiation and median survival was 7 months. Whole brain treatment did not improve survival or local control, but it did reduce the risk of new cerebral metastasis. Grob *et al.* [33] reported on 35 patients treated with SRS alone for melanoma metastatic to the brain. Local control rates were high, as in other series. Median survival for four patients with solitary metastases was 22 months. In patients with solitary or few cerebral metastases of suitable size, SRS without whole brain irradiation is a reasonable option, particularly if there is disease at other sites.

Should whole brain irradiation be added in the treatment of cerebral metastases? This is an important issue because of the late effects, particularly cognitive impairment, of the treatment in those who survive for long periods. Data from surgical series [27,28] suggest that we should continue to recommend whole brain irradiation but data from radiosurgical series are less clear. Successful salvage may be feasible, but for those few patients with true solitary metastasis who may have prolonged survival, detailed discussion of the risks and benefits is required on an individual basis until relevant randomized trials are reported.

Soft tissue disease

Most of the data reviewed above in relation to dose per fraction comes from a series of patients irradiated for nodal or soft tissue recurrence. Clearly, high rates of local control are achievable. In patients with disseminated disease, hypofractionated regimens may well be appropriate in view of response rates and convenience. Inevitably, normal tissue tolerance will need to be considered. Sause *et al.* [18] observed a slight increase in complications in the hypofractionated arm, but commented that many patients did not survive long enough for late complications to be evident. Rounsaville *et al.* [11] noted moderate to severe fibrosis in two patients treated with 24 Gy in three fractions over 21 days for in-transit lesions in the thigh. Overgaard *et al.*'s trial [9] suggests that increasing the dose above 5 Gy does not impart any additional benefit. Sause *et al.*'s data [18] indicate that 50 Gy in 20 fractions produces satisfactorily high response rates and may therefore be a useful conventionally fractionated regimen, particularly where survival may be prolonged and normal tissue tolerance a relevant consideration. Where hypofractionated regimens may be useful, 30–33 Gy in six fractions over 2–3 weeks may be appropriate—calculated to be equivalent, at an $\alpha:\beta$ ratio of 2 Gy, to 50 Gy in 20 fractions. If fewer visits are advantageous, particularly if survival is unlikely to be prolonged, 24 Gy in three fractions as in the 0, 7, 21 day regimen [8] may be useful.

Mucosal melanoma

Melanoma arising in the mucosa is rare, accounting for little over 1% of all melanomas. Of these, just over half arise in the head and neck with female genital tract, anus and rectum accounting for most of the others [34].

For head and neck primaries, the local recurrence rate remains high and overall survival is poor. A number of authors recommend radical surgery followed by postoperative radiotherapy [35–38]. These are generally small series where retrospective review suggests that those receiving radiotherapy may have slightly prolonged disease-free intervals and occasionally improved overall survival. Nandapalan *et al.* [36] found 259 cases of which 36 received combined surgery and radiotherapy. The tumour-specific survival was 45% at 5 years. On the basis of these data they recommend postoperative radiotherapy. Kingdom & Kaplan [37] reviewed 17 cases, seven of whom had postoperative radiotherapy. The whole group had a local recurrence rate of 85%, but those treated with radiotherapy had longer disease-free intervals and longer survival. On this basis, they recommend postoperative radiotherapy irrespective of margins. However, Lund *et al.* [39] found no difference in survival or local control from the addition of radiotherapy. Five-year survival was only 28% and it is not clear how cases were selected for radiotherapy. Loree *et al.* [40] found 20% 5-year survival among 28 patients and recommended aggressive surgical resection without radiotherapy. They noted that only two of 17 patients who underwent surgery died of local disease. Where disease is not resectable, radiotherapy may be considered as primary treatment. Nandapalan *et al.* [36] found it ineffective but Gilligan & Slevin [41] treated 28 cases and achieved 49% local disease-free survival.

For gynaecological sites, Irvin *et al.* [42] reported on seven cases of vaginal melanoma. Two of these were treated with wide local excision and radical radiotherapy and remained locally disease-free. Petru *et al.* [43] reviewed 14 cases of whom nine received radiotherapy, either alone or after surgery. Three of their cases were alive at 5 years. All had small primaries, ≤3 cm. Two were treated by radiotherapy alone, one by radiotherapy following wide local excision. These data may be of importance in suggesting that wide excision followed by radiotherapy is a satisfactory alternative to radical and mutilating surgery in patients with a poor prospect of long-term survival.

Data are even scarcer of anorectal melanoma. Shank *et al.* [44] noted that AP resection, sometimes in combination with radiotherapy, was the only treatment reported to lead to long-term survival. Presant [45], on the other hand, found no survival benefit from an aggressive surgical approach. However, there are no data on whether local control is equivalent with more conservative surgery and radiotherapy.

Curative radiotherapy for cutaneous melanoma

Primary treatment

Lentigo maligna and its invasive counterpart, lentigo maligna melanoma, are diseases predominantly of the elderly, frequently occurring on the face. The morbidity of surgical procedures required to achieve adequate clearance margins in this population has led many centres to treat such cases with conventional radiotherapy. A number of authors have published series of such patients. Harwood & Cummings [8] from Toronto reported 88% (15/17) lentigo malignas and 91% (21/23) lentigo maligna melanomas adequately controlled by 32.5 Gy in five fractions or 45 Gy in 10 fractions using orthovoltage radiotherapy—in doses similar to those used for non-melanoma skin cancer. Christie & Tiver [46] reported prolonged local control in seven lentigo malignas using 100 kV radiography and conventional fractionation (44 Gy in 11 treatments to 57.5 Gy in 23 treatments). Schmid-Wendtner *et al.* [47] in Munich treated 42 lentigo malignas and 22 lentigo maligna melanomas with superficial radiotherapy. In all the lentigo maligna melanoma cases, the nodular lesion was excised prior to radiotherapy. They reported no recurrence in lentigo maligna and only two of 22 in lentigo maligna melanoma, both salvaged by surgery. Pannizon [48] reported local control in 98% (127/129) of cases of lentigo maligna and in 92% (25/27) of cases of lentigo maligna melanoma treated with superficial radiography. He compared this favourably with a surgical series of age- and stage-matched controls in which 84% control was achieved. There seems little doubt of a role for radiotherapy, particularly in those unsuitable for surgery.

Adjuvant radiotherapy for primary lesions

Local recurrence remains a problem even with wide excision margins for particular groups of melanoma. O'Brien *et al.* [49] found 24% local recurrence from melanomas ≥4 mm thick. Others have reported high rates of local failure after surgery, particularly with desmoplastic neurotropic melanomas where the local recurrence rate may be as high as 50% [50]. Although there are no randomized studies, a number of authors have reported the effects of radiotherapy to the primary. Harwood & Cummings [8] reported six cases of superficial spreading melanoma treated with radiotherapy either after biopsy only or with involved margins after local excision. All six cases remained disease-free, albeit at a relatively short interval after treatment. Harwood *et al.* [10] also reported local control in 14 of 15 cases irradiated after local excision from head and neck site. Nitter [51] reported on 135 patients treated with postoperative radiotherapy after excision biopsy and Dickson reviewed 121 patients similarly treated [52]. Both authors noted outcomes to be as good as those achieved with radical surgery as then practised. More recently, Ang [4] has updated the MD Anderson experience. One hundred and eighteen patients with high-risk primaries were irradiated postoperatively to the primary site and nodes. Locoregional failure was seen in 14%. Stevens *et al.* [53] irradiated 32 cases with high-risk features for local relapse: close or positive margins; neurotropic desmoplastic histology or recurrence with perineural spread; or early or multiple recurrence. Local recurrence rates of the 32 cases, plus 142 patients irradiated following nodal surgery, were 11%, well below published rates for high-risk disease.

None of these data should support changes in surgical practice in terms of treatment of the primary. It seems unlikely that a randomized trial would be feasible to address this issue. However, where surgical clearance remains in doubt after maximal surgery, it is not unreasonable to consider postoperative radiotherapy. No conclusions are possible about what regimens of treatment may be optimal and the question will be addressed in the next section on adjuvant regional treatment.

Adjuvant therapy following nodal recurrence

Lee *et al.* [54] from Roswell Park recently reviewed patterns of failure in patients undergoing complete lymph node dissection with pathologically involved nodes. They found 338 patients between 1970 and 1996. Seventy-five per cent had therapeutic node dissection for clinically involved nodes and 25% had elective lymph node dissection. No patients were irradiated. Disease-specific survival at 10 years was 36% and nodal basin recurrence was 30%. Risk of recurrence in cervical lymph nodes was 43% with axillary and inguinal involvement at 28 and 23%, respectively. On multivariate analysis, extracapsular extension and site of involvement were predicted for further regional recurrence. Both size and number of nodes were associated with increasingly high rates of further regional recurrence, but were also associated with poorer overall survival. They concluded that patients with cervical involvement, extracapsular spread, more than three positive nodes, or nodes >3 cm—all features individually associated with nodal failure rates of 40% or more—should be considered for adjuvant radiotherapy.

Other authors have found similar risks. Shen *et al.* [55] found that, while overall recurrence was only 14%, this rose to 31% recurrence in the neck at 5 years in those with extracapsular spread. Number of nodes or presence of palpable nodes did not increase the risk. O'Brien *et al.* [49] reported 34% neck recurrence after therapeutic neck dissection, while Byers found a rate of 50% [56].

Does adjuvant radiotherapy reduce these published rates of recurrence? A randomized trial has been published by Creagan *et al.* [57] looking at patients with cutaneous primaries in the head and neck. This showed no advantage in either local control or overall survival. However, the radiation regimen was not optimal—it was a split course treatment with small dose per fraction and long overall treatment time.

Harwood & Cummings [8] reported local control in 82% (18/22) of patients irradiated with 24 Gy in three fractions over 21 days. Their patients had extracapsular spread or nodes >3 cm. Late fibrosis with neuropathy in two cases does give cause for concern about the fractionation. Ross & Meyer [58] reported on 21 patients treated with adjuvant radiotherapy to the axilla after complete nodal dissection without gross residual disease. All patients had either extracapsular spread, multiple nodes or recurrence after a previous node dissection. Most were treated with 30 Gy in five fractions over 2.5 weeks. Only one of these 21 patients relapsed in the axilla, a local control rate of 95%. Lymphoedema was reported in 18%, but no patients had functional impairment in the arm. Rounsaville *et al.* [11] reported permanent local control in 78% (14/18) patients irradiated for either positive surgical margins, multiple recurrence or large or multiple lymph nodes. The majority of sites were treated with conventional fractionation. As local recurrence was seen in 23% it is not clear that these data support the use of adjuvant radiotherapy.

Geara & Ang [38] have reported the MD Anderson experience for head and neck sites. This has recently been updated by Ang [4]. Thirty-nine patients after first neck dissection for positive nodes, and 67 patients with fully resected locoregional recurrence, were irradiated with 30 Gy in five treatments. Locoregional failure was 8% in the first group and 12% in the second, which compares favourably with published data for high-risk disease. There were few late complications: one case of moderate neck fibrosis, one case of mild hearing impairment and one case of transient exposure of cartilage. Their results compare favourably with O'Brien *et al.* [59] who reported a 7% locoregional failure rate after radiotherapy following neck dissection. More recently, Stevens *et al.* [53] reported on 142 patients irradiated following lymph node dissection, either at first nodal metastasis (107 patients) or following second recurrence. Indications in the group irradiated initially included positive margins, extracapsular spread, multiple nodes, large nodes, perineural or vascular invasion, or parotid involvement. Fifty-five per cent of patients had neck irradiation, 34% had treatment to the axilla, 8% to the inguinal region and 3% had more than one site treated. Most received 33 Gy in six fractions over 3 weeks. Overall local failure rate was 11%. There was significant morbidity in those treated in the axilla with 10 of 17 two-year survivors developing lymphoedema requiring some degree of treatment. Of interest is the observation that patients treated in an overall treatment time of < 18 days had a 4% failure rate, compared with 15% of those treated over > 18 days.

The above data suggest that there may be a role for adjuvant radiotherapy, particularly following nodal recurrence with high-risk features on histology, but possibly also for those with high-risk features on resection of primary disease. The issue needs to be addressed in randomized trials. One such is currently running within the Eastern Cooperative Oncology Group (ECOG). This trial uses a hypofractionated regimen as used in the MD Anderson series and includes all three main regional nodal basins. However, there are still no clear randomized data suggesting that hypofractionated treatment is superior to conventional fractionation, and the only randomized trial to address this issue, in a palliative setting, showed no advantage to 32 Gy in four fractions of 8 Gy each, compared to 50 Gy in 20 fractions of 2.5 Gy each.

Conclusions

Radiotherapy has often been viewed as inappropriate in the treatment of melanoma. The data reviewed above show that there is a clear if limited role for the modality and that randomized trials are needed more than ever to delineate this further.

References

1 Paterson R. The radical X-ray treatment of the carcinomata. *Br J Radiol* 1936; **106**: 671–9.
2 Ellis F. The radiosensitivity of malignant melanoma. *Br J Radiol* 1939; **12**: 327–52.
3 Cascinelli N, Clemente C, Belli F. Cutaneous melanoma. In: Peckham M, Pinedo H, Veronesi U, eds. *Oxford Textbook of Oncology*. Oxford: Oxford University Press, 1995: 902–28.
4 Ang KK. Radiotherapy for melanoma. In: de Vita V, Hellman S, Rosenberg SA, eds. *Cancer: Principles and Practice of Oncology*. Philadelphia: JB Lippincott, 1997.
5 Hornsey S. The relationship between total dose, number of fractions and fraction size in the response of malignant melanoma in patients. *Br J Radiol* 1978; **51**: 905–9.
6 Overgaard J. Radiation therapy of malignant melanoma. *Int J Radiat Oncol Biol Phys* 1980; **6**: 41–4.
7 Overgaard J, Overgaard M, Vejby-Hansen P, *et al.* Some factors of importance in the radiation treatment of malignant melanoma. *Radiother Oncol* 1986; **5**: 183–92.
8 Harwood AR, Cummings BJ. Radiotherapy for malignant melanoma: a re-appraisal. *Cancer Treat Rev* 1981; **8**: 271–82.
9 Overgaard J, van der Maase H, Overgaard M. A randomised study comparing two high dose per fraction radiation schedules in recurrent or metastatic malignant melanoma. *Int J Radiat Oncol Biol Phys* 1985; **11**: 1837–9.
10 Harwood AR, Dancuart F, Fitzpatrick P, Brown T. Radiotherapy of non-lentiginous melanoma of the head and neck. *Cancer* 1981; **48**: 2599–605.
11 Rounsaville MC, Cantril ST, FontanesiJ, Vaeth JM, Green JP. Radiotherapy in the management of cutaneous melanoma: effect of time, dose and fractionation. *Front Radiat Ther Oncol* 1988; **22**: 62–78.
12 Lobo PA, Liebner EJ, Chao JJH, Kanji AM. Radiotherapy in the management of malignant melanoma. *Int J Radiat Oncol Biol Phys* 1981; **7**: 21–6.
13 Trott KR, von Lieven H, Kummermehr J, *et al.* The radiosensitivity of malignant melanomas. Part II: clinical studies. *Int J*

Radiat Oncol Biol Phys 1981; **7**: 15–20.
14 Fenig E, Eidelevich E, Njuguna E, *et al.* Role of radiation therapy in the management of cutaneous malignant melanoma. *Am J Clin Oncol Cancer Clin Trials* 1999; **22**: 184–6.
15 Dewey DL. The radiosensitivity of melanoma cells in culture. *Br J Radiol* 1971; **44**: 816–17.
16 Barranco SC, Romsdahl MM, Humphrey RM. The radiation response of human malignant melanoma cells grown *in vitro*. *Cancer Res* 1971; **31**: 830–3.
17 Rofstad EK. Radiation biology of malignant melanoma. *Acta Radiol Oncol* 1986; **25**: 1–10.
18 Sause WT, Cooper JS, Rush S, *et al.* Fraction size in external beam radiation therapy in the treatment of melanoma. *Int J Radiat Oncol Biol Phys* 1991; **20**: 429–32.
19 Hilaris BS, Raben M, Calabrese AS, *et al.* Value of radiation therapy for distant metastases from malignant melanoma. *Cancer* 1963; **16**: 765–73.
20 Konefal JB, Emani B, Pilepich MV. Malignant melanoma: analysis of dose fractionation in radiation therapy. *Radiology* 1987; **164**: 607–10.
21 Kirova YM, Chen J, Rabarijaona LI, Piedbois Y, Le Bourgeois JP. Radiotherapy as palliative treatment for metastatic melanoma. *Melanoma Res* 1999; **9**: 611–13.
22 Katz HR. The results of different fractionation schemes in the palliative irradiation of metastatic melanoma. *Int J Radiat Oncol Biol Phys* 1981; **7**: 907–11.
23 McQuay HJ, Collins SL, Carroll D, Moore RA. Radiotherapy for the palliation of bone metastases. *Cochrane Database Syst. Rev.* 2000; (2): CD001793.
24 Ziegler JC, Cooper JS. Brain metastases from malignant melanoma: conventional vs. high dose per fraction radiotherapy. *Int J Radiat Oncol Biol Phys* 1986; **12**: 1839–42.
25 Loeffler JS, Barker FG, Chapman PH. Role of radiosurgery in the management of central nervous system metastases. *Cancer Chemother Pharmacol* 1999; **43** (Suppl.): 11–14.
26 Lavine SD, Petrovich Z, Cohen-Gadol AA, *et al.* Gamma knife radiosurgery for metastatic melanoma: an analysis of survival, outcome and complications. *Neurosurgery* 1999; **44**: 59–64.
27 Skibber JM, Soong S, Austin L, *et al.* Cranial irradiation aftre surgical excision of brain metastases in melanoma patients. *Ann Surg Oncol* 1996; **3**: 118–23.
28 Hagen WA, Cirrincione C, Thaler HT, De Angelis LM. The role of radiation therapy following resection of single brain metastases from melanoma. *Neurology* 1990; **40**: 158–60.
29 Chidel MA, Suhl JH, Reddy CA, Chao ST, Lundbeck MF, Barnett GH. Application of recursive partitioning analysis and evaluation of whole brain irradiation among patients treated with stereotactic radiosurgery for newly diagnosed brain metastases. *Int J Radiat Oncol Biol Phys* 2000; **47**: 993–9.
30 Sneed PK, Lambourn KR, Forstner JM, *et al.* Radiosurgery for brain metastases: is whole brain radiotherapy necessary? *Int J Radiat Oncol Biol Phys* 1999; **43**: 549–58.
31 Seung SK, Sneed PK, McDermott MW, *et al.* Gamma knife radiosurgery for malignant melanoma brain metastases. *Cancer J Sci Am* 1998; **4**: 103–9.
32 Mori Y, Kondziolka D, Flickinger JC, Kirkwood JM, Agarwala S, Lunsford LD. Stereotactic radiosurgery for cerebral metastatic melanoma: factors affecting local disease control and survival. *Int J Radiat Oncol Biol Phys* 1998; **42**: 581–9.
33 Grob JJ, Regis J, Laurans R, *et al.* Radiosurgery without whole brain radiotherapy in melanoma brain metastases. *Eur J Cancer* 1998; **34**: 1187–92.
34 Chang AE, Karnell LH, Menck HR. The national cancer database report on cutaneous and noncutaneous melanoma: a summary of 84 836 cases from the past decade. *Cancer* 1998; **83**: 1664–78.
35 de Meerleer GO, Vermeersch H, van Eijkeren M, *et al.* Primary sinonasal mucosal melanoma: three different therapeutic approaches to inoperable local disease or recurrence and a review of the literature. *Melanoma Res* 1998; **8**: 449–57.
36 Nandapalan V, Roland NJ, Helliwell TR, Williams EMI, Hamilton JW, Jones AS. Mucosal melanoma of the head and neck. *Clin Otolaryngol* 1998; **23**: 107–16.

37 Kingdom TT, Kaplan MJ. Mucosal melanoma of the nasal cavity and paranasal sinuses. *Head Neck* 1995; **17**: 184–9.
38 Geara FB, Ang KK. Radiation therapy for malignant melanoma. *Surg Clin North Am* 1996; **76**: 1383–98.
39 Lund VJ, Howard DJ, Harding L, Wei WI. Management options and survival in malignant melanoma of the sinonasal mucosa. *Laryngoscope* 1999; **109**: 208–11.
40 Loree TR, Mullins AP, Spellman J, North JH, Hicks W. Head and neck mucosal melanoma: a 32 year review. *Ear Nose Throat J* 1999; **78**: 372–5.
41 Gilligan D, Slevin NJ. Radical radiotherapy for 28 cases of mucosal melanoma in the nasal cavity and sinuses. *Br J Radiol* 1991; **64**: 1147–50.
42 Irvin WP Jr, Bliss SA, Rice LW, Taylor PT Jr, Andersen WA. Malignant melanoma of the vagina and locoregional control: radical surgery revisited. *Gynecol Oncol* 1998; **71**: 476–80.
43 Petru E, Nagele F, Czerwenka K, *et al.* Primary melanoma of the vagina. *Gynecol Oncol* 1998; **70**: 23–6.
44 Shank B, Cohen A, Kelsen D. Anorectal melanoma. In: de Vita V, Hellman S, Rosenberg SA, eds. *Cancer: Principles and Practice of Oncology*. Philadelphia: JB Lippincott, 1993: 1018–19.
45 Presant CA. Malignant melanoma of mucosal sites. In: Constanzi JJ, ed. *Malignant Melanoma*. Boston: Martinus Nijohoff, 1982; 55–83.
46 Christie DRH, Tiver KW. Radiotherapy for melanotic freckles. *Australas Radiol* 1996; **40**: 331–3.
47 Schmid-Wendtner MH, Brunner B, Konz B, *et al.* Fractionated radiotherapy of lentigo maligna and lentigo maligna melanoma in 64 patients. *J Am Acad Dermatol* 2000; **43**: 477–82.
48 Pannizzon RG. Radiotherapy of lentigo maligna and lentigo maligna melanoma. *Skin Cancer* 1999; 203–7.
49 O'Brien CJ, Coates AS, Petersen-Schaefer K, *et al.* Experience with 998 cutaneous melanomas of the head and neck over 30 years. *Am J Surg* 1991; **162**: 310–14.
50 Beenken S, Byers R, Smith JL, *et al.* Desmoplastic melanoma. *Arch Otolaryngol Head Neck Surg* 1989; **115**: 374–9.
51 Nitter L. The treatment of malignant melanoma with special reference to the possible effect of radiotherapy. *Acta Radiol* 1956; **46**: 547–62.
52 Dickson RJ. Malignant melanoma: a combined surgical and radiotherapeutic approach. *Am J Roentgenol* 1958; **79**: 1063–70.
53 Stevens G, Thompson JF, Firth I, O'Brien CJ, McCarthy WH, Quinn MJ. Locally advanced melanoma: results of postoperative hypofractionated radiation therapy. *Cancer* 2000; **88**: 88–94.
54 Lee RJ, Gibbs JF, Proulx GM, Kollmorgen DR, Jia C, Kraybill WG. Nodal basin recurrence following lymph node dissection for melanoma: implications for adjuvant radiotherapy. *Int J Radiat Oncol Biol Phys* 2000; **46**: 467–74.
55 Shen P, Wanek LA, Morton DL. Is adjuvant radiotherapy necessary after positive lymph node dissection in head and neck melanomas? *Ann Surg Oncol* 2000; **7**: 554–9.
56 Byers RM. The role of modified neck dissection in the treatment of cutaneous melanoma of the head and neck. *Arch Surg* 1986; **12**: 1338–41.
57 Creagan ET, Cupps RE, Ivins JC, *et al.* Adjuvant radiation therapy for regional nodal metastases from malignant melanoma: a randomised prospective study. *Cancer* 1978; **42**: 2206–10.
58 Ross M, Meyer JL. Management of the regional lymph nodes in malignant melanoma: surgery, radiotherapy or observation. *Front Radiat Ther Oncol* 1994; **28**: 226–34.
59 O'Brien CJ, Petersen-Schaefer K, Ruark D, *et al.* Radical, modified and selective neck dissection for cutaneous malignant melanoma. *Head Neck* 1995; **17**: 232–41.

21: What should we tell patients about hormones after having melanoma?

Stephen R.D. Johnston

Introduction

Controversy continues about the possible association of malignant melanoma with steroid hormones, in particular oestrogen. Several questions may arise, not least whether any hormonal factors are associated with the risk of getting melanoma or may influence a patient's subsequent outcome. For example, women and their doctors may worry that taking the oral contraceptive pill may increase their individual risk of developing melanoma. After a previous diagnosis of an early stage melanoma, many younger women may wish to continue use of the oral contraceptive pill, while older women may merit consideration of hormone replacement therapy (HRT)—are there data to reassure us that their use in this setting is safe?

The incidence of melanoma is increasing in women, with the average age at presentation being around 45 years [1]. With the increasing tendency to delay having children until the fourth to fifth decade, pregnancy may coincide with a diagnosis of melanoma. Is the prognosis for such women worse, and can melanoma arising in pregnancy spread to the fetus? Equally, can a woman have another baby following a diagnosis of melanoma, and if so when?

This chapter aims to address each of these questions by reviewing the available published evidence, and to conclude by providing practical advice to both patients and clinicians who are faced with any of these difficult issues.

Do women have the same prognosis as men?

Epidemiological evidence has suggested that prognosis from malignant melanoma is better in women than in men. Initially, it was suggested that this could relate to associated clinical factors which are known to be more common in women, such as thinner lesions at presentation which may be distributed more frequently on the lower limbs. However, subsequent multivariate analyses which account for these prognostic variables have consistently demonstrated a female survival advantage. In a US study of 6383 patients with melanoma there was a 34% improvement in overall survival advantage for women compared with men, with a 28% improvement in disease-free survival [2]. On multivariate analysis which accounted for age, site, tumour thickness, Clark level and histological type, sex appeared to be an independent prognostic factor. In a German study of 5093 patients which accounted for other known prognostic variables, there was a similar highly significant ($P<0.0001$) survival advantage for women [3].

The better prognosis in women has been interpreted as evidence to suggest that oestrogens may in fact inhibit melanoma growth. The 5-year survival figures in premenopausal women have been reported to be significantly better than in postmenopausal women [4], while case reports exist of melanoma diagnosed in premenopausal women only metastasing many years later (>10) once in the postmenopausal period [5]. These data, if anything, may imply that endogenous oestrogens have a protective effect on melanoma—is there any biological evidence for such an interaction?

Are there experimental data to suggest that hormones influence melanoma growth?

The early clinical data prompted several laboratory investigations to examine the influence of steroid hormones on melanoma growth. Some studies of melanomas transplanted into mice suggested that female hormones may have an inhibitory effect on growth; for example, the growth rate of B16 melanomas was noted to be slower in female than in male mice, but following oophorectomy the growth rate was similar in females to the uncastrated males [6]. Another group demonstrated that while neither oestradiol or the antioestrogen tamoxifen influenced human melanoma cell growth *in vitro*, an inhibitory effect of oestradiol could be demonstrated on growth of the same melanoma cells transplanted into athymic mice *in vivo* [7]. Others have demonstrated that transplantable B16 melanomas may be significantly growth-inhibited by administration of glucocorticoids [8]. The mechanism of any growth inhibitory effect by steroid hormones in these animal models remains unclear.

There are conflicting reports in the literature regarding the expression of oestrogen receptors (ER) in human melanomas. Initial reports described high-affinity intracytoplasmic oestrogen-binding activity, similar to that seen in breast cancer [9]. A subsequent eight studies all used different methodologies and reported expression of oestrogen-binding activity in 12–43% of human melanomas [10–17]. However, sucrose density gradients failed to demonstrate a distinct 8S peak consistent with the identifiable classical species of oestrogen receptor seen in breast carcinomas [18]. It now transpires that in these early studies most of the binding of oestrogen to putative 'receptors' may represent non-specific binding to the enzyme tyrosinase [19]. More recent immunocytochemical studies with monoclonal ER antibodies have failed to detect true ER in human melanomas [20,21]. It appears therefore that any endocrine effect of steroid hormones–in particular, oestrogen—on the biological behaviour of melanoma cannot be explained by the classical oestrogen receptor pathway.

Does a woman's menstrual or reproductive history influence her risk of getting melanoma?

During the 1980s several studies examined whether hormonal factors were associated with an increased risk of malignant melanoma. Some showed a weak association with reproductive factors, including late age at first birth [22] and number of live births [23]. Other studies failed to demonstrate any effect of age, either at first birth or menarche, on melanoma risk [24,25]. It is important to recognize that other lifestyle factors which may be linked to reproductive history could have an influence on melanoma risk. For example, in one study where an inverse association was shown between number of live births and melanoma, this was lost when corrected for education and sun exposure [26].

In a Danish case–control study of 280 cases and 536 controls, there was no association between risk of melanoma and various menstrual factors, including age at menarche, menopausal status, age at natural menopause and number of reproductive years [27]. Similar findings were reported in a larger, more recent Swedish case–control study of 400 cases and 640 controls [28]. Both studies failed to show any significant association between parity factors and melanoma risk (Table 21.1), although a trend for decrease in melanoma risk with greater number of live births was seen in the Swedish study. Overall, there appears to be little evidence from these epidemiological studies for any association of melanoma risk with a woman's menstrual or reproductive history.

Does use of the oral contraceptive pill increase risk of melanoma?

Most of the early studies which examined the effect of oral contraceptive use and risk of malignant melanoma failed to show any association [23–27,29,30]. There were some reports which implied an association between duration of oral contraceptive use and increased risk [22,31], although these were often non-significant and had not been corrected for sun exposure. The most recent Swedish case–control study showed that oral contraceptive use was not associated with increased melanoma risk [28]. The adjusted odds ratio which accounted for both host factors and sun exposure was 1.6 (95%

Table 21.1 Odds ratios (95% CI) for developing malignant melanoma in relation to parity factors

	Danish study [27]	Swedish study [28]
Pregnancies (n)		
0	1.0	1.0
1–2	1.0 (0.6–1.6)	1.0 (0.6–1.7)
3–4	0.8 (0.5–1.3)	0.7 (0.4–1.3)
≥5	0.9 (0.4–1.9)	0.8 (0.3–2.0)
	P=0.362	*P*=0.4
Age at first pregnancy		
<25		1.0
25–29	1.3 (0.8–1.9)	1.1 (0.6–1.7)
≥30	1.0 (0.6–1.8)	1.2 (0.7–1.9)
	P=0478	*P*=0.5
Live births (n)		
0	1.0	1.0
1–2	1.1 (0.7–1.7)	0.8 (0.5–1.4)
≥3	1.0 (0.6–1.6)	0.6 (0.3–1.0)
	P=0.32	*P*=0.01

CI=0.9–2.8) for ever using oral contraceptives vs. never used. The duration of pill use, age a first use and timing of oral contraceptive use in relation to first child was not associated with any increased risk.

One previous study of 289 women had suggested an influence of oral contraceptive use on the pattern and thickness or primary melanoma in stage I disease [32]. Women who had taken oral contraceptives at any time before diagnosis, presented with significantly thinner tumours than women who had not, while women who used oral contraceptives in the year before melanoma was diagnosed had thinner lesions than those who stopped use more than a year before. Overall, in that study oral contraceptives did not effect survival, possibly because of the higher incidence of truncal lesions. Indeed, none of the case–control studies of melanoma have been large enough to assess site-specific location (trunk vs. extremities vs. head) in relation to oral contraceptive use, and thus the clinical significance of any association of melanoma site with oral contraceptive use remains unclear.

More recently, there have been two large systematic reviews of the literature which have suggested that overall there is no evidence for oral contraceptive use in the development of melanoma. A meta-analysis analysed 18 case–control studies published between 1977 and 1996 involving 3796 cases with 9442 controls [33], and showed that there was no evidence for any association of oral contraceptive use with the occurrence of primary cutaneous malignant melanoma (odds ratio of 0.95, 95% CI=0.87–1.04). A recent second sytematic review came to a similar conclusion [34].

Is it safe to prescribe either the pill or HRT to a women with a previous history of melanoma?

The package inserts for oral contraceptives continue to include a history of melanoma as a contraindication to its use. There are very few data on whether subsequent pill use influences outcome in women with a previous history of primary melanoma. It is quite likely that until recently general concern about a possible adverse influence of the pill on risk of recurrence prevented its widespread use. However, at the present time there remains no convincing argument to deny the use of the oral contraceptive pill to women who have had melanoma.

The situation regarding HRT has been less well studied. In terms of HRT use and risk of developing primary melanoma, early published case–control studies suggested no evidence for any association [23,24,31,35]. In the larger, more recent Danish and Swedish case–control studies the adjusted relative risk for ever having used HRT were 1.1 (95% CI=0.7–1.7) and 1.0 (95% CI=0.5–1.8), respectively [27,28]. As observed with oral contraceptives, no associations were found for duration of HRT use, age at first use, or type of replacement therapy used (oestrogen alone, or opposed oestrogen).

The question as to whether subsequent HRT use following a previous diagnosis of melanoma influences prognosis has not been studied. With an increasing number of women wishing to take HRT, clinical studies in women previously treated for melanoma are urgently required in this area. However, as with the pill, at present there are no data to deny women with a prior history of melanoma HRT if required on either symptomatic grounds or for prevention of osteoporosis.

Is it safe to become pregnant following a diagnosis of melanoma, and if so when?

The impact of subsequent pregnancies on prognosis and outcome from melanoma has been assessed in at least two studies. In the Scottish case–control study, there was no difference in survival or time to progression for women who became pregnant after a diagnosis of melanoma, or those treated for melanoma between pregnancies, compared with those who had completed all pregnancies before melanoma was diagnosed [36]. In a previous study, 43 women who became pregnant within 5 years of diagnosis with stage I melanoma were compared with a control group of 337 women of childbearing age who did not become pregnant or have a recurrence within 2 years of diagnosis [37]. There was no difference in disease-free interval or survival, and pregnancy within 5 years of diagnosis was not a significant adverse prognostic factor on either multivariate or univariate regression analyses.

In spite of this reassuring evidence, it is common clinical practice to recommend to women who wish to become pregnant after apparently successful excision of primary melanoma that they wait at least 2 years after diagnosis and surgery. This is empirical timing based on the fact that over 65% of melanoma recurrences occur within this time period, and irrespective of pregnancy status which for early stage disease does not appear to alter the prognosis [38].

Does melanoma arising in pregnancy have a worse outcome?

Early anecdotal evidence suggested that melanoma arising in pregnancy was associated with a poorer prognosis [39,40]. Numerous subsequent case reviews and uncontrolled studies continued to imply that pregnancy may induce or worsen the prognosis of malignant melanoma. However, there have been five well-controlled studies that have addressed the issue as to whether pregnancy during or after diagnosis of melanoma affects the outcome following appropriate management (reviewed in [41]). The conclusion from all of these studies was that if pregnant patients had American Joint Commission of Cancer (AJCC) stage I or II melanoma (primary site only with any tumour thickness) diagnosed during pregnancy and managed appropriately, the prognosis (survival) from her melanoma was unaltered compared with non-pregnant age-matched controls. In two of the studies [37,42] there did appear to be a significantly shorter disease-free interval in the pregnant cohort. However, in both studies tumours were significantly thicker in pregnant vs. non-pregnant women, although on multivariate regression analysis both tumour thickness and pregnancy were independent prognostic factors on disease-free survival. In the other three studies which involved a total of 181 cases, there was no impact of pregnancy on either survival or disease-free interval [36,43,44].

Increased tumour thickness in pregnancy-associated melanomas is well recognized. In the Scottish study of 388 women with stage I primary cutaneous melanoma during their child-bearing years, 85 had received treatment prior to pregnancy, 92 during pregnancy, 143 after completing all pregnancies, and 68 between pregnancies [36]. Mean tumour thickness was significantly higher ($P=0.002$) in those with pregnancy-associated melanoma (2.38 mm) vs. melanoma prior to pregnancy (1.49 mm), after pregnancy (1.96 mm) or between pregnancy (1.48 mm). When corrected for tumour thickness, there was no effect of pregnancy on disease-free or overall survival. In a more recent US study of 465 women of reproductive age with melanoma, 45 were identified with pregnancy-associated melanoma [45]. Again, tumour thickness was significantly greater (2.28 vs. 1.22 mm, $P<0.007$), but there was no adverse effect of pregnancy on prognosis when corrected for thickness.

The biological basis for increased tumour thickness remains unclear. It has been accepted that during pregnancy benign melanocytic naevi may enlarge, or new naevi develop, possibly in association with an increase in hormonally regulated circulating growth factors released during early stages of pregnancy. However, a recent study followed 22 women with benign naevi during the first trimester of pregnancy [46]. In total only 8/129 (6%) of naevi changed, challenging the widely held belief that hormonal changes in such lesions are common and suggesting that any enlarging or changing naevi in a pregnant women still require dermatological advice.

While prognosis may be unaffected in those presenting with early stage I–II disease during pregnancy, the situation may be very different for those women with melanoma recurrence during pregnancy involving either the regional lymph nodes (AJCC stage III) or distant metsatases (AJCC stage IV). One previous study from the Memorial Sloan Kettering Cancer Centre has shown significantly reduced 5-year survival for pregnant patients with regional lymph node recurrence of melanoma compared with nulliparous women or parous women with no disease recurrence during pregnancy (29 vs. 55%, $P<0.05$) [47].

Should melanoma arising in pregnancy be treated differently?

There are specific therapeutic considerations regarding the management of such patients [48]. For those with early stage I–II primary melanomas, standard surgical excision with margins appropriate for tumour thickness should be performed. This may often be under local anaesthetic without any increased risk to the developing fetus.

For those patients presenting with either regional (stage III) or metastatic disease (stage IV) during pregnancy, treatment decisions are more difficult. While therapeutic lymph node dissections may still be performed for stage III disease, the role of adjuvant interferon in improving the prognosis of high-risk disease in pregnant patients is unclear. Fetuses born to women who receive interferon during pregnancy may be small-for-dates, although no other serious congenital abnormalities have been noted to date [38].

In women with very aggressive or advanced disease developing during the first trimester, the issue of termination of pregnancy has been raised as a therapeutic 'hormonal' manoeuvre. Despite early anecdotal reports of tumour regression after delivery of the fetus [49], no studies have shown a consistent positive influence of therapeutic abortion or spontaneous delivery on maternal tumour regression [50,51]. The more difficult ethical debate relates to whether the mother with advanced disease should receive conventional systemic treatment at the risk of harming the developing fetus [52]. The expectant mother may become seriously ill before term, putting the life of the fetus at risk, or she may die soon after delivery leaving a child without a mother. If the prognosis for the mother is so poor that further treatment is unlikely to influence the outcome, should fetal survival be placed above maternal outcome? The gestational age at which the problem develops may influence treatment decisions with regard to fetal risk. Dacarbazine is the single most active chemotherapeutic agent in melanoma and can be given safely during the second and third trimesters of pregnancy [53], without risk of long-term effects in the children exposed *in utero* [54].

Can advanced melanoma arising in pregnancy spread to the baby?

An additional consideration is the risk of transplacental spread of melanoma to the fetus. Several case reviews have highlighted the risk of subsequent infant mortality from malignant melanoma in situations where placental involvement is noted postpartum in women with disseminated disease [55,56]. Although overall the risk is considered low [57], the chance of infants developing metastatic melanoma—mainly skin and liver—may be up to 25% in situations where there is histological evidence of melanoma cells within the placenta (Fig. 21.1). These issues need to be considered when counselling women who develop regional or metastatic recurrence of melanoma during pregnancy.

Are hormone therapies used to treat advanced melanoma?

Despite the lack of recent laboratory studies to support an ER-dependent steroid hormone growth pathway, clinical trials with the non-steroidal antioestrogen tamoxifen have been performed. Following some initial case reports, Phase II studies were undertaken in patients with metastatic melanoma using doses of between 20 and 100 mg tamoxifen daily. Overall, the objective

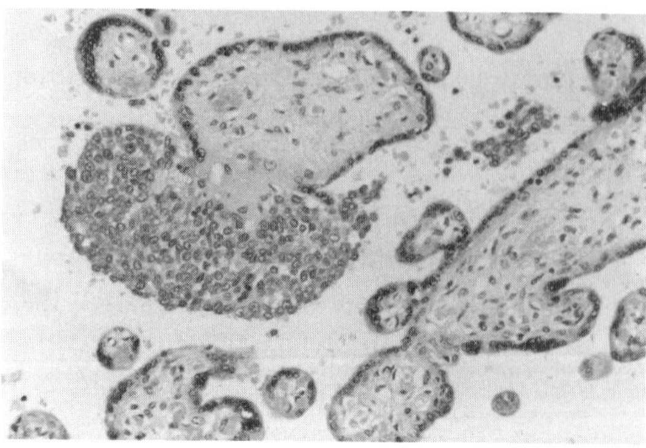

Fig. 21.1 Placenta showing deposits of malignant melanoma within the intervillous space, invading into villous core.

response rates were low in the range 4–6% [58–60]. Likewise, some clinical activity has been seen in patients with advanced melanoma treated with progestins [61,62]. In a prospective randomized trial of adjuvant megestrol acetate vs. observation in patients with high-risk resected stage I–II melanoma, a longer disease-free interval and overall survival was seen in the treatment arm, although this did not reach statistical significance [63].

Recent clinical investigations have examined the combination of tamoxifen with chemotherapy, on the basis of experimental data suggesting that tamoxifen could synergize with cisplatin in killing melanoma cells *in vitro* [64]. A variety of Phase II non-randomized trials adding tamoxifen to cytotoxic agents, including dacarbazine, cisplatin, and carmustine, suggested improved response rates which range from 13 to 55% [65]. The true effect of adding tamoxifen to chemotherapy has been addressed in a total of four randomized clinical trials [66–69]. These show an added therapeutic benefit of tamoxifen to single agent dacarbazine (28 vs. 12% response rate [66]), but little added benefit when given in combination chemotherapy regimens [67–69]. It is of interest that the maximal benefit of adding tamoxifen to single agent dacarbazine was seen in female patients [66].

Conclusions and practice points

The overall message is generally very reassuring, namely that hormones probably have a negligible role in the aetiology of the disease and do not appear to adversely influence the outcome.

The following 10 practice points can be made on the basis of current knowledge:

1 Women diagnosed with melanoma have a better prognosis than men, irrespective of known differences in site of disease.

2 Recent data show no evidence for oestrogen receptors in melanoma.

3 There is no evidence that parity or menstrual history is associated with an increased risk of melanoma.

4 There is no evidence that use of either the oral contraceptive pill or HRT increases the risk of melanoma.

5 There are no data to deny women with a previous history of melanoma subsequent use of either the pill or HRT.

6 There are as yet no data to suggest that subsequent pregnancy following a prior history of melanoma adversely affects outcome; most clinicians advise a remission-free interval of 2 years before becoming pregnant.

7 Women who are diagnosed with melanoma during pregnancy have thicker lesions, but their survival corrected for this is identical to non-pregnant women.

8 Recurrence of advanced disease during pregnancy may be associated

with a poorer outcome, although rare transplacental spread of systemic disease can occur.

9 In general, treatment of melanoma during pregnancy is the same as for a non-pregnant patient; there is no clinical evidence for therapeutic termination of pregnancy, but difficult issues in relation to fetal well-being vs. maternal prognosis in advanced disease may need to be faced.

10 Hormone therapy (tamoxifen) is sometimes used in advanced disease; response rates to single agent therapy are low, and most of the evidence for its use is in the potentiation of chemotherapy.

References

1 MacKie RM. Pregnancy and exogenous hormones in patients with cutaneous malignant melanoma. *Curr Opin Oncol* 1999; **11**: 129–31.

2 Stidham KR, Johnson JL, Seigler HF. Survival superiority of females with melanoma. *Arch Surg* 1994; **129**: 316–24.

3 Garbe C, Buttner P, Bertz J, *et al.* Primary cutaneous melanoma: identification of prognostic groups and estimation of individual prognosis for 5093 patients. *Cancer* 1995; **75**: 2484–91.

4 Shaw HM, Milton GW, Farago G, McCarthy WH. Endocrine influences on survival from malignant melanoma. *Cancer* 1978; **42**: 669–77.

5 Raderman D, Giler S, Rothem A, Ben-Basset M. Late metastases (beyond 10 years) of cutaneous malignant melanoma. *J Am Acad Dermatol* 1986; **15**: 374–8.

6 Proctor JW, Auclair BG, Stokowski L. Endocrine factors and the growth and spread of B16 melanoma. *J Natl Cancer Inst* 1976; **57**: 1197–8.

7 Fuecht KA, Walker MJ, DasGupta TK, Beattie CW. Effect of 17β-estradiol on the growth of estrogen receptor-positive human melanoma *in vitro* and in athymic mice. *Cancer Res* 1988; **48**: 7093–101.

8 Bhakoo HS, Paolini NS, Milholland RJ, *et al.* Glucocorticoid receptors and the effect of glucocorticoids on the growth of B16 melanoma. *Cancer Res* 1981; **41**: 1695–701.

9 Fisher RI, Neifeld JP, Lippman ME. Oestrogen receptors in human malignant melanoma. *Lancet* 1976; **ii**: 337–9.

10 Neifeld JP, Lippman ME. Steroid hormone receptors and melanoma. *J Invest Dermatol* 1980; **74**: 379–81.

11 Rumke P, Persijn JP, Korsten CB. Oestrogen and androgen receptors in melanoma. *Br J Cancer* 1980; 41: 652–6.

12 Creagan ET, Ingle JN, Woods JE, *et al.* Estrogen receptors in patients with malignant melanoma. *Cancer* 1980; **46**: 1785–6.

13 Karakousis CP, Lopez R, Bhakoo HP, *et al.* Estrogen and progesterone receptors and tamoxifen in malignant melanoma. *Cancer Treat Rep* 1980; **64**: 819–27.

14 Bhakoo HS, Milholland RJ, Lopez R, *et al.* High incidence and characterization of glucocorticoid receptors in human malignant melanoma. *J Natl Cancer Inst* 1981; **66**: 21–5.

15 Kokoschka EM, Spona J, Knobler R. Sex steroid hormone receptor analysis in malignant melanoma. *Br J Dermatol* 1982; **107** (Suppl. 23): 54–9.

16 Walker MJ, Beatie CW, Patel MK, *et al.* Estrogen receptor in malignant melanoma. *J Clin Oncol* 1987; 5: 1256–61.

17 Ferno M, Borg A, Erichsen C, *et al.* Estrogen and progesterone receptors in melanoma metastases with special reference to analytical methods and prognosis. *Anticancer Res* 1989; **4**: 179–82.

18 Neifeld JP. Endocrinology of melanoma. *Semin Oncol* 1996; **12**: 402–6.

19 Hakim AA. Correlation between tyrosine hydroxylase activity, melanogenesis and estradiol binding in human melanoma cells. *Res Exp Med (Berl)* 1982; **180**: 99–115.

20 Lecavalier MA, From L, Gaid N. Absence of estrogen receptors in dysplastic nevi and malignant melanoma. *J Am Acad Dermatol* 1990; **23**: 242–6.

21 Flowers JL, Seigler HF, McCarthy KS, SrKonrath J, McCarthy KS Jr. Absence of estrogen receptor in human melanoma as evaluated by a monoclonal antiestrogen receptor antibody. *Arch Dermatol* 1987; **123**: 764–5.

22 Holly EA, Weiss NS, Liff JM. Cutaneous melanoma in relation to exogenous hormones and reproductive factors. *J Natl Cancer Inst* 1983; **70**: 827–31.

23 Gallagher RP, Elwood JM, Hill GB, Coldman AJ, Threlfall WJ, Spinell JJ. Reproductive factors, oral contraceptives, and risk of malignant melanoma. *Br J Cancer* 1985; **52**: 901–7.

24 Holman CDJ, Armstrong BK, Heenan PJ. Cutaneous malignant melanoma in women: exogenous sex hormones and reproductive factors. *Br J Cancer* 1984; **50**: 673–80.

25 Green A, Bain C. Hormonal factors and melanoma in women. *Med J Austr* 1985; **142**: 446–8.

26 Zanetti R, Franceschi S, Rosso S, Bidoli E, Colonna S. Cutaneous malignant melanoma in females: the role of hormonal and reproductive factors. *Int J Epidemiol* 1990; **19**: 522–6.

27 Osterlind A, Tucker MA, Stone BJ, Jensen OM. The Danish case–control study of cutaneous malignant melanoma. III. Hormonal and reproductive factors in women. *Int J Cancer* 1988; **42**: 821–4.

28 Westerdahl J, Olsson H, Masback A, Ingvar C, Jonsson N. Risk of malignant melanoma in relation to drug intake, alcohol, smoking and hormonal factors. *Br J Cancer* 1996; **73** (9): 1126–31

29 Bain C, Hennekens CH, Speizer FE, Rossner B, Willet W, Belanger C. Oral contraceptive use and malignant melanoma. *J Natl Cancer Inst* 1982; **68**: 537–9.

30 Helmrich SP, Rosenberg L, Kaufman D, *et al.* Lack of elevated risk of malignant melanoma in relation to oral contraceptive use. *J Natl Cancer Inst* 1984; **72**: 617–20.

31 Beral V, Ramcharan S, Faris R. Malignant melanoma and oral contraceptive use among women in California. *Br J Cancer* 1977; **36**: 804–9.

32 Lederman JS, Lew RA, Koh HK, Sober AJ. Influence of estrogen administration on tumor characteristics and survival in women with cutaneous melanoma. *J Natl Cancer Inst* 1985; **74**: 981–5.

33 Gefeller O, Hassan K, Wille L. Cutaneous malignant melanoma in women and the role of oral contraceptives. *Br J Dermatol* 1998; **138**: 122–4.

34 Pfahlberg A. Systematic review of case–control studies: oral contraceptives show no effect on melanoma risk. *Public Health Rev* 1997; **25**: 309–15.

35 Adam SA, Sheaves JK, Right NH, Mosser G, Harris R, Vessey MP. A case–controlled study of the possible association between oral contraceptives and malignant melanoma. *Br J Cancer* 1981; **44**: 45–50.

36 MacKie RM, Hole D, Hunter JAA, Rankin R, Evans A, McLaren K. Cutaneous malignant melanoma in Scotland: incidence, survival, mortality, 1979–94. *Br Med J* 1997; **315**: 1117–21.

37 Reintgen OS, McCarthy KS, Vollmer R. Malignant melanoma and pregnancy. *Cancer* 1985; **55**: 1340–4.

38 MacKie RM, Bufalino R, Morabito A, Sutherland C, Cascinelli N. Lack of effect of pregnancy on outcome of melanoma. *Lancet* 1991; **337**: 653–5.

39 Pack GT, Scharnagel IM. The prognosis for malignant melanoma in the pregnant woman. *Cancer* 1951; **4**: 324–34.

40 Conybeare RC. Malignant melanoma and pregnancy. *Obstet Gynaecol* 1964; **24**: 451–4.

41 Grin CM, Discoll MS, Grant-Kels JM. Pregnancy and prognosis of malignant melanoma. *Semin Oncol* 1996; **23** (6): 734–6.

42 Singluff CL, Reintgen DS, Vollmer RT, Seigler HF. Malignant melanoma arising during pregnancy: a study of 100 patients. *Ann Surg* 1990; **211**: 552–9.

43 McManamny DS, Moss ALH, Pocock PV, *et al.* Melanoma and pregnancy; a long-term follow-up. *Br J Obstet Gynaecol* 1989; **96**: 1419–23.

44 Wong DJ, Strassner HT. Melanoma in pregnancy. *Clin Obstet Gynaecol* 1990; **33** (4): 782–91.

45 Travers RL, Sober AJ, Berwick M, Mihm MC, Barnhill RL, Duncan LM. Increased thickness of pregnancy-associated melanoma. *Br J Dermatol* 1995; **132** (6): 876–83.

46 Pennoyer JW, Grin CM, Driscoll MS, *et al.* Changes in size of melanocytic nevi during pregnancy. *J Am Acad Dermatol* 1997; **36**: 378–82.

47 Shiu MH, Schottenfeld D, Maclean B,

Fortner JG. Adverse effect of pregnancy on melanoma. *Cancer* 1976; **37**: 181–7.
48 Ross MI. Melanoma and pregnancy: prognostic and therapeutic considerations. *Cancer Bull* 1994; **46**: 412–7.
49 Byrd BF, McGanity WJ. The effect of pregnancy on the clinical course of malignant melanoma. *South Med J* 1954; **47**: 196–200.
50 Colbourn DS, Nathanson L, Belilios E. Pregnancy and malignant melanoma. *Semin Oncol* 1989; **16**: 377–87.
51 Kjems E, Krag C. Melanoma and pregnancy. *Acta Oncol* 1993; **32**: 371–8.
52 Johnston SRD, Broadley K, Henson G, Fisher C, Henk M, Gore ME. A difficult case: management of metastatic melanoma during pregnancy. *Br Med J* 1998; **316**: 848–51.
53 Harkin KP. Case report: dacarbazine for metastatic melanoma during pregnancy. *Ir Med J* 1990; **83**: 116–17.
54 Aviles A. Long-term follow-up of 43 children exposed to chemotherapy *in utero*. *Am J Haematol* 1991; **36**: 243–8.
55 Anderson JF, Kent S, Machin GA. Maternal malignant melanoma with placental metastasis: a case report with literature review. *Pediatr Pathol* 1989; **9**: 35–42.
56 Baergen RN, Johnson D, Moore T, Benirschke K. Maternal melanoma metastatic to the placenta. *Arch Pathol Lab Med* 1997; **121**: 508–11.
57 Wong JH, Sterns EE, Kopald KH, Nizze JA, Morton DL. Prognostic significance of stage I melanoma. *Arch Surg* 1989; **124**: 1227–31.
58 Wagstaff J, Thacher N, Rankin E, Crowther D. Tamoxifen in the treatment of metastatic malignant melanoma. *Cancer Treat Rep* 1982; **66**: 1771.
59 Telhaug R, Klepp O, Bormer O. Phase II study of tamoxifen in patients with metastatic malignant melanoma. *Cancer Treat Rep* 1982; **66**: 1437.
60 Creagan ET, Ingle JN, Green SJ, *et al.* Phase II study of tamoxifen in patients with disseminated malignant melanoma. *Cancer Treat Rep* 1980; **64**: 199–201.
61 Beretta G, Tabiadon D, Fossati P. Clinical evaluation of medroxyprogesterone acetate in malignant melanoma. *Cancer Treat Rep* 1979; **63**: 1200.
62 Creagan ET, Schu AJ, Ahmann DL, Green SJ. Phase II study of high-dose megestrol acetate in patients with advanced malignant melanoma. *Cancer Treat Rep* 1982; **66**: 1239–40.
63 Creagan ET, Ingle JN, Schutt AJ, Schaid DJ. A prospective, randomized controlled trial of megesterol acetate among high-risk patients with resected malignant melanoma. *Am J Clin Oncol* 1989; **12**: 152–5.
64 McClay EF, Albright KA, Jones JA, *et al.* Tamoxifen modulation of cisplatin sensitivity in human malignant melanoma cells. *Cancer Res* 1993; **53**: 1571–6.
65 McClay EF, McClay M-ET. Tamoxifen: is it useful in the treatment of patients with metastatic melanoma? *J Clin Oncol* 1994; **12**: 617–26.
66 Cocconi G, Bella M, Calabresi F, *et al.* Treatment of metastatic melanoma with dacarbazine plus tamoxifen. *N Engl J Med* 1992; **327**: 516–23.
67 Ferri W, Agarwala SS, Kirkwood JM, *et al.* Carboplatin and dacarbazine with/without tamoxifen for metastatic melanoma. *Proc Am Soc Clin Oncol* 1994; **13**: A1341.
68 Legha S, Ring S, Bedikian A, *et al.* Lack of benefit from tamoxifen added to a regimen of cisplatin, vinblastine, DTIC and α-interferon in patients with metastatic melanoma. *Proc Am Soc Clin Oncol* 1993; **12**: A1325.
69 Rusthoven JJ, Quirt IC, Iscoe NA, *et al.* Randomized double-blind placebo-controlled trial comparing the response rates of carmustine, dacarbazine, and cisplatin with/without tamoxifen in patients with metastatic melanoma. *J Clin Oncol* 1996; **14**: 2083–90.

Index

Note: Page references in **bold** refer to Tables; those in *italics* refer to Figures